Competitive Managed Care

Competitive Managed Care

The Emerging Health Care System

John D. Wilkerson

Kelly J. Devers

Ruth S. Given

Editors

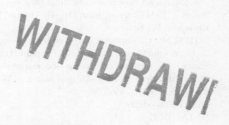
Jossey-Bass Publishers • San Francisco

Substantial discounts on bulk quantities of Jossey-Bass books are available to corporations, professional associations, and other organizations. For details and discount information, contact the special sales department at Jossey-Bass Inc., Publishers (415) 433–1740; Fax (800) 605–2665.

For sales outside the United States, please contact your local Simon & Schuster International Office.

 Manufactured in the United States of America on Lyons Falls Pathfinder Tradebook. This paper is acid-free and 100 percent totally chlorine-free.

Library of Congress Cataloging-in-Publication Data

Competitive managed care : the emerging health care system / John D.
  Wilkerson, Kelly J. Devers, Ruth S. Given, editors.
    p.   cm.—(Jossey-Bass health series)
    Includes bibliographical references and index.
    ISBN 0-7879-0309-4 (alk. paper)
    1. Managed care plans (Medical care)—Economic aspects—United
States.   I. Wilkerson, John D.   II. Devers, Kelly J.   III. Given,
Ruth S.   IV. Series.
    [DNLM: 1. Managed Care Programs—economics—United States.
2. Economic Competition.   3. Prepaid Health Plans—economics—United
States.   4. Group Purchasing—economics—United States.   5. Delivery
of Health Care—trends—United States.   W 130 AA1 C68 1997]
RA413.5.U5C66   1997
362.1'0973—dc20
DNLM/DLC
for Library of Congress   96-24679

HB Printing   10 9 8 7 6 5 4 3 2 1   FIRST EDITION

Contents

Preface

We are like a big fish that has been pulled from the water and is flopping wildly to find its way back in. In such a condition the fish never asks where the next flip or flop will bring it. It senses only that its present condition is intolerable and that something else must be tried.
ANONYMOUS QUOTED IN LINK, P. "CHINA IN TRANSFORMATION." *DAEDALUS*, SPRING 1993, P. 201.

Less than three years ago, the president and Congress were poised to pass comprehensive national health reform legislation. The Health Security Act, introduced by President Clinton in 1993, was an attempt to blend private market forces with government oversight to provide universal health care coverage to all U.S. citizens and legal residents while controlling health care costs. A variant of Alain Enthoven's "managed competition," the plan called for the government to regulate competition among private prepaid health plans for privately and publicly funded enrollees. Had it passed, the act would have required health care plans to offer the same basic package of benefits to all enrollees. The quality of the health care services they provide would have been monitored and that information shared with consumers. Payments to health care plans would have been based on the health care needs of their enrollees, and overall health care spending would have been limited.

But one year later, comprehensive government-led health care reform was completely discredited politically. And, like a fish out of water, policymakers and employers searched for an alternative solution to an intolerable situation. The solution, many hoped, lay in the fact that many large employers were achieving cost savings through increased free-market competition among managed care organizations.

Although managed care has existed for decades, it came to the forefront nationally with the introduction of President Clinton's Health Security Act. The acceleration in the growth of managed care that occurred in part in anticipation of national health care reform, and the subsequent rise of more aggressive purchasers of health insurance, fueled competition on the basis of price. This increased emphasis on price competition among private prepaid health care plans forms the basis of this book. It examines the profound and rapid changes that are occurring in the health care marketplace and their potential consequences for health care practitioners, policymakers, and the public.

Proponents of managed care argue that these changes will produce a more efficient health care system—overutilization and excess capacity will be reduced or eliminated, prevention and health promotion will be emphasized, and costs will decline. We believe, however, that many of the popular arguments extolling the virtues of increased market competition in health are based on a superficial understanding of textbook economics. Economic theory suggests that free-market mechanisms allocate goods and services efficiently—but only under a specific set of conditions. Economic theory also suggests that when one or more of these conditions is not present, other mechanisms besides a free market may lead to more efficient allocations. Furthermore, economic theory values improved efficiency at the expense of other goals, such as equity, that a society may be just as (or more) concerned with promoting. The disjuncture between economic theory and the popular rhetoric about markets provides the primary motivation for this book. What does economic theory suggest are the central obstacles to promoting economic efficiency, as well as other values, in the health care marketplace? How are these challenges being addressed, if at all, and which are likely to have the greatest impact on the future of health care delivery and financing in the United States?

Overview of the Contents

Because economic theory is helpful for understanding both the advantages and disadvantages of free-market competition, we use it as a framework for our examination of competitive managed care. In Part One, "Understanding Competitive Managed Care," the authors provide a brief introduction to recent changes in the health care marketplace and discuss what the theory of perfect competition tells us about the potential and limits of market-based approaches to health care reform. Because the focus of much of the debate about recent changes has been on efficiency, Chapter Two, by Harold S. Luft, considers what efficiency means in the health care context and examines the evidence for it in managed care organizations.

In Part Two, "Private Sector Initiatives and Responses," the authors examine developments in the private sector that are shaping the competitive managed care marketplace and its effects. In Chapter Three, Linda Bergthold and Loel Solomon consider some of the challenges purchasers face in their efforts to reduce costs and increase efficiency through competition. They discuss and assess the important role employers and purchasing cooperatives are playing in limiting their own health care costs. In Chapter Four, Helen Halpin Schauffler and Tracy Rodriguez describe one purchasing group's efforts to get competing managed care organizations to focus on prevention. In Chapter Five, Andrew Bindman discusses the challenges in ensuring that plans do not sacrifice quality in their efforts to lower costs.

The next two chapters offer insights into the consequences for practitioners of recent changes in the health care environment. In Chapter Six, Edward O'Neil and Leonard Finnocchio consider the impact of competitive managed care on the changing demand for different types of health care professionals. In Chapter Seven, Howard Waitzkin and Jennifer Fishman offer an insider's perspective on how increased competition is affecting relationships between providers and their patients at a very personal level.

Part Three, "Public Sector Initiatives and Responses," examines the roles governments are playing, and the challenges they face, in attempting to structure this emerging market to promote efficiency as well as other values. In Chapter Eight, Ruth Given looks at the important role government regulators must play in deciding when increased consolidation in the health care industry is economically beneficial and when it is economically harmful. Tom Buchmueller reports in Chapter Nine on California's effort to create a market for insurance for small employers through a state-sponsored purchasing cooperative. In Chapter Ten, Michael Sparer describes how states are looking to the market and managed care as a way to stretch limited Medicaid dollars at a time of increasing demand for services.

The three other chapters in Part Three illustrate the political challenges and risks to the government and the public of using market-based approaches. In Chapter Eleven, Kelly Devers describes the political, organizational, and technical challenges that have been encountered in Colorado's recent effort to introduce competitive managed care principles into its Medicaid mental health program. In Chapter Twelve, John Wilkerson describes how free-market rhetoric was used in the 104th Congress to conceal changes to the Medicare program that had nothing to do with improving the program's efficiency. In Chapter Thirteen, Donald Light discusses the positive and negative lessons of Britain's five years of experience with managed care and reflects on the relevance of those lessons for the United States.

In the Conclusion, "The Potential and Limits of Competitive Managed Care," we consider what this emerging competitive managed care system may mean, not only for the future of the health care system in the United States but also for the health of all Americans.

Audience for the Book

This book is targeted at four primary audiences: health care practitioners, purchasers and consumers of health care, policymakers and analysts, and graduate students in health policy, public policy, public health, and health services management.

Health Care Practitioners

The U.S. health care industry, which makes up about one seventh of the national economy, is undergoing radical change. Indemnity insurance firms, freestanding hospitals, and small specialty medical practices are being replaced by large prepaid health plans (health maintenance organizations), multihospital or integrated delivery systems, and large, multispecialty physician practices. Managers in the health care industry are interested in better understanding how these changes may affect their organizations. What will the industry's future business environment look like, and what factors will be most important in terms of their ability to compete and succeed in this changed environment? Members of the health care labor force, including physicians, nurses, physician assistants, pharmacists, and mental health clinicians, are interested in better understanding how these changes are likely to affect the demand for their skills and the nature of their work.

Purchasers and Consumers of Health Care

Public and private purchasers of health care benefits and direct consumers of health care services are also extremely interested in how these changes may affect access to affordable coverage and quality care in the future. At the moment, large group purchasers appear to be controlling and even actually reducing costs through the forces of the market. Many questions remain about the future, however. Purchasers are aware that the strength of their bargaining position—and thus their recent gains in controlling costs—may be threatened by the rapid consolidation now occurring throughout all sectors of the health care industry. Also, because this is an industry in which quality measurement and monitoring systems are still very primitive, both purchasers and direct consumers have a considerable interest in the expected effect on quality of care of an increasingly price-competitive environment.

Policymakers and Analysts

Governments are rethinking their roles as providers, purchasers, and regulators of health care services. State and federal governments provide the safety net when markets fail to yield a socially acceptable distribution of health care services. What is the impact on the health of Americans of treating health care increasingly as a market commodity? How is it likely to affect access to care in traditionally underserved areas and for the uninsured? How will it affect government health programs that provide health care for the poor and the elderly or support medical teaching, research, and public health programs? What new regulatory challenges will state and local governments face as these responsibilities are shifted increasingly from the federal to the local level?

Graduate Students

In contrast to many collections of essays, this volume has a well-defined theme. Each of the empirical chapters explores and illustrates key concepts drawn from a basic theoretical framework, that of efficiency in the economic theory of markets, presented in Chapter One. We believe that this approach offers readers the most accessible introduction to economic theory—and its applicability to health care markets—available anywhere. Students in public policy courses may find it useful to analyze the case of health care to evaluate the strengths and limits of market-based approaches. Students in health services management courses can discover how the health care delivery environment is changing, preparing them to debate the consequences of ongoing changes for specific segments of the industry. Finally, students in public health courses will better understand how these changes are likely to affect health care services for special populations and how they will affect efforts to prevent disease and promote better health in the general population.

Acknowledgments

This volume was prepared while the editors were in residence at the University of California, Berkeley, as Robert Wood Johnson Foundation Scholars in Health Policy Research. We are grateful to the Robert Wood Johnson Foundation and the School of Public Health at the University of California, Berkeley, for providing us with the opportunity to pursue this and other research projects. We are also grateful to Hal Luft at the Institute for Health Policy Studies, University of California, San Francisco, for his support and judgment, and to Richard Scheffler for establishing the Scholars program at Berkeley, which made this collaboration possible. The views expressed are the authors' and not necessarily those of the institutions with which they are now affiliated.

In addition to the contributors, many people have helped to make this book possible and better. We would especially like to thank our shepherd at Jossey-Bass, Barbara Hill, who kept us moving and in the right direction. For their advice and reactions to drafts of various chapters, we would like to thank Franci Duitch, Susan Giaimo, Peter May, Jon Oberlander, Mark Rom, and Michael Schoenbaum.

Finally, this collaborative project would not have been possible without the assistance, support, and tolerance of Barbara Simonsen, Kristin Carman, Jim Given, and Margaret, Mary, and Robert Shepard.

September 1996

John D. Wilkerson
Seattle, Washington

Kelly J. Devers
Washington, D.C.

Ruth S. Given
San Francisco, California

Competitive Managed Care

Part One

Understanding Competitive Managed Care

Free-market competition among managed care organizations has been promoted as the primary strategy of private and public sector purchasers for controlling their health care costs without reducing coverage or quality. In Chapter One, John Wilkerson, Kelly Devers, and Ruth Given introduce this emerging system and examine what economic theory actually says about the potential for a free market to provide health care services efficiently. Economic theory predicts that a free market for health care services will not operate efficiently because it does not conform to the conditions assumed by such theory. The explanations for the sources of inefficiency inherent in health care markets provide the thread that ties the rest of this volume together. How can efficient outcomes be promoted in health care markets? Where do other goals besides efficiency, such as equity, fit in?

In Chapter Two, Hal Luft explores the meaning of efficiency in the health care context and in managed care in particular. Although efficiency seems like a simple concept from the perspective of economic theory, it proves much less simple when seen from the differing perspectives of participants in the health care system. In the current price-competitive environment, it is important to understand that reduced costs alone do not signal greater efficiency if accompanied by reductions in quality or coverage.

Chapter One

The Emerging Competitive Managed Care Marketplace

John D. Wilkerson, Kelly J. Devers, Ruth S. Given

America's health care system is undergoing a transformation that will have major consequences for the health care industry and the people who benefit from it. Price has become an increasingly important component of employers' health insurance purchasing decisions. This increased emphasis on price has benefited health care plans that are more successful at controlling costs—the "alphabet soup" of insurer-provider organizations popularly known as managed care (Weiner and de Lissovoy, 1993). Managed care organizations integrate the financing and delivery of medical care by contracting with selected physicians and hospitals, by controlling utilization and quality, and by giving patients financial incentives to use providers and facilities associated with them (Iglehart, 1994).

This chapter has two main objectives. The first is to describe briefly some of the changes that are occurring in the financing and delivery of health care that we believe are setting the stage for a new health care system. The second is to provide a framework for thinking about the consequences of these changes. Because much of the popular rhetoric surrounding health care reform focuses on the alleged advantages and drawbacks of free-market competition, we focus on the economic theory of perfect competition. This theory is helpful for identifying not only the circumstances under which health care markets are likely to succeed but also where they are most likely to fail. In the chapters that follow, economists, sociologists, political scientists, and health care practitioners examine different aspects of the emerging competitive managed care market to assess its future implications for the health care industry and the public.

The Evolution of Managed Care

Until recently, several features characterized health care financing and delivery in the United States. Most of the health insurance purchased in the private market was purchased by employers for their employees. Insurers exercised little control over the prices providers charged or patients' utilization of services. Whether privately or publicly funded, insurers reimbursed physicians and hospitals in proportion to the quantity of services they provided—providers who performed more services were paid more. Providers and their patients, not insurers, decided whether a treatment or service was appropriate.

This "fee-for-service" system implicitly valued higher volumes of technologically sophisticated health care services. Patients were usually free to see any provider they preferred. Because most insurance arrangements paid what providers charged, doctors and hospitals competed for patients by offering the most up-to-date technologies and the most attractive practice settings.

Although managed care plans have existed for decades in some regions of the country, they were at a disadvantage in this environment of quality rather than price competition. Individuals who were covered by insurance plans that allowed them to choose their own doctor or hospital saw little benefit in joining a plan that would restrict those choices. And most providers saw little benefit in joining a managed care organization that might restrict their potential income or alter their style of practice.

Managed care began to attract more attention during the 1970s as government and industry became increasingly concerned with rising health care costs. In 1973 President Nixon signed the Health Maintenance Organization Act to encourage the formation and expansion of prepaid health care plans. The act provided more than $200 million in financial subsidies for health maintenance organizations (HMOs) and required that businesses with twenty-five or more employees offer their employees an HMO if one was available in their area (Starr, 1982, p. 401; Iglehart, 1994, p. 233). The act fell far short of its stated objective of creating 1,700 HMOs to serve forty million members by 1976 (Iglehart, 1994, p. 233). Only 174 HMOs had formed by 1976, serving six million Americans (U.S. Public Health Service, 1995, p. 242), and by the end of the decade, HMO enrollment still remained below ten million.

The managed care industry, which had smoldered for decades, began to catch fire during the 1980s. Health care costs continued to increase at double-digit rates, at a time when economic growth had slowed and business competition was increasing both domestically and internationally (Bureau of National Affairs, 1986). Rising health care costs were particularly problematic for large corporations that included health care benefits in their retirement packages and for small companies, which already had difficulty affording these benefits. For many, managed care offered a less expensive alternative to traditional fee-for-service insurance plans. Between 1981 and 1987, HMO enrollment tripled from ten million to almost thirty million (Kraus, Porter, and Ball, 1991, p. 52).

Managed care came to the forefront nationally in the early 1990s. As businesses continued to curtail benefits, increasing numbers of Americans found themselves having to pay more out of their own pocket for health care, or they lost their coverage altogether. Adopting a strategy that his campaign strategist, James Carville, had used successfully to help elect U.S. Senator Harris Wofford (D-Penn.), Democratic presidential nominee Bill Clinton made health care "security" a prominent part of his platform. Once elected, Clinton promised that health care reform was at the top of his legislative agenda.

The Health Security Act, introduced in the fall of 1993, promised universal coverage without higher costs. Expanded coverage would be achieved by improving the efficiency of the health care system through a variant of "managed competition" (Enthoven and Kronick, 1989). The government would sanction a limited number of large, prepaid health care plans to compete for enrollees within different regions across the nation. Competition among the plans would be regulated by the government to ensure that they competed on a level playing field. Each plan would be required to offer the same standard set of benefits. The government would monitor the plans and provide consumers with information on the quality of care they provide. The government would also risk-adjust payments to the plans to remove the incentive to lower expenses by attracting healthier enrollees. And finally, although it was not a feature of Enthoven's original proposal, the government would place a cap on total health care expenditures to ensure that the expected savings would be realized, even if the market mechanisms in the act failed to do so.

A widespread presumption that Democratic control of the presidency and Congress would lead to some kind of reform accelerated transformations that were already occurring within the health insurance industry. The president's initiative clearly favored large insurers with access to widespread networks of providers. Mergers between insurers and managed care plans increased (Kenkel, 1992; Loomis, 1994). Managed care plans and other insurers sought out contracts with physicians and hospitals, whose patients they hoped to enroll. Physicians and hospitals formed increasingly large networks (Miller, 1996; Gillies and others, 1993; Shortell, Gillies, and Anderson, 1994; Shortell and others, 1996).

The presumption turned out to be incorrect, of course. National health care reform failed, and it contributed to the election of a Republican majority in Congress (for the first time in forty years) and in many statehouses that had planned to piggyback local reform onto expected federal efforts. Although the problems that had led the public and many employers to support some version of reform remained unaddressed, government-led comprehensive reform had become politically infeasible.

It was apparent that employers could not depend on the government for a solution to health care costs; thus they increasingly turned to the market and new provider arrangements that had developed in anticipation of national health care reform. Between 1987 and 1992, HMO enrollment had increased by about 1 million persons per year, from 30 million to 36 million. Between 1992 and 1995, HMO enrollment increased by about 3 million per year (from 36 million to 58 million), with another 8.1 million Americans enrolled in less tightly controlled versions of managed care (Zelman, 1996, Chapter 1). For the first time in a decade, some employers saw their health care costs stabilize or even decline (Service, 1995; Findlay and Meyeroff, 1996).

Managed care's apparent success at squeezing the inefficiency out of the health care system captured the imagination of policy-makers looking for ways to stretch shrinking health care budgets during an era of expanding need. More states requested federal Medicaid waivers to encourage private managed care plans to provide services to Medicaid enrollees. At the national level, congressional Republicans passed Medicare reforms designed to shift the program away from a government-dominated fee-for-service program toward a voucher system for the purchase of private health insurance.

Managed Care Today

Managed care used to refer primarily to four different arrangements between health care plans and physicians (Miller and Luft, 1994). In a staff-model HMO, the health plan employs its physicians directly. In a group-model HMO, the health plan contracts for the exclusive services of one or more large group practices. In a network-model HMO, the plan contracts with one or more large groups, but the relationship is not exclusive. Finally, some HMOs negotiate contracts with individual practitioners or small-group practices through an intermediary known as an independent practice association (IPA).

These four models are not as useful for describing the managed care environment today. The largest growth in recent years, in terms of both the number of plans and enrollment, has been in "mixed" plans that offer enrollees the option of seeing an out-of-network provider (so long as they are willing to pay more for that option). Between 1990 and 1994, enrollment in mixed plans grew from 10 to 30 percent of all managed care enrollees, while enrollment in IPA plans declined from 40 to 38 percent and enrollment in traditional group- and staff-model HMOs declined from 50 to 32 percent. It should be noted that much of the dramatic increase in enrollment in mixed plans resulted from the reclassification of many traditional MHOs into the mixed category with their addition of an out-of-network option.

Increasingly, health plans are shifting their financial risks to the physicians and medical groups with whom they contract. Capitation (where providers are paid a fixed amount to provide all the care that an enrollee may require) and withholding (where physicians are given a financial incentive to limit referrals to specialists or hospitals) are becoming more common, particularly in markets where HMO penetration is high (Robinson and Casalino, 1995; Zelman, 1996, Chapter 2). Capitation removes the incentive to provide unnecessary services to increase revenues, but the low monthly payment to provide all the care an enrollee may require provides an incentive to "turf" patients who require expensive care to specialists or hospitals in order to avoid incurring the costs of their treatment (Trauner and Chesnutt, 1996, p. 162). Withholding and total capitation, where physicians are at risk for the cost of all medically necessary services, are two tactics increasingly used to deal with this problem. In 1994, fifty-seven percent of network and IPA HMOs reported having capitation arrangements with their primary physicians, and nearly 80 percent of those also withheld funds (or offered bonuses) as an incentive to limit referrals (Gold and others, 1995).

This combination of increased consumer flexibility and choice (albeit at higher cost) with increased financial pressures on providers appears to stem from the competing concerns of employers. From the standpoint of controlling costs, many employers would prefer to see their employees enroll in less costly, tightly managed plans. But from the standpoint of promoting employee satisfaction, employers also desire plans that offer freedom of choice. Such freedom is especially important to employers who want to encourage their employees to "migrate" into prepaid plans without forcing them to terminate their existing doctor-patient relationships (Loomis, 1994; Eaton, 1996).

Several recent studies have concluded that current HMO enrollment will double (at least) between 1995 and 2000, to include more than one hundred million Americans (Zelman, 1996, Chapter 2). This expansion will be accelerated to the extent that state governments respond to shrinking federal Medicaid funds by encouraging (or forcing) large numbers of beneficiaries into prepaid plans and to the extent that the federal government responds similarly to the impending fiscal challenges facing Medicare.

The major evidence for an emerging competitive managed care system comes from California. According to a recent study in *Health Affairs,* "health care costs in California are declining, and market forces are driving a widespread effort by providers to innovate in ways that will have a positive impact on cost, quality and access" (Enthoven and Singer, 1996b, p. 40; see also Trauner and Chesnutt, 1996). Competition among managed care plans has reduced premiums for large private and public purchasers in California by as much as 10 percent in a single year. National purchasers, including the Federal Employees Health Benefits Program and Medicare, have also benefited from increased competition in California (Enthoven and Singer, 1996b, p. 42).

Is California's experience with increased price competition among managed care organizations relevant to the future of health care delivery and financing in other parts of the nation? We believe that it is, primarily because the potential financial savings to private and public purchasers of insurance and health care services—and the potential profits for health care plans—are dramatic. According to recent figures, hospitalization rates, which contribute considerably to overall health care costs, are substantially lower in California than in the nation as a whole. Commercial HMO enrollees in California averaged 133 inpatient hospital days per thousand enrollees in 1995 (O'Neil, 1996). Nationally, commercial HMO enrollees averaged 486 hospital days per thousand enrollees—over three times as high. For the Medicare population, California plans averaged 960 inpatient hospital days per thousand, compared with 2,927 per thousand nationally. Other recent research supports the existence of this variation in hospitalization rates across the country, with the lowest rates occurring in West Coast metropolitan areas. Among fifteen metropolitan areas surveyed, there appears to be a strong inverse relationship between the percentage of the population enrolled in managed care and the rate of inpatient hospital days (Duke, 1996).

Competitive managed care is raging like wildfire in California. It has flared up in other sections of the country as well, and it is likely to sweep across much of the nation. Evidence that practices in California are being adopted in other regions of the nation is now starting to emerge (Johnsson, 1995a, 1995b; Zelman, 1996; Rosenthal, 1996). No one really knows what the consequences will be for America's health care system—will it lead to a wasteland of low-cost, low-quality care, or will it lead to renewed innovation that succeeds in finally achieving the goals of the 1973 Health Maintenance Organization Act?

Although it is clear that increased price competition among managed care plans in California and a number of other areas has reduced premiums for both large and small employer purchasing groups, it is less clear whether these lower costs demonstrate the superiority of market-based health care reform, as many now suggest. Are lower premiums evidence of increased efficiency? Are they the result of a greater emphasis on preventing illness and reducing inappropriate care, as proponents of the 1973 act envisioned? Or are they the result of shifting costs to purchasers who lack market power or of reducing coverage, access, and the quality of care?

Over the long term, the answers to these and related questions will depend on how a new health care system that is now in its infancy develops. We do not feel qualified to make any predictions at this point. There is, however, a framework that is extremely helpful for thinking about the advantages and disadvantages of markets in general and of health care markets in particular. The economic theory of perfect competition lies at the heart of contemporary claims about the superiority of markets as mechanisms for allocating goods and services, including health care. This theory offers lessons about the strengths—as well as the limitations—of free markets as a means for allocating health care and promoting health.

The Economic Theory of Perfect Competition

Suppose someone claims that a private package-delivery service is more efficient because it delivers the same package from Seattle to Denver for a lower price than the U.S. Postal Service. This claim is based on the assumption that everything but price is the same. It might not be true if, for example, the Postal Service were legally required to provide affordable delivery services to customers in remote areas and to offset those costs by charging more for deliveries in more profitable, urban areas. As a health care–related example, consider the price of hospital services in the United States. Hospitals have historically shifted some of the costs of caring for uninsured patients to the insured by charging more for insured services than they actually cost. A recent article in the *New York Times* reported that some health care plans, in an effort to offer lower premiums to employers, are attempting to end this "cross-subsidization" (Preston, 1996). By ending such cross-subsidization, health care plans can shift costs back to the uninsured or to the government and thus lower their premiums. One might debate whether those who purchase insurance ought to be subsidizing care for the uninsured. But it is clear, in any case, that savings to employers from the elimination of cross-subsidization would have more to do with a redistribution of resources than with any efficiency gains from increased market competition.

We begin with a simple example, a market for tomatoes, to illustrate the central conditions for an efficient market. We then consider health care markets and the extent to which they meet these conditions, as well as the potential consequences when they do not.

Textbook economic theory tells us that perfectly competitive markets are desirable because they lead to the most efficient outcomes. Thus, free-market mechanisms for the financing and delivery of health care would seem to provide an intuitive and reasonable solution to the problem of rising health care costs. Real-world markets do not always correspond to the assumptions of such theory, however. And even if they do, a society may wish to promote values that conflict with those resulting from free-market competition.

The appeal of free-market competition relies on two very important assumptions. The first is that increasing economic efficiency is necessarily more desirable than other social objectives. The second is that the relevant market is, in fact, perfectly competitive. When either of these assumptions is not true for a particular market, economic theory suggests that other, nonmarket mechanisms, including various forms of government intervention, may lead to either more efficient outcomes or outcomes that are better in other ways.

What is efficiency? Economists define market efficiency in terms of the benefit a consumer derives from purchasing a particular good or service; in an efficient market, it just equals the cost of producing and selling that good or service (Stiglitz, 1988, p. 65). This is best illustrated through our necessarily simplified example, a market for tomatoes. Imagine a market in which many growers are interested in selling some tomatoes and many other people are interested in buying some tomatoes. Each grower knows that, all other things being equal, she will be able to sell more tomatoes if she charges a lower price. Each buyer also knows that, all other things being equal, he will be able to buy more tomatoes if he is willing to pay a higher price than other buyers. These two pieces of information can be used to predict how many tomatoes will be bought and sold in the market and at what price.

Figure 1.1 shows how consumers and producers interact in a market for tomatoes. The line labeled "Supply" represents the total number of tomatoes that all of the growers combined are willing to produce and sell at different prices. The line indicates that growers are willing to produce and sell more tomatoes at higher prices than they are at lower prices. The other line ("Demand") represents the total number of tomatoes that all buyers in the market are willing to buy at different prices. Buyers are willing to buy more tomatoes as the price goes down.

An efficient outcome results when a market meets a set of conditions that make it perfectly competitive (discussed below). The price determined by the intersection of the supply and demand curves is considered the efficient price because it represents that combination of price and quantity where the value to the consumer of purchasing a tomato just equals the cost of production for the grower. This is point A in Figure 1.1, where one thousand tomatoes can be bought and sold at the efficient price of $0.50 per tomato. To reinforce why this single price-quantity combination is most efficient, we provide two counterexamples, points B and C, and demonstrate why buyers and sellers (and society) are better off moving from either of these points to point A.

At point B, the price of $0.25 per tomato is lower than the efficient price of $0.50 per tomato. For this price, there will be an undersupply of tomatoes relative to what consumers would value. In a free market (where prices can fluctuate to equalize supply and demand), consumers would bid up the price toward $0.50. This rise in price would cause the growers to increase output, ultimately leading to the efficient price-quantity combination (point A). Alternatively, at point C the price of $0.75 per tomato is higher than the efficient price. In this instance there would be insufficient demand. In a perfectly competitive market, the tomato producers would compete against one another and reduce their prices to the level

Figure 1.1. Efficiency and Inefficiency in a Market for Tomatoes.

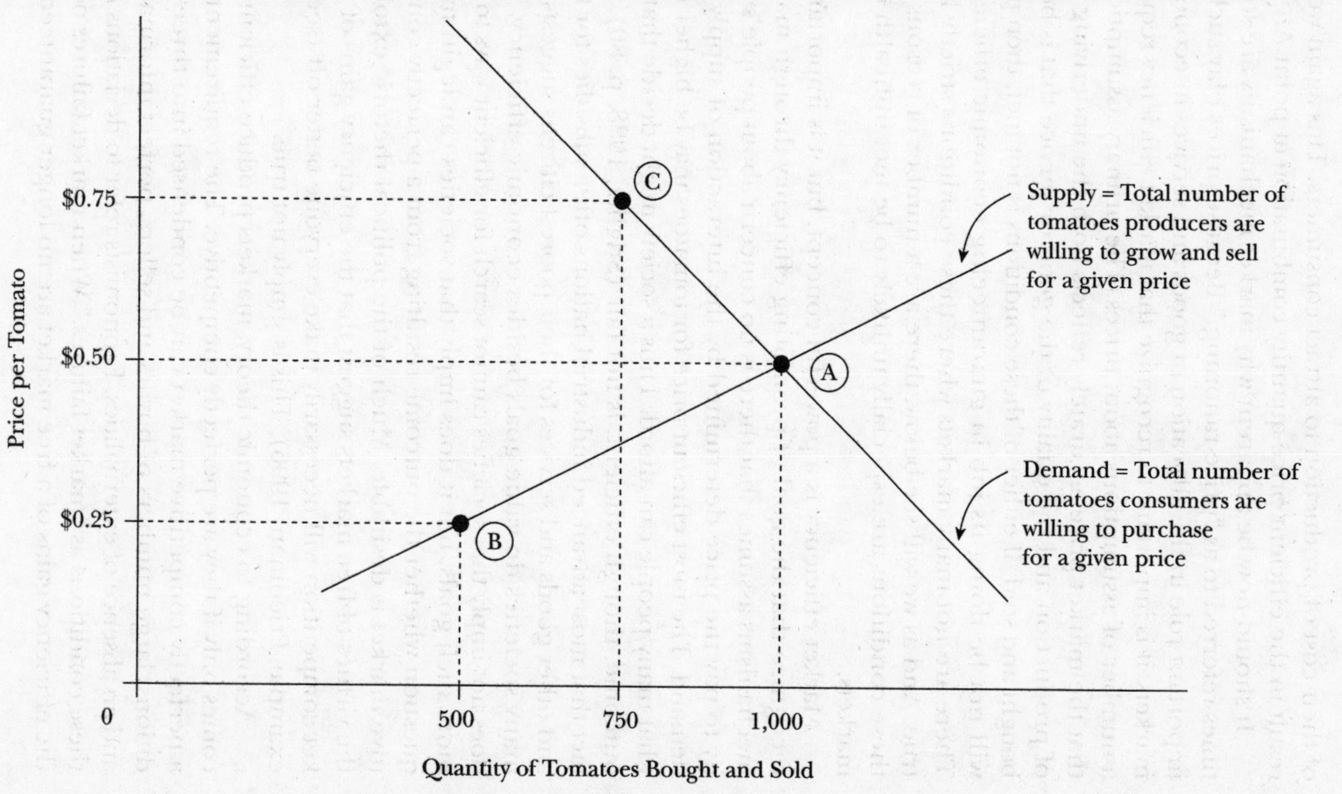

of their cost of production to attract consumers. This again would result in the efficient price-quantity combination at point A.

It should now be apparent why market mechanisms are sometimes referred to as "price rationing." Because prices play such an important role in the allocation of goods and services in economic markets, it is important to recognize that market efficiency requires a number of assumptions about prices. The primary assumption is that the market price accurately reflects both the underlying cost of production and the quality of the good or service that is being bought and sold. If either of these conditions is not met, then price will not be doing its job in guaranteeing economic efficiency. There are not many markets where these conditions strictly hold true. And as we will see below, there are a number of reasons why these conditions are especially unlikely to be met in health care markets.

Market efficiency is a powerful concept, but it is important to recognize that the goal of promoting efficiency through market mechanisms assumes that there is no concern about people's ability to pay the price determined by the interaction of supply and demand. The most efficient price for tomatoes may be higher than what many people can afford. Thus a society might decide that this outcome, though efficient, is not fair (Stiglitz, 1988, p. 80). The fact that most advanced industrial nations offer subsidies for food and other goods and services for their poorest citizens suggests that many societies do value goals besides economic efficiency. This does not imply that societies cannot search for efficient ways to promote such goals, but it does imply that societies can legitimately question whether the outcome resulting from a perfectly competitive market is desirable. Much of the political rhetoric extolling the virtues of free markets suggest that the efficiency gains of market competition will necessarily make everyone better off (see, for example, Friedman, 1996). This is simply not true.

According to economic theory, markets produce efficient outcomes only if they are perfectly competitive. The requirements for a perfectly competitive market can be condensed into three conditions: large numbers of buyers and sellers, perfect information, and an absence of externalities. Economists refer to deviations from these conditions as "market failures." When market failures occur, the efficiency gains of a free market are no longer guaranteed.

Large Numbers of Buyers and Sellers

In a perfectly competitive market, large numbers of buyers and sellers compete freely for goods and services, and no particular buyer or seller is able to influence the market price by reducing the supply or demand for a product. In our example, individual growers must decide only whether they are willing to sell their tomatoes for what buyers are willing to pay, and individual buyers must decide only whether they are willing to pay what sellers are asking.

A familiar example of the failure of a market to meet this condition is if all of the tomatoes in our market were supplied by one grower (a monopoly) or a small number of growers (an oligopoly). In this situation, the grower or growers could raise the price of tomatoes by restricting their supply. Although this would limit the number each could sell, higher prices charged would result in higher profits.

Whether a monopoly grower would be able to sustain an excessive profit margin over the long term depends on other characteristics of the market. How difficult is it for other growers to enter the market? Although it takes money and time to grow tomatoes, it may be relatively easy to transport them from another location. How committed are buyers to consuming the tomatoes grown by the monopoly producer? How willing would they be to switch to another vegetable or even another type of food?

Good Information About Price and Quality

In a perfectly competitive market, producers and consumers are able to accurately judge how much a product or service is worth to them. The price of a product or service is assumed to be a perfect indicator of its quality or value, both for the seller and for the purchaser. If this is not true, then the buyer may end up buying more or less of a product than he actually prefers, and the seller may end up selling it for too little or too much.

A consumer might be willing to pay a higher price for shiny red tomatoes on the assumption that red and shiny on the outside mean sweeter and juicier on the inside. But if this assumption is not correct, the consumer ends up purchasing too few tomatoes for a given price.

Producers of sweet and juicy tomatoes thus have a financial incentive to help consumers identify and select their product (by labeling them, for example, or offering free samples). Producers of bland tomatoes have a financial incentive to mislead consumers into purchasing their products by imitating the products of sweet and juicy producers to the extent that they can. Anyone who has purchased an expensive but flavorless bright red tomato in winter understands the perils of imperfect information.

Absence of Externalities

In a perfectly competitive market, the selling price of a product is assumed to reflect the total costs of producing it, and the price that a buyer is willing to pay for it is assumed to reflect its total value. Economists refer to the difference between the selling price of a product and its true costs or benefits to society as *externalities*. Externalities lead to inefficient outcomes, because (as in the case of imperfect information) either too much or too little of a product is sold than would be sold if its true value were reflected in its selling price.

If a farmer uses pesticides to reduce infestations, for example, he may generate additional, indirect health and environmental costs to society ("Drinking Water in Midwest . . . ," 1995). If the price of tomatoes is not increased to reflect these additional social costs (through a tax on pesticides, for example), then more tomatoes will be produced and sold than is socially efficient. On the other hand, even if growing tomatoes has other social benefits (such as reducing carbon dioxide and producing oxygen), too few may be grown to realize these benefits if consumers do not value them or they do not play a part in their purchasing decisions. If the positive externalities outweigh the negative ones, it might be economically efficient to subsidize tomato production to increase the supply available.

Failures in Health Care Markets

Addressing the failures of health care markets has been a central justification for past government interventions. In the discussion that follows, we consider how health care markets can fail and how such failures might be addressed to improve economic efficiency. As in our tomato market example, health care markets can fail when there is reduced competition, when there is imperfect information, and when they exhibit significant positive or negative externalities. The examples we use have been selected not because we believe that they are the only ones (or the most egregious ones) but because they are particularly helpful for illustrating health care market failures. When appropriate, we will also highlight chapters in this volume that are particularly relevant to the conditions being discussed.

Reduced Competition

In health care markets, the assumption that there will be a large number of buyers and sellers is most likely to be violated on the sellers' (supply) side. For example, hospitals require a large initial investment for equipment and facilities and must treat a high volume of patients to recoup this investment. In many localities, the population is not large enough to support more than one hospital (Eisenstadt, 1994). In an unregulated market, a "natural" monopoly of this kind can make it possible for the hospital to charge more for its services than it could if it were forced to compete for its patients.

Both the federal government and state governments have historically intervened in the hospital industry to encourage hospitals to locate in rural areas (through subsidies or by building hospitals themselves) and to discourage monopoly pricing behavior in private hospitals (through price controls). In the past a number of state governments regulated hospital prices, either for treating state clients or for treating the general public. Governments also use tax incentives to encourage nonprofit private hospitals, on the assumption that they are less likely to engage in such behavior.

Recent changes in the health care industry are leading to an unprecedented volume of mergers among insurers, hospitals, physicians, and drug companies. Health plans recognize that their attractiveness to large employers increasingly depends on their ability to offer a wide range of services over as large a geographic area as possible. In addition to mergers among similar institutions, increasingly large alliances are also forming among providers who provide complementary services. Hospitals and physicians recognize that forming large (even national) networks improves their negotiating positions with insurers and positions them to market their services directly to employers. Mergers can increase efficiency (for example, through economies of scale), but they can also reduce efficiency by making markets less competitive. Governments will play a central role in deciding where to strike a balance between these positive and negative consequences of increased consolidation (see Chapter Eight).

Information-Related Problems

There are a wide range of information-related problems in health care markets. These can be categorized according to who is affected (the consumer-purchaser or the provider-insurer) and how they are affected. (This is demonstrated in Table 1.1. The various causes and consequences of market failure detailed in the table are explained in greater detail below.) Consumers might be uncertain about their own future health care needs, or they may know less than a provider about the value of a service. Providers might be uncertain about the most efficient way to treat a patient or deliver a service, or they may know less than the consumer about the value of that service to the consumer.

Consumer Uncertainty, Moral Hazard, and Overutilization

Health care purchases are different from many other kinds of purchases. Most people can expect to remain relatively healthy for most of their lives. However, each of us faces a small chance of becoming seriously ill and incurring large health care costs. Economists assume (and there is empirical evidence) that people are *risk averse*. When offered a choice, most individuals prefer a certain but small financial loss to an uncertain but potentially large financial loss. An insurance premium that is based on a consumer's expected health care costs is efficient because it allows individuals to trade a gamble for a sure thing, the premium (Arrow, 1963).

However, possessing health insurance can also increase the amount of health care services consumers use, by changing their economic calculations. An insured consumer pays only part (or

Table 1.1. Information-Related Health Care Market Failures and Their Consequences.

	Type of Problem	
Groups Affected	General Uncertainty	Informational Disadvantage
Consumers-Purchasers	The small probability of high medical care expenses together with *risk aversion* leads to the demand for health insurance. Low out-of-pocket payments under health insurance result in *moral hazard,* which causes overutilization of services with minimal benefits.	The *principal-agent* relationship between patient and provider (or enrollee and HMO) means that the consumer has less information on quality and reasonableness of price than does the seller. Consumer ignorance can lead to consumers' receiving poorer quality of care or paying too high a price.
Providers-Insurers	The general uncertainty about the most appropriate treatment leads to underuse or overuse of particular procedures and treatments. The result is less efficient or poorer quality of care.	Consumers who know of their own above-average health care risk or costs are more likely to purchase insurance or to purchase more generous insurance. *Adverse selection* causes a collapse of the market for individual insurance policies. *Risk selection* results in "cream skimming" rather than true price competition.

none) of the costs of a service directly, and the cost to the insurance company for that service is distributed evenly among all its subscribers instead of being charged directly back to the individual consumer. For the same reason that equally dividing a dinner check might lead some diners to also order dessert, having insurance can lead some consumers to use health care services that they would not have purchased directly. This change in behavior, observed when insurance coverage shields consumers from the true costs of the services they receive, is called *moral hazard.*

Some policymakers and economists believe that overutilization due to insurance is the most important explanation for why medical care costs have risen much more rapidly than general inflation over the past several decades and for why increasing numbers of Americans are unable to afford basic health insurance. Controlling health care utilization was at the center of President Clinton's Health Security Act as well as recent Republican proposals in Congress to reform Medicare (see Chapter Twelve). Both reform efforts sought to limit unnecessary utilization through increased cost sharing, increased use of private prepaid or managed care organizations, and the establishment of overall spending caps.

Consumer Informational Disadvantages and Provider Abuse

We seek out health care professionals because they know more about health, illness, and treatment than we do. Like many situations where knowledge or experience is not equally shared (car repair comes to mind), individuals can benefit by paying for others' expertise. However, the possibility exists that those whom we rely on do not really know what they are doing or will take advantage of our ignorance to overcharge us. We may choose to go under the knife of an inattentive or incompetent surgeon based on the mistaken belief that he or she is competent, or we may not question a hospital bill that includes unreasonably high charges. Economists refer to this general informational inequality in contracting as the *principal-agent* problem, where the principal (the patient) has less information about the value of a service than the agent (the physician).

The potential for physicians to betray their patients' trust is one rationale for the Hippocratic oath. That potential also exists for other service providers, from insurers to pharmacists to telemarketers. Historically, governments have intervened to help discourage provider abuse by requiring them to satisfy state or federal requirements for licensure, by regulating business practices, by permitting consumers to sue providers in civil court, and by prosecuting providers for violations of criminal laws.

Recent changes in the health care market are creating new challenges in this area. Under fee-for-service medicine, a major area of concern was that providers were prescribing services that were profitable but promised little real benefit to the patient (and sometimes caused real harm). These incentives are typically reversed under managed care arrangements. Because the provider receives a fixed payment for all the services an enrollee might need, the primary concern is that unscrupulous providers will attempt to avoid providing care that is more expensive. This concern is at the heart of recent controversies surrounding decisions by some health care plans to pay for only one day of inpatient care for new mothers, to refuse patients' requests to receive care from specialists outside their network (Herbert, 1996), or to limit what doctors can tell their patients about treatment options (see Chapter Seven).

Provider Uncertainty and Inefficient Practice Patterns

Health care services are also different from many other kinds of services in that providers themselves are sometimes uncertain about which treatments are best for their patients. If providers choose less appropriate forms of care because they lack good information, then the health care market operates less efficiently than it could. More effective treatments may be underprescribed while less effective treatments are overprescribed. Phelps and Mooney (1993) have shown that practice patterns vary considerably across the United States; they suggest that these variations are explained in part by an absence of good information on the relative effectiveness of different treatments. The federal government has historically played a role in this area by requiring pharmaceutical companies to provide evidence of the safety and efficacy of their products. More recently, the government has attempted to subsidize the collection and dissemination of information and research on the effectiveness of other types of treatment ("AHCPR Drops Guideline Development," 1996).

Under fee-for-service reimbursement systems, providers have a financial incentive to err on the side of providing treatment even if it may have only minimal benefits. The fixed payments associated with managed care, on the other hand, give providers a financial incentive to err on the side of not providing a treatment if they are uncertain about whether it will prove beneficial to a patient. This switch in incentives creates new risks for patients and new monitoring challenges for businesses and governments seeking quality health care at low cost (see Chapters Four and Five).

Insurer Informational Disadvantages and Adverse Selection

As described above, the primary reason consumers purchase insurance is to reduce the probability of a large financial loss. In addition, consumers who know that they are at high risk for costly health problems are more likely to seek insurance coverage. Their potential insurers lack this information, however. Because individual insurance coverage is purchased disproportionately by those who expect to incur large expenses, its underlying cost (and thus its price) is very high.

Adverse selection refers to the tendency of sicker individuals to shop for plans with more comprehensive coverage (Akerlof, 1970). In the most extreme cases, adverse selection can cause a market for individual insurance coverage to collapse. This occurs through a process known in the insurance industry as the "death spiral," where insurers respond to rising health costs by raising premiums, which leads more healthy individuals to drop their coverage. Premiums continue to spiral upward until the insurance becomes unaffordable (Enthoven and Singer, 1996a). *Risk selection* refers to the efforts of insurers to design their policies or their marketing efforts to deter purchase by unhealthy individuals and attract healthy ones. Insurers can also try to attract better risks through (among other things) preexisting condition exclusions, additional benefits (such as health club memberships), and advertising campaigns that portray enrollees as vigorous and healthy (as opposed to ill but well cared for). They can also reduce their risk by insuring only large groups and not individuals. (Another important reason to do this, of course, is lower per capita administrative costs.)

The expectation that individuals will sort themselves according to their health status helps explain why millions of people are unable to purchase affordable health coverage in the individual insurance market. The threat of a "death spiral" may produce a race to the bottom, in which insurers compete to make their policies less comprehensive and less attractive to the unhealthy— severely limiting consumers' range of insurance options in the process. Adverse selection can be discouraged by making it more difficult for individuals to base their purchasing decisions on their anticipated health care usage; risk selection can be discouraged by making it more difficult for insurers to market to and thus attract only the healthiest enrollees. Governments can do this by requiring all insurers to offer the same set of standard benefits, by requiring insurers and individuals to contract for long enrollment periods, by prohibiting insurers from excluding individuals based upon health-related characteristics and requiring them to offer the same benefits-premium package to all prospective purchasers, and by risk-adjusting premiums in order to fairly compensate health plans for enrolling higher-risk populations.

Many of the techniques described above for dealing with the related problems of adverse selection and risk selection were incorporated into the version of managed competition proposed by the Clinton administration. Although they did not become national policy, many of these techniques have been adopted and applied on a limited basis by private and public health benefit purchasers, such as large private employers and state-sponsored purchasing coalitions (see Chapters Three and Nine).

Externalities in Health Care Markets

Health care markets also often fail to conform to the assumption that the market price of a product reflects its total social costs and benefits. If a product's selling price does not reflect all of the social costs involved in producing or consuming it, more of it will be produced and sold than is socially efficient. On the other hand, if consumers do not recognize all of the benefits of a product and do not acknowledge them in the price they are willing to pay, less of it will be produced and consumed than is socially efficient.

Externalities are common in health care markets—especially underinvestments in programs that produce social benefits. The most obvious examples are those programs that are either provided or subsidized by various levels of government. One major category of health-related expenditures with a substantial external benefit is that related to traditional public health activities such as sanitation and control of infectious disease. Another is the production of information. Unlike other goods and services, once information is produced, it is often difficult to charge for its use. Activities that produce health care–related information, such as basic scientific and clinical research, have been heavily subsidized, mainly by the federal government. The government can also promote the private production of information with social benefits through intellectual property laws, such as patents, that encourage innovation by allowing companies to behave as temporary monopolies in order to recoup initial investments in research and development.

Ideally, managed care organizations have an incentive to focus on maintaining health rather than treating illness and to provide cost-effective care for those who do require treatment (Breslow, 1996). This way of thinking may be unfamiliar to many practicing physicians, and the information needed to assess the cost-effectiveness of different approaches to care is often not available. One might also argue that it is more important today for consumers to have access to objective information about the performance of different plans. It is costly to collect the kind of information needed to measure cost-effectiveness and performance, however, and the benefits of such information do not necessarily go only to those who collect it (see Chapters Four and Five). The same may be true for training practitioners to operate in a managed care environment, if plans cannot ensure that the providers they train will not work elsewhere (see Chapter Six).

Social Values Besides Increased Economic Efficiency

Americans do seem willing to make a distinction between health care and other goods and services. Most do not object to insurance companies' charging substantially more for automobile insurance for drivers with bad records, but most would object to their charging more for health insurance for diabetics or hemophiliacs. The distinction many would make is that people have much more control over their driving record than they do over their health. People who drive poorly *deserve* to pay more for their auto insurance, but hemophiliacs should not have to pay more for their health insurance, because they are not responsible for their own health status.

Obviously, the notion of responsibility begins to blur when certain health conditions (such as lung cancer, heart disease, and acquired immunodeficiency syndrome) are considered. The important point is that most Americans agree that health care should not be allocated solely according to the consumer's ability to pay, even though this may conflict with the goal of increased efficiency. When a society values resource distributions other than those based on ability to pay, it cannot rely on perfectly competitive markets to provide them; it typically requires social intervention into the market. In recent decades, the federal government has been the central player in efforts to make health care more available to the very poor and elderly through the Medicare and Medicaid programs. Efforts by the federal government to make affordable health care available to all Americans have repeatedly failed, however.

The changes occurring in the health care market are not likely to resolve the long-standing debate over whether all Americans should have access to affordable health care. The number of uninsured and underinsured Americans continues to increase, and governments are proposing to reduce future spending on health programs that benefit the poor, disabled, and the elderly (Somerville, 1995). Although advocates of market-based health care reform suggest that efficiency gains from increased competition will make it possible to reduce program costs for Medicare and Medicaid beneficiaries without reducing choice, coverage, or quality, there is little evidence to date to support this assertion (see Chapters Ten and Eleven).

Conclusion

The rejection of President Clinton's Health Security Act set the stage for a privately led reform movement emphasizing price competition among managed care organizations. This world of "competitive managed care" seems destined to produce a health care system unlike any other in the United States or any other nation. In this chapter we have presented a framework for identifying some of the central economic issues that will shape how health care financing and delivery will evolve in the United States. We have pointed out that the theory underlying popular rhetoric about the superiority of free markets is more complex than many advocates of market-based reform would have us believe. Economic theory guarantees efficient outcomes only when a market meets a set of specific conditions. If these conditions are not met, we are no longer assured that the efficiency gains of a free market will be realized. As noted in this chapter, an unrestricted health care market would fail to meet many of these conditions. In addition, Americans support goals other than the efficient allocation of health care services according to the consumer's willingness and ability to pay. These two characteristics of health care markets—the existence of market failures and the importance of other social goals—imply that other arrangements besides unconstrained market forces may lead to a better collective outcome.

However, even though government intervention may appear to be justified by the presence of market failures, there is no guarantee that such public action will lead to greater efficiency. Some market failures are not easily solved by government or any other entity (Schultze, 1977; Stiglitz, 1988). Government interventions can also fail because policy responses are developed through a political process of consensus building, which introduces many problems not previously considered (see Chapters Twelve and Thirteen). For a proposal to become law, it often must be modified to address the concerns of those who may be adversely affected. And even if a proposal makes it through the legislative process more or less intact, similar political forces come into play during its implementation as agencies, private entities, and ultimately the courts offer their own interpretations about the law's intent and the best approaches for accomplishing it (see Chapter Eleven).

Society must ultimately decide how it will balance competing values (Freudenheim, 1996). In the case of market-based health care reform, the ultimate question concerns how much efficiency

Americans are willing to give up in order to promote a more equitable distribution of health care or how much inequality they are willing to accept in order to promote a more efficient health care system.

References

"AHCPR Drops Guideline Development." *HSR Reports,* June 1996, p. 4.

Akerlof, G. "The Market for Lemons: Quality Uncertainty and the Market Mechanism." *Quarterly Journal of Economics,* 1970, *84,* 488–500.

Arrow, K. J. "Uncertainty and the Welfare Economics of Medical Care." *American Economic Review,* 1963, *53,* 941–973.

Breslow, L. "Public Health and Managed Care: A California Perspective." *Health Affairs,* 1996, *15*(1), 92–99.

Bureau of National Affairs. *Health Care Costs: Where's the Bottom Line?* Washington, D.C.: Bureau of National Affairs, 1986.

"Drinking Water in Midwest Has Pesticides, Report Says." *New York Times,* October 18, 1995, p. A13.

Duke, K. S. "Hospitals in a Changing Health Care System." *Health Affairs,* 1996, *15*(2), 49–61.

Eaton, L. "Aetna to Buy U.S. Healthcare in Big Move to Managed Care." *New York Times,* April 2, 1996, pp. A1, C1.

Eisenstadt, D. "Hospital Competition and Costs: The Carilion Case." In J. E. Kwoka and L. J. White (eds.), *The Antitrust Revolution: The Role of Economics.* (2nd ed.) New York: HarperCollins, 1994

Enthoven, A. C., and Kronick, R. "A Consumer-Choice Health Plan for the 1990s." *New England Journal of Medicine,* 1989, *320*(1), 29–37.

Enthoven, A. C., and Singer, S. J. "Health Care Markets: What to Regulate and by Whom?" In H. J. Aaron (ed.), *The Problem That Won't Go Away: Reforming U.S. Health Care Financing.* Washington, D.C.: Brookings Institution, 1996a.

Enthoven, A. C., and Singer, S. J. "Managed Competition and California's Health Care Economy." *Health Affairs,* 1996b, *15*(1), 39–57.

Evans, R. G., Barer, M. L., and Marmor, T. R. (eds.). *Why Are Some People Healthy and Others Not? The Determinants of Health of Populations.* Hawthorne, N.Y.: Aldine de Gruyter, 1994.

Findlay, S., and Meyeroff, W. J. "Health Costs: Why Employers Won Another Round." *Business and Health,* Mar. 1996, pp. 49–51.

Folland, S., Goodman, A. C., and Stano, M. *The Economics of Health and Health Care.* New York: Macmillan, 1993.

Freudenheim, M. "Health Care in the Era of Capitalism." *New York Times,* April 7, 1996, p. E6.

Friedman, M. "A Way Out of Soviet-Style Health Care." *Wall Street Journal,* April 17, 1996, p. A20.

Frist, B. "The Future of Medicare: One Senator's Vision." *Health Affairs,* 1995, *14*(4), 82–88.

Gillies, R. R., and others. "Conceptualizing and Measuring Integration: Findings from the Health Systems Integration Study." *Hospital and Health Services Administration,* 1993, *38*(4), 467–489.

Gold, M., and others. *Arrangements Between Managed Care Plans and Physicians: Results from a 1994 Survey of Managed Care Plans.* Washington, D.C.: Mathematica Policy Research, 1995.

Herbert, B. "Torture by HMO." *New York Times,* March 15, 1996, p. A29.

Iglehart, J. K. "The American Health Care System: Managed Care." In P. R. Lee and C. L. Estes (eds.), *The Nation's Health.* Boston: Jones & Bartlett, 1994.

Johnsson, J. "West Meets East: Philadelphia HMOs Follow California into Price War." *American Medical News.* Feb. 13, 1995a, pp. 1, 7.

Johnsson, J. "HMO Price War Hits the East Coast." *American Medical News.* Nov. 11, 1995b, p. 7.

Kenkel, P. J. "Smaller, Struggling HMOs Lure Suitors." *Modern Healthcare,* August 10, 1992, p. 33.

Kraus, N., Porter, M., and Ball, P. *The Interstudy Edge—Managed Care: A Decade in Review 1980–1990.* Excelsior, Minn.: InterStudy, 1991.

Loomis, C. "The Real Action in Health Care." *Fortune,* July 11, 1994, pp. 149–157.

Miller, R. H. "Health System Integration: A Means to an End." *Health Affairs,* 1996, *15*(2), 92–106.

Miller, R. H., and Luft, H. S. "Managed Care Plan Performance Since 1980: A Literature Analysis." *Journal of the American Medical Association,* 1994, *271*(19), 1512–1518.

O'Neil, E. H. "Overview of Forces Driving Health Care Change." Paper presented to Blue Cross Washington and Alaska, Seattle, Wash., March 8, 1996.

Phelps, C. E., and Mooney, C. "Variations in Medical Practice Use: Causes and Consequences." In R. J. Arnould, R. F. Rich, and W. D. White (eds.), *Competitive Approaches to Health Care.* Washington, D.C.: The Urban Institute Press, 1993.

Preston, J. "Hospitals Look on Charity Care as Unaffordable Option of Past." *New York Times,* April 14, 1996, p. A1.

Robinson, J. C., and Casalino, L. P. "The Growth of Medical Groups Paid Through Capitation in California." *New England Journal of Medicine,* 1995, *333*(25), 1684–1687.

Robinson, J. C., and Luft, H. "Competition, Regulation, and Hospitals' Costs, 1982 to 1986." *Journal of the American Medical Association,* 1988, *260*(18), 2676–2681.

Rosenthal, E. "Panels See New York City Hospital Closings." *New York Times,* Apr. 7, 1996, p. A14.

Schultze, C. L. *The Public Use of Private Interest.* Washington D.C.: Brookings Institution, 1977.

Service, M. "Why Health Costs Got Smaller in 1994." *Business and Health,* Mar. 1995, pp. 20–28.

Shortell, S. M., Gillies, R. R., and Anderson, D. A. "The New World of Managed Care: Creating Organized Delivery Systems." *Health Affairs,* 1994, *13*(5), 46–64.

Shortell, S. M., and others. *Remaking Health Care in America: Building Organized Delivery Systems.* San Francisco: Jossey-Bass, 1996.

Somerville, J. "Uninsured Number Up as Politicians Argue over Solutions." *American Medical News,* Sept. 18, 1995, p. 4.

Starr, P. *The Social Transformation of American Medicine.* New York: Basic Books, 1982.

Stiglitz, J. E. *Economics of the Public Sector.* (2nd ed.) New York: Norton, 1988.

Trauner, J. B., and Chesnutt, J. S. "Medical Groups in California: Managing Care Under Capitation." *Health Affairs,* 1996, *15*(1), 159–170.

U.S. Public Health Service. *Health, United States, 1994.* Washington, D.C.: U.S. Government Printing Office, 1995.

Weiner, J. P, and de Lissovoy, G. "Razing a Tower of Babel: A Taxonomy for Managed Care and Health Insurance Plans." *Journal of Health Politics, Policy, and Law,* 1993, *18*(1), 75–103.

Zelman, W. A. *The Changing Health Care Marketplace: Private Ventures, Public Interests.* San Francisco: Jossey-Bass, 1996.

Chapter Two

Perspectives and Evidence on Efficiency in Managed Care Organizations

Harold S. Luft

Managed care organizations (MCOs) have moved to center stage in the health care delivery arena. Managed care played an important role in the Clinton health reform proposal, and despite that policy's legislative failure, it has become the marketplace's preferred solution to rising health care costs. Headlines and news stories about managed care appear almost daily, including reports that health insurance premiums are falling for perhaps the first time in recorded history ("HMO Coverage Cost Less in '95," 1996). Health care providers are reporting enormous cost-containment pressures imposed by MCOs, and hospitals are announcing mergers and closures, again attributed to managed care. On the other hand, there are also reports about the refusal of HMOs to cover certain treatments and the high administrative costs and profits in some plans (Larson, 1996; Schulte and Bergal, 1995).

While it is clear that the health care system is perceived to be in the midst of a major upheaval, it is more difficult to know whether this is really the case. For example, hospital-merger waves have occurred in previous decades; new types of health care providers, such as physician assistants, were introduced in the 1970s; health insurance premiums are known to follow a cyclical pattern; and general inflation in the economy has subsided. Thus, slower growth in health insurance costs may just be part of the larger picture. Identifying what is real from what is public relations and posturing by special interest groups is difficult at best. Furthermore, the very notion of efficient health care is not very clear as soon as one moves away from theoretical constructs and into the real world.

This chapter will attempt to address issues related to managed care efficiency by first discussing what the term *efficiency* means and why the varying definitions of it (or *cost containment*) may lead to diametrically opposed answers, depending on the perspective of the observer. The second section reviews some of the most recent evidence on resource use for patient care—one important component of efficient production of services. This is followed by a discussion of enrollee assessments of the value of managed care plans—that is, patients' perception of quality. It also examines some of the places one might look to "follow the dollars" to see why various actors have differing perspectives on the efficiency of MCOs. Finally, the effects of MCOs on the costs of the overall health care system will be discussed.

Varying Perspectives on Efficiency

Economists use the term *efficiency* in two related ways. The first concerns whether consumers, given their preferences and incomes, are consuming the mix of goods and services that maximizes their individual well-being, given their income and wealth. (Most economic theorists do not consider whether a redistribution of resources should occur or whether individuals benefit from knowing that others are better off [see, for example, Ferber and Nelson, 1993]). Subsidized goods and services are generally not allocated efficiently, because people are induced to buy more of them than they would if they had to pay the full cost of the resources used. This is especially likely to be the case in the health care arena because of the role of insurance and the tax-exempt status of health insurance benefits paid for by an employer. Workers tend to prefer health insurance benefits over a comparable amount of money in wages, because cash income is subject to tax but the amount employers contribute for health insurance premiums is not. Also, insurance alters the perceived price of medical care at the time of consumption—often to zero—while the costs are borne widely through increased insurance premiums, to be paid later and largely by others. These aspects of inefficiency are often the focus of proposals by market-oriented economists who propose ways either to eliminate the tax subsidy or to increase patient price sensitivity through medical spending accounts (Pauly and Goodman, 1995).

The second notion of economic efficiency concerns whether firms are combining inputs optimally to achieve the desired outcomes. For example, are health care providers using the best mix of inpatient and outpatient care and specialists versus generalists to produce a given amount and quality of health care? Again, one might believe that the U.S. health care system, with its orientation toward more comprehensive coverage of inpatient services and its bias in training toward specialists, might be less efficient in this regard than might be the case in a perfect world of resource allocation.

Even at this relatively theoretical level, there are important complications that need to be raised in a discussion of efficiency. Perhaps most important is the question of the product or service desired by the consumer. Although some people may actually seek medical care for its own sake (the most extreme example is the very rare Munchausen's Syndrome, in which a person feigns illness to receive treatment), most people are really interested only in maintaining a functional level of good health. That is, they would be just as happy (or happier) if their health plan offered fewer services and prevented illness. Although this concept makes sense to most people, it creates enormous practical problems because it would require valid and reliable measures of potential enrollees' health status in order to assess whether the end results offered by various health plans were comparable. Such broad-based measures are not available currently, so we are often left with comparisons of the efficiency with which different plans deliver services, often measured in quite narrow and conventional categories. (This point will arise again in the discussion concerning enrollee assessments of plans, below.)

Assuming, for the sake of discussion, that not too much is lost in the current policy debate by focusing on relatively conventional medical care, it is still the case that it is difficult to develop comprehensive measures of the quality of care. Various components may be measured, such as technical proficiency in performing certain procedures, mortality rates for certain conditions, and enrollee satisfaction with certain aspects of the treatment process or the steps required to obtain care. Unfortunately, however, such measures are difficult to obtain, of limited scope, and impossible to aggregate. Even if one had accurate measures of various aspects of quality for a set of health care plans, different consumers might assess them differently. Some may be more concerned about avoiding the rare disastrous outcome, others may focus on waiting time in the office, and others may be most sensitive to the nature of their personal interactions with providers.

The first notion of efficiency, which focuses on consumer choice, is most easily applied to very simple commodities such as milk and bread. Once one shifts to far more complex goods and services, such as medical care, the assessment of comparability by an outsider becomes almost impossible. Thus, in the face of an absence of data, most people change the focus from a broad notion of efficiency to a narrow examination of costs. That is, if MCOs offer services comparable to those offered by other health plans, then lower costs for MCOs would be considered an indication of their greater efficiency.

Focusing just on costs simplifies the matter, but there is the additional question of perspective. Figure 2.1 may help in this regard. Just to the right of the vertical dotted line is the mix of services used by an MCO to produce medical care for its enrollees. These would be measured in terms of hospital admissions and patient days, physician office visits, pharmaceuticals, and so on. To the extent that an MCO or other entity must undertake certain administrative functions, those activities also need to be included as resource requirements. Added to this are any services that people purchase outside the plan because of limitations in benefits, lack of convenience, or other factors. (These are shown below the horizontal line.) That is, a plan should not be assessed only by how much it covers but also by what people feel they need to purchase to supplement its benefits.

Multiplying these inputs by their respective economic costs and summing the results give the cost from a societal perspective. The economic costs used in this calculation are the "opportunity costs," or the value of the resources in their next best use. For example,

Figure 2.1. Components of Health Care Costs from Various Perspectives.

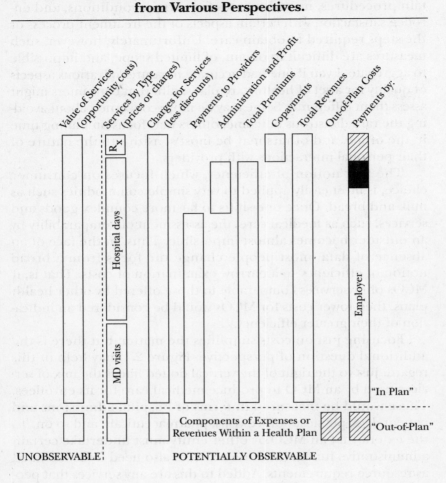

UNOBSERVABLE   POTENTIALLY OBSERVABLE

= copayments for covered services

= enrollee share of premium (not paid by employer)

if physicians have been able to maintain artificially high incomes due to restrictions on entry to the profession, then their true cost would be the hourly wage similarly qualified persons could earn in another job. The payments above opportunity cost level are considered "economic rents" and reflect an existing level of market power; these may be eliminated without a true cost to society. If an anesthesiologist is able to earn $200 per hour and the next best job he or she could get is at $100 per hour, then any wage of $100 or more would keep the individual working as an anesthesiologist, and that is all that his or her services are worth from a societal perspective. Likewise, administrative costs need to be calculated in terms of opportunity costs, and profits should be no higher than those found in other industries in order to maintain capital investment.

The problem with this notion of "social cost" is that opportunity costs are not observable in the real world. Instead, the best one can do is observe prices, charges, or transactions. Thus, one could apply charges, or list prices, to the various inputs to approximate what one would have to pay for them, at least on a full-charge, or "retail," basis. It is important to recognize that these prices may bring substantial economic rents and profit margins. They may also be inflated, because few people pay retail. For example, with the exception of cars such as the Saturn, most dealers routinely negotiate prices, and the sticker price is merely a starting point for the bargain. It would be silly to assume that the value of automobiles sold in the United States is equal to the sum of all cars sold times their respective sticker prices.

One important aspect of MCOs is that they often contract with providers (including hospitals) for lower fees. An MCO's costs for providing health care services to its enrollees thus reflect these discounts. Sometimes payments to providers are actually below opportunity cost levels, in the sense that they do not cover the costs of replacing capital or other base expenses. (One can easily see why some providers are less than enthusiastic about MCOs.) In addition to payments to providers for services to enrollees, MCOs must add in administrative costs and profit. Some people argue that administrative costs are unproductive and the true cause of high health care expenditures in the United States (Woolhandler and Himmelstein, 1991). While this may be true in some regards (for example, with respect to enrollment and marketing costs, which could be avoided in a system of universal coverage), some administration is necessary for the coordination of activities and resources. Likewise, some profit is necessary to encourage private investment in the system. These components of cost, however, are political "hot buttons."

MCO revenues are derived largely from premiums and copayments. The latter are paid entirely by the enrollee, whereas premiums are often split by the employer and the employee. Out-of-plan costs are also paid entirely by the enrollee. The splitting of premium costs between employer and employee is important in the debate about MCOs. In contrast to conventional fee-for-service (FFS) or even preferred provider organization (PPO) coverage, MCOs tend to rely much less on copayments and more on internal controls over costs and utilization. They may also have a broader benefit package, with better coverage for preventive services, and thus less out-of-plan costs than is the case with FFS or PPO coverage. With MCOs, therefore, more of the total bundle of services is included in the premium, and less is included in out-of-pocket expenses. To the extent that the employer pays a fixed percentage of its employees' premiums or a fixed amount that fully covers an HMO's premium, one can see how the shifting of expenses into the benefit package and premium may increase the employer's absolute costs (and certainly its share of the total), even if total resource use is less in an MCO. Thus, it is quite possible for MCOs to be more efficient, offer a better package of coverage and services to enrollees, and yet cost employers more.

A final perspective takes an even broader view, focusing not on, say, the efficiency of MCOs versus conventional FFS programs but on the efficiency of a world with MCOs versus one without them. For example, suppose that MCOs develop more efficient ways of providing certain services of comparable quality. In the short run these efficiencies might be translated into resource and cost savings for a limited population. In the long run, however, they might lead FFS providers to adopt similar production patterns and become similarly efficient. A comparison of the two systems would then demonstrate no advantage for the MCOs, yet this would simply be because everyone's efficiency would be greater due to the presence of the MCO. It might also be the case that competition among MCOs and between MCOs and FFS programs would lead to a decrease in demand for certain types of provider services, which would then rapidly erode long-standing rents and excess profits among providers. While this might drive charges (or payments) closer to opportunity costs, differential efficiencies might not be detectable. Thus, one also needs to ask whether the growth and development of MCOs and the competition they engender alter the overall cost of health care in a market area. This, in fact, is probably the perspective that comes closest to answering whether MCOs can bring U.S. health care costs more in line with those of other developed nations.

Evidence on Resource Use, Quality, and Costs

As the preceding discussion has illustrated, it is impossible to estimate the true opportunity costs associated with medical care use, and charge-based information may be wildly misleading. Instead, therefore, this section will focus on the evidence concerning the use of particular types of medical inputs, as well as the available information with respect to quality of care. While it is far from a "bottom line" (or even one of the many "bottom lines" described in the preceding section), the focus on inputs allows attention to whether there is evidence of differences in practice that should be observable if true differences in efficiency exist. If none can be detected, then "bottom line" differences most likely reflect more aggressive negotiations about price and a transfer of rents from some parties to others.

This section is also limited in that it focuses almost entirely on health maintenance organizations (HMOs) and mostly on the more established plans. There is little published evidence in peer-reviewed journals on some of the new or hybrid plans that include point-of-service options to allow people to use out-of-network providers with partial coverage. In part this reflects the rapid development of the marketplace and the lag time required to design, carry out, and publish research. In part it reflects a greater willingness on the part of traditional HMOs to undertake or open themselves to research. Miller and Luft (1994) reviewed the published literature on various aspects of HMO performance between

1980 and 1993; that material will only be summarized here, along with any major new information that has become available in the ensuing two years.

Resource Use

In general, the evidence going back to a paper I published in 1980 has shown consistently lower hospital use for enrollees in HMOs. However, there seems to be a change in the pattern of how those utilization differences occur. In the earlier period, it seemed to be the case that admission rates were lower for people in HMOs, but there was little evidence of consistent differences in length of stay. In the more recent period, the admission rate results are somewhat more mixed, with some HMOs exhibiting higher admission rates, but not significantly higher rates. At the same time, the more recent length of stay results are more consistently showing shorter stays for HMOs in contrast to comparison (largely FFS) enrollee groups.

Stearns, Wolfe, and Kindig (1992) presented data from a small population of Wisconsin government employees who were patients of a group of physicians whose payment basis changed from fee for service to capitation between 1983 and 1984. The research design holds constant the patient and physician pools, thus addressing many of the concerns people have about biased selection. While the sample is small and the differences appear to be insignificant, there was a reduction in admissions, a small increase in length of stay, and an overall decline in inpatient days.

Most of the research findings focus on overall measures of hospital use, but some recent studies examine use for narrowly defined conditions. For example, Pearson and his colleagues (1994) reported on the admission rates for patients presenting to Brigham and Women's Hospital in Boston with the complaint of chest pain. Admission rates for those at high risk of having had a heart attack were the same across payer categories. For patients at low risk of having had an infarction, those belonging to Harvard Community Health Plan had a significantly higher rate of hospital admission than others, even after accounting for their risk factors. One possible explanation offered by the authors for this counterintuitive finding was the more extensive information accompanying the HMO patients when referred by their HMO physicians, which may have made it more difficult for the attending physicians not to admit those patients.

A common assumption about HMOs has been that they tend to shift care from inpatient to outpatient settings, both because of providers' financial incentives and because HMO patients face a lower financial barrier to outpatient treatment due to the absence of significant deductibles and copayments. The more recent studies reported in Miller and Luft (1994) do not show a consistent pattern of more physician use in HMOs, perhaps because cost-containment pressures affect all types of use. Consistent with their data's being relatively old, the Stearns, Wolfe, and Kindig study (1992) demonstrates significantly higher use of physician services after capitation.

One important concern in almost all the studies of managed care plans is the potential for biased selection, whereby the people choosing HMOs are somehow different from those remaining in FFS. There is substantial evidence of such selection, and it is often in the direction of lower-risk people enrolling in the HMOs, although this is not always the case. (See, for example, Luft and Miller, 1988; Hellinger, 1995.) The recent effort by the Department of Defense to implement managed care for the dependents of military personnel under its CHAMPUS program offers an important quasi-experimental example addressing this problem. CHAMPUS eligibles in Hawaii and California were forced to choose between a PPO option and an independent practice association (IPA)–type HMO, although both had substantially better benefit packages in terms of lower copayments. Data were available for sites in those two states prior to the experiment, as well as in matched sites in states in which the traditional FFS program was still available. Two studies (Goldman, Hosek, Dixon, and Sloss, 1995; Goldman, 1995) reported the findings of this experiment. After controlling for the factors that might lead people to choose the HMO or the PPO, Goldman found that people in the HMO were far more likely to access the system and had an increase in ambulatory visits, probably due to the improved coverage. No significant differences were found in inpatient use, but the sample size may have been too small to detect an effect.

Other studies indicate lower resource use by HMOs for selected procedures. For example, Kukendall, Johnson, and Geraci

(1995) examined the use of coronary revascularization for patients admitted to California hospitals for coronary atherosclerosis. Controlling for various risk factors, HMO enrollees were about as likely to undergo either coronary artery bypass graft (CABG) or percutaneous transluminal coronary angioplasty (PTCA) as were Medicare beneficiaries, but they were less likely to do so than those covered by private health insurance. Much of this difference was in the use of the less expensive, but less definitive, PTCA rather than in the use of CABG.

As part of the Medical Outcomes Study, an extensive study of patient outcomes, Sturm and his colleagues (1995) focused on depressed patients. They found that, controlling for health status, depressed patients in prepaid settings were significantly, but only slightly, less likely (.50 probability versus .56) to see a mental health provider during a six-month period, but their intensity of use (9 visits versus 14) was markedly lower.

Miller and Luft (1994) reported on several studies indicating lower rates of cesarean section among women covered by HMOs. Tussing and Wojtowycz (1994) examined obstetric deliveries in New York State in 1986. They found that the probability of a C-section is lower for HMO enrollees (although the differences they found were smaller than those reported in some other studies, particularly studies from California). The results for IPA enrollees indicate an even smaller differential. Furthermore, HMO enrollees are more likely than women with FFS coverage to have dystocia (a risk factor for C-section) reported, thereby increasing the risk-adjusted difference—but HMO physicians are less likely to use this as a reason for a C-section. Part of these findings is due to the authors' inclusion of HMO market share as an explanatory variable, which captures part of the HMO effect.

In general, the existing literature provides strong evidence of lower utilization of services by HMO enrollees than by people with conventional FFS coverage. This is true both for overall measures of resource use, controlling as best as one can for differences in risk factors, and for the use of specific services for more narrowly defined populations. The latter studies, while more limited, are more convincing both because of their more detailed approach to risk adjustment and because they indicate how HMOs are substituting lower-cost for higher-cost interventions, especially when there is little evidence of differences in overall effectiveness. In some cases the results are counterintuitive, such as the greater differential for the use of the lower-cost PTCA than for the higher-cost CABG. However, CABG is often seen as a more definitive intervention, and it may be the case that the HMOs are more likely to avoid hospitalizing those patients with marginal indications.

Quality and Satisfaction

The question of whether HMOs lower medical care use cannot be considered apart from whether the quality of care and service they offer is comparable. If lower use leads to poorer quality, then HMOs might or might not provide a better value in medical care coverage—it would depend on how much lower was the cost and how much poorer was the quality. Some individuals would consider almost any diminution of quality unacceptable, regardless of the savings, yet in the real world these people usually make all sorts of similar trade-offs, accepting slightly lower quality for markedly lower prices. Except for the very rich, most people choose to fly coach rather than pay for first class. While the service is definitely better in first class, the safety record and on-time records are the same. An issue of major importance is the importance of the differences in quality between HMOs and FFS systems. (That is, to continue with the airline analogy, which are they comparable to—safety records, on-time arrivals, or cuisine?)

Miller and Luft's review (1994) suggested that the quality of medical care for enrollees in HMOs was usually comparable or better than for those in FFS settings. A few more recent studies continue the pattern of somewhat mixed results. A study of the treatment of non-Hispanic white women with breast cancer in Orange County, California, suggested that those with localized cancers had a significantly higher than average mortality rate if initially treated in an HMO hospital (Lee-Feldstein, Anton-Culver, and Feldstein, 1994). (Much of this difference was associated with patients presenting before 1988; in the period from 1989 to 1990 there was no difference for women in HMO hospitals.) Survival rates for women with regional breast cancer were no different for those treated in HMO hospitals. Recent findings from the Medical Outcomes Study, which analyzed patient outcomes in Boston, Los

Angeles, and Chicago in various delivery settings, indicate no meaningful differences in disease outcomes for patients with hypertension or non-insulin-dependent diabetes, despite lower resource use by the HMOs for those patients (Greenfield and others, 1995).

Patient assessments of the quality of care offered by HMOs tend to be more negative (Miller and Luft, 1994). For example, a survey of randomly selected Medicare beneficiaries indicated significantly lower satisfaction among HMO enrollees than among FFS patients in regard to measures of technical quality (for example, "your doctor is very careful to check everything when examining you" and "your doctor has a complete understanding of the things that are wrong with you") of their usual source of care. Similar but not significant differences appeared for disabled patients on Medicare (Adler, 1995). The differences by type of plan were even smaller for the "interpersonal" aspects of care, such as "your doctor seems to be in a hurry" and "your doctor often does not explain your medical problems to you."

A study comparing people who chose FFS coverage over managed care, people who chose managed care over FFS, and people who have managed care and did not have a choice showed marked differences in enrollee satisfaction (Davis, Collins, Schoen, and Morris, 1995). While managed care enrollees were typically more dissatisfied than those with FFS coverage (except in regard to paperwork and out-of-pocket costs), those enrolled in managed care because they had no other option were the most dissatisfied. (Unfortunately, the survey did not include people in FFS plans without a choice of managed care.)

This leads to the more general question of self-selection, a very important issue both in terms of measurement and policy implications and with respect to the implementation and assessment of managed care. When people have a choice of plans, it is reasonable to assume that many will have substantial reasons for choosing one option over another. These may reflect differences in consumers' need for, or preferences about, various types of medical care, their ability to select their health care providers, and the financial costs associated with the various options. In the past, most HMOs required that employers and the government offer a FFS option along with their health plan, thus heading off concerns (including legal requirements) about choice of physician. This policy had the additional effect of ensuring that people dissatisfied with their HMO would be able to leave during the next open season; it provided a mechanism for people to "vote with their feet," and, simultaneously, it enhanced the reported satisfaction of those remaining in the HMO.

It is now increasingly common for employers, especially smaller employers, to offer only a managed care plan. Thus many people in HMOs today may feel that they were forced into a setting they do not want (especially those who had to sever preexisting physician relationships). This trend toward offering only managed care may lead not only to dissatisfaction but also to poorer quality care if continuity of care is threatened. Attributing these problems to the managed care plan may be unfair, however, if it is the employer or government program that forces individuals into this situation.

The issue of selection is more commonly addressed in the growing literature on risk assessment and adjustment with respect to differences in enrollees among various plans (Luft and Miller, 1988; Hellinger, 1995). For example, if people choosing HMOs tend to be less sick than those staying in FFS (perhaps because those with chronic illnesses choose to stay with their current provider), then comparisons of utilization and cost figures between HMOs and FFS are likely distorted, favoring HMOs. Some of the studies reviewed above attempt to adjust for this problem with state-of-the-art risk assessment, but most make only admittedly crude adjustments. Furthermore, the distribution of medical care expenditures is highly skewed; a very small number of cases account for a substantial fraction of total health care costs, and this small group of people may be difficult to detect in many studies (Berk and Monheit, 1992). This issue is a major concern for proposals to fix capitation payments or sponsor contributions across plans. On the other hand, it is not likely to account for the very consistent patterns of cost and utilization observed in the existing studies. Furthermore, as more and more people are being denied the choice of a FFS option, the issue of selection in these studies becomes less important, although it is still an issue for comparisons among various HMOs.

Costs as Viewed by Various Parties

While it seems to continue to be the case that HMOs use fewer resources than FFS providers and insurers, this does not necessarily mean that HMO costs are lower. To determine whether this is likely to be the case, one needs to understand the relationship between costs from various perspectives. As indicated in Figure 2.1, if HMOs use fewer medical care resources, such as inpatient and outpatient services, *and if their administrative costs are not enormously higher than in FFS,* then the overall societal costs are lower. There are numerous articles in the lay press, as well as some in the refereed literature (Woolhandler and Himmelstein, 1991), that indicate that substantially higher proportions of total revenues go to administration and profit in MCOs than in FFS insurers. Unfortunately, these numbers are not as simple to assess as it seems.

For example, suppose that an MCO develops a new clinical information system that keeps track of patient visits, diagnoses, and lab values, and the system allows the MCO to identify those patients with diabetes or congestive heart failure who are not taking their medications appropriately. This information is somewhat expensive to collect and maintain, yet it enables practitioners to intervene to help patients manage their illness, and it prevents unnecessary hospitalizations. An external assessment of such a system would find that medical care expenditures are lower than in the uncoordinated FFS system, administrative costs are higher, and, obviously, the ratio of administration to total is much higher. Furthermore, the comparison would be even more biased if the HMO were to charge the total cost of its information system against current income (which it may be allowed to do for tax purposes), even if the system will be available for several years and is truly an investment.

The above was obviously an example favorable to HMOs, but there are others suggesting that the reported administrative cost figures may be too low. For example, HMOs that contract with medical groups for capitated care incur relatively little in the way of direct administrative costs. These are borne by the medical groups and passed along to the HMO through the capitation payments, so the figures reported by the HMO as "medical care" actually overstate the true amount of medical services provided.

Likewise, reported figures for "profit" may be highly misleading. For example, suppose a radiologist owns an imaging facility and gets paid both for professional services and for the services of the facility, which she owns. The latter figure probably includes a substantial return on investment above and beyond the risk price of capital and might be considered profit, yet it would in a FFS environment be considered part of the medical care provided. If our radiologist sells her practice to an organization in exchange for a share of the plan and receives a base salary plus a share of the profits (and perhaps some stock options to provide extra incentives for improved future performance), then it will appear that medical care has gone down and profits up, yet this may not be the case.

The issue of how to conceptualize profit is an important one. Economists typically view profit as a return to risk taking, in the sense that those who gamble on ventures are entitled to a large return on those ventures that do pay off, because many do not. In the long run, if the rate of profit is unusually high and if there are no barriers to entry, then new competitors will drive the rate of profit down in each industry, although this does not mean that individuals may not report very high profits in any particular year. If barriers to entry exist, either through licensure, patent protection, or other external means, then profits may be routinely higher in an industry. (For example, there is lively debate over whether the pharmaceutical industry typically obtains a "higher than normal" rate of return.) Likewise, some people argue that physicians earn incomes substantially higher than is justified by their training and effort and that this is due to the restrictions on entry due to licensure and the relatively noncompetitive way in which prices have been set under fee for service with third-party reimbursement. If this argument is true, and if the growth of managed care merely means that excess profits are being transferred from physicians to HMO administrators and stockholders, then this shift in wealth may be very upsetting (or welcome) to some—but it has little to do with efficiency. In fact, if the easier entry of administrators is more likely to lead to "normal" salaries and profits than has been the case for physicians, then in the long run there will be less distortion in these markets than has been the case in the past.

One might feel on firmer ground in asserting that advertising and marketing costs have no place in medical care and are a dead-weight loss. That is, even if "sharing the profit" might be an accounting fiction (or even if it can play a valuable role in creating incentives), what social benefit derives from media expenditures to lure patients into one plan or another? While some of these expenditures certainly are excessive, it needs to be determined whether competition among health plans leads to increased costs or increased efficiencies. This question will be addressed below.

In addition to all these conceptual issues involving how to measure profits and administrative costs, there are other important issues in assessing perceptions of costs. On the right-hand side of Figure 2.1, it is apparent that while much of the revenue received by a health care plan can be represented by premium dollars (the remainder is copayments), the premium may be borne in varying degrees by the subscriber and the sponsor (usually the employer or government). Making the issue more complex is the fact that HMO copayments are typically relatively minor, while FFS deductibles are usually substantial, and there are additional FFS copayments. Furthermore, the typical HMO benefit package covers services such as well-baby care and physician exams, which may be excluded from the typical FFS insurance package. Thus, while the HMO may end up using fewer medical services for its enrollees, because it has to cover the costs of more services, its premiums may be higher than that of an FFS insurer with high out-of-pocket costs. Thus, the shift of enrollees from FFS to HMOs could simultaneously lower resource costs, lower costs for enrollees, yet increase employer costs.

The preceding example assumed that the people switching into HMOs are a random sample of those in FFS programs. In fact, there is substantial evidence that HMOs often (but not always) attract enrollees with lower than average risk (Luft and Miller, 1988; Hellinger, 1995). This has two important implications. The first is that it is often very difficult to assess whether, even if HMO premiums are lower than those of FFS insurers, this is due to efficiencies that are being passed on, or whether the HMOs are merely attracting low-risk enrollees. Second, to the extent that low-risk people are migrating to HMOs, the FFS plans will have an increasingly high-risk enrollee population, thereby forcing up their premiums. As many employers have until recently tied their contribution levels to FFS premiums, this would lead to an even faster increase in employer costs.

Numerous recent reports from benefits consultants indicate that HMO premiums have been rising more slowly than FFS premiums, or even falling in absolute dollars (KPMG Peat Marwick, 1993). As indicated above, it may be difficult to determine whether this is due entirely to resource savings; thus these reports need to be considered with a good deal of skepticism. Nonetheless, the impression recently is that employers seem to be increasingly satisfied with the cost of HMOs relative to FFS insurance, although some feel that HMOs should be able to constrain costs further.

The Global Perspective

One problem with the studies reviewed above is that they focus on relatively limited aspects of the impact of managed care, largely because of the problem of designing a feasible study that is empirically valid. Thus, most consider differences in cost, use, quality, or satisfaction between enrollees in a managed care plan and those in FFS. If managed care were a simple uniform intervention comparable to a new drug, then such studies would be helpful in choosing among the two options. However, managed care plans vary enormously in their design, their financial incentives, and the people involved. Thus, it is impossible to generalize from one plan to another, even if they are of the same type. Furthermore, the comparison group—FFS insurance—is not uniform. Sometimes people have a choice between the two types of plans; other times they do not. In some locations managed care is so commonplace that people in FFS programs are probably there because they know they do not want managed care; in other locations managed care is a new phenomenon, and those in FFS include many who might be just as happy in managed care. Thus it is not surprising that some reports that draw from various sites, such as the Medical Outcomes Study, indicate differing results across communities.

More comprehensive studies that include large numbers of sites would be needed to address some of the more global questions about managed care as a policy option rather than an enrollee choice. From a policy perspective, managed care is potentially important not just as another way for people to obtain their medical care but as a possible means to slow the rate of growth in health care costs and improve the quality of care. The logic behind this view is that competition between managed care and FFS and among managed care plans will lead to improvements in efficiency, perhaps lower provider economic rents and excess profits, and improved outcomes as plans take on responsibility for defined populations. In the very long run, pressures by managed care plans on manufacturers of new drugs and devices to demonstrate the value of their products should also shape the rate of growth in, and orientation of, new medical technologies.

Focusing on the policy importance of whether the development of managed care lowers the rate of growth in overall community medical care costs avoids the problems of selection bias. That is, as long as one controls in a reasonable fashion for regional differences in delivery, socioeconomic factors, and demographic factors, and if one can capture costs at the community level, then it does not matter whether HMOs have attracted low- or high-risk people. While these studies are an improvement over simple reports on trends in premiums, which for the last few years have been reporting slower rates of growth in HMOs than in FFS plans, the evidence is still incomplete. If HMOs are experiencing increasingly favorable selection, that could explain the diverging premiums. In many instances, moreover, these premium surveys do not control for changes in benefit design or other important factors.

Several recent studies, however, shed important information on the overall effects of HMOs on premiums and costs. Feldstein and Wickizer (1995) used data from ninety-five employers insured by a single large company (see also Wickizer and Feldstein, 1995). They found that conventional insurance premiums grew significantly more slowly for groups in areas with higher HMO penetration. For example, if the HMO share were 12.5 percent, instead of 10 percent, the estimated rate of growth for conventional insurance would be 5.9 percent rather than 7 percent per year. Wholey, Feldman, and Christianson (1995) examined HMO premiums in various market areas across the nation in the period from 1988 to 1991. In contrast to Feldstein and Wickizer, their focus is primarily cross-sectional rather than on the rate of growth in premiums, and they found that increased competition, as measured by the number of HMOs in an area, is associated with lower HMO premiums. At the same time, they found that higher HMO market penetration is associated with higher premiums. They attribute this to a reflection of selection bias—in low-penetration areas, HMOs tend to attract the lower-risk individuals, but as their market share increases, they must reach deeper into the pool of high-risk persons.

Baker and Corts (1995) examined the effects of HMO market share on conventional insurance premiums using cross-sectional data for 1991. They found that conventional insurance premiums increase with HMO market share for shares above 10 percent, but in many instances the results are only marginally significant. These results suggest that the market-disciplining effects of HMOs on insurance premiums may be outweighed by the market-segmentation effects. Contrary evidence on this issue is offered by Baker (1995) with respect to the Medicare market. In his study, Baker examined the effects of overall HMO enrollment on the expenditures of FFS Medicare beneficiaries using pooled data from 1986 to 1990. Baker used various functional forms and models because of the difficulties raised by omitted variables and simultaneity. In general, his results indicate lower expenditures in counties with higher HMO market shares, although in some models expenditures increase with market share at the low end of the range.

While reconciling these conflicting findings is beyond the scope of this chapter, several points are important to keep in mind. HMOs are not randomly located around the nation—they generally originate and grow in response to market opportunities, and there is substantial evidence that they have often begun in areas in which medical care use is high. Furthermore, various employer characteristics, such as a willingness to provide relatively high health benefits contributions, are associated with HMO market penetration. Insurers are also responsive to market conditions. Premiums may diverge more from costs in more, rather than less, competitive markets. While this seems counterintuitive, the spread between premium and medical expenditures includes not only profit but also marketing, administrative, and underwriting costs. If HMO entry leads to more plan switching, underwriting, and marketing, then premiums may increase while medical expenditures fall (or at least rise less rapidly).

Yet another issue is the distinction between cross-sectional and time-series analyses. While cross-sectional studies offer the advantages of many more observations and increased variability, they suffer more from endogeneity and specification errors. Time-series analyses suffer more from the misattribution of external events, and they focus on things that happen over only a short period of time. In particular, health insurance premiums are known to follow a cyclical pattern of overshooting and undershooting the rate of growth in medical expenditures. This pattern has been analyzed largely at a national level, and there may well be regional differences of a year or two in the cycle. Thus short time-series analyses may occasionally reflect the premium cycle rather than true differences in long-term trends.

While premiums may be the initial focus of competitive strategies, long-term gains from HMOs should be assessed using more global measures, such as overall resource use. Robinson (1991) found slower rates of growth in hospital costs located in areas with larger HMO market shares. Chernew (1995) extended this to a national analysis, using metropolitan area data to assess the impact of changes in non-IPA enrollment on hospital capacity and use between 1982 and 1987. He found that a 10 percent increase in market share is associated with a 4 percent reduction in the number of hospitals and a 5 percent reduction in hospital days and beds.

A more global but more limited assessment is offered by Melnick and Zwanziger (1995), who focused both on hospital expenditures in California as a function of local competitiveness among hospitals and on overall expenditures for hospitals, physicians, and drugs at the state level for the period 1980 to 1991. They found that while California hospitals in more competitive markets had nearly 14 percent higher total net revenue than those in less competitive markets in 1980 to 1982, by 1989 to 1990 they averaged 1.6 percent lower revenue. It is likely that this was the result of pressures from HMOs. More importantly, their analysis of state-level data show that while overall real per capita expenditures for the United States grew by 63 percent between 1980 and 1991, in California the figure was only 39 percent. It is possible that these differences in the rate of growth in expenditures are associated with differences in policy and other factors unrelated to HMO competition, but this theory will require further examination of the data.

Conclusion

There is an ever-increasing body of evidence on HMO performance and a slowly growing accumulation of information on other
types of managed care. It is becoming more difficult to weigh and
assess this evidence, however, because of the changing medical care
market and changing medical technologies. It used to be the case
that HMOs fit into fairly well-defined types such as group- or staff-
model plans and relatively open IPA models. Plans used to collect
fairly comprehensive—albeit crude—measures of inpatient and
outpatient use, and premiums used to be set on the basis of community rating, so all employers faced essentially the same premium
from a given HMO. The world is now quite different. More medical care is taking place in outpatient settings, with quite complicated and intensive treatments being provided at home. Although
this may represent some savings in resource use, it is definitely not
appropriate to focus just on the savings in inpatient days. Yet, as
health plans are increasingly passing on the responsibility and risk
for services to medical groups and IPAs as part of a capitation contract, the plans may no longer be getting the utilization data from
the groups, even though the groups may have the information.
Thus, reported statistics become increasingly suspect.

As market competition has become more intense, premium
setting and pricing decisions are more important. No longer can
one assume that premium information available for one enrollee
group is representative of that quoted to another. Furthermore,
biased selection, especially among competing health plans, may be
an increasingly important component of observed differences.

Some of the reported evidence may be misleading, or at least
not reflective of the questions being asked. As indicated in Figure
2.1, there are many different "costs," and which are relevant may
depend on who is asking the question and why. Thus, resource use
may be lower, but costs to employers may be higher even in a stable, long-term environment. To the extent that real-world data
reflect information drawn from snapshots, with strategic pricing
decisions, short-term cross-subsidies, and similar distortions, dis-
cerning the long-term bottom line is almost impossible.

On the other hand, it is difficult to believe that all this is just
smoke and mirrors. Much of the best evidence is from large, well-

established group- and staff-model plans, with stable enrollments and little evidence that they benefit substantially from favorable selection. Furthermore, many of the studies are now able to focus in detail on selected conditions and their treatment. Thus, while a plan may have a somewhat lower-than-average risk-enrollee mix, and this may affect its overall hospital use rates, selection bias is not likely to explain why the plan is able to treat patients with appendicitis, stroke, or heart attack more efficiently or effectively.

Thus, on balance, the evidence suggests that for the plans studied in the time frame examined, costs and utilization are lower for HMO enrollees, while quality is at least comparable. Whether these lower resource costs are passed on to employers is a different issue, and there the evidence is less clear. At the same time, enrollees' perceptions of their treatment by HMOs have been less favorable. Implicit in these assessments are several crucial caveats. Little is known about newer types of HMOs that have broadly dispersed networks of providers linked by protocols, utilization management, and various types of individually based financial incentives. We also know little about how even the old-line plans will perform in a far more competitive market. While there is reason to believe that increased pricing pressures may lead to corner cutting, this need not be the case. Some plans are focusing on reengineering how they organize and deliver services. Some purchasers are making it clear that they are willing to pay more for high-quality care and better patient outcomes—if superior performance can be demonstrated. Thus outcome-focused competition could lead to marked improvements in both quality and cost. Whether purchasers direct the basis of competition in that direction is a question for the future; the answer to that question will probably determine the future performance of MCOs.

References

Adler, G. "Medicare Beneficiaries Rate Their Medical Care: New Data from the MCBS." *Health Care Financing Review,* 1995, *16*(4), 175–187.

Baker, L. C. *HMOs and Fee-for-Service Health Care Expenditures: Evidence from Medicare.* National Bureau of Economic Research Working Paper No. 5360. Cambridge, Mass.: National Bureau of Economic Research, November 1995.

Baker, L. C., and Corts, K. S. *The Effects of HMOs on Conventional Insurance Premiums: Theory and Evidence.* National Bureau of Economic Research Working Paper No. 5356. Cambridge, Mass.: National Bureau of Economic Research, November 1995.

Berk, M. L., and Monheit, A. C. "The Concentration of Health Expenditures: An Update." *Health Affairs,* 1992, *11*(4), 145–149.

Chernew, M. "The Impact of Non-IPA HMOs on the Number of Hospitals and Hospital Capacity." *Inquiry,* 1995, *32*(2), 143–154.

Davis, K., Collins, K. S., Schoen, C., and Morris, C. "Choice Matters: Enrollees' Views of Their Health Plans." *Health Affairs,* 1995, *14*(2), 99–112.

Feldstein, P. J., and Wickizer, T. M. "Analysis of Private Health Insurance Premium Growth Rates, 1985–1992." *Medical Care,* 1995, *33*(10), 1035–1050.

Ferber, M. A., and Nelson, J. A. (eds.). *Beyond Economic Man: Feminist Theory and Economics.* Chicago: University of Chicago Press, 1993.

Goldman, D. P. "Managed Care as a Public Cost-Containment Mechanism." *RAND Journal of Economics,* 1995, *26*(2), 277–295.

Goldman, D. P., Hosek, S. D., Dixon, L. S., and Sloss, E. M. "The Effects of Benefit Design and Managed Care on Health Costs." *Journal of Health Economics,* 1995, *14*(4), 401–418.

Greenfield, S., and others. "Outcomes of Patients with Hypertension and Non-Insulin-Dependent Diabetes Mellitus Treated by Different Systems and Specialties: Results from the Medical Outcomes Study." *Journal of the American Medical Association,* 1995, *274*(18), 1436–1444.

Hellinger, F. J. "Selection Bias in HMOs and PPOs: A Review of the Evidence." *Inquiry,* 1995, *32*(2), 135–142.

"HMO Coverage Cost Less in '95." *San Jose Mercury News,* Jan. 31, 1996, p. 3D.

KPMG Peat Marwick. *Trends in Health Insurance: HMOs Experience Lower Rates of Increase than Other Plans.* Washington, D.C.: KPMG Peat Marwick, 1993.

Kukendall, D. H., Johnson, M. L., and Geraci, J. M. "Expected Source of Payment and Use of Hospital Services for Coronary Atherosclerosis." *Medical Care,* 1995, *33*(7), 715–728.

Larson, E. "The Soul of an HMO." *Time,* Jan. 22, 1996, p. 44.

Lee-Feldstein, A., Anton-Culver, H., and Feldstein, P. J. "Treatment Differences and Other Prognostic Factors Related to Breast Cancer Survival: Delivery Systems and Medical Outcomes." *Journal of the American Medical Association,* 1994, *271*(15), 1163–1168.

Luft, H. S. "Assessing the Evidence on HMO Performance." *Milbank Memorial Fund Quarterly/Health and Society,* 1980, *58*(4), 501–536.

Luft, H. S., and Miller, R. H. "Patient Selection in a Competitive Health Care System." *Health Affairs,* 1988, *7*(2), 97–119.

Melnick, G. A., and Zwanziger, J. "State Health Care Expenditures Under Competition and Regulation, 1980 through 1991." *American Journal of Public Health,* 1995, *85*(10), 1391–1396.

Miller, R. H., and Luft, H. S. "Managed Care Plan Performance Since 1980: A Literature Analysis." *Journal of the American Medical Association,* 1994, *271*(19), 1512–1518.

Pauly, M. V., and Goodman, J. C. "Tax Credits for Health Insurance and Medical Savings Accounts." *Health Affairs,* 1995, *14*(1), 125–139.

Pearson, S. D., and others. "The Impact of Membership in a Health Maintenance Organization on Hospital Admission Rates for Acute Chest Pain." *Health Services Research,* 1994, *29*(1), 59–74.

Robinson, J. C. "HMO Market Penetration and Hospital Cost Inflation in California." *Journal of the American Medical Association,* 1991, *266*(19), 2719–2732.

Schulte, F., and Bergal, J. "The Medicaid HMO Game: Poor Care, Big Profits." (Four-part series.) *Miami Sun-Sentinel,* Nov. 26–29, 1995.

Stearns, S. C., Wolfe, B., and Kindig, D. A. "Physician Responses to Fee-for-Service and Capitation Payment." *Inquiry,* 1992, *29*(4), 416–425.

Sturm, R., and others. "Mental Health Care Utilization in Prepaid and Fee-for-Service Plans Among Depressed Patients in the Medical Outcomes Study." *Health Services Research,* 1995, *30*(2), 319–340.

Tussing, A. D., and Wojtowycz, M. A. "Health Maintenance Organizations, Independent Practice Associations, and Cesarean Section Rates." *Health Services Research,* 1994, *29*(1), 75–92.

Wholey, D., Feldman, R., and Christianson, J. B. "The Effect of Market Structure on HMO Premiums." *Journal of Health Economics,* 1995, *14*(1), 81–105.

Wickizer, T. M., and Feldstein, P. J. "The Impact of HMO Competition on Private Health Insurance Premiums, 1985–1992." *Inquiry,* 1995, *32*(3), 241–251.

Woolhandler, S., and Himmelstein, D. U. "The Deteriorating Administrative Efficiency of the U.S. Health Care System." *New England Journal of Medicine,* 1991, *324*(18), 1253–1258.

Part Two

Private Sector Initiatives and Responses

Demand-Side Challenges and Initiatives

The impetus for market-based reform and price-competitive managed care comes largely from the demand side of the health care market—that is, from large purchasers of health benefits. A key element of price-competitive managed care is the enhancement and use of bargaining power by large purchasers. In Chapter Three, Linda Bergthold and Loel Solomon provide a broad overview of employer purchasing groups, including a discussion of their history, their various forms and functions, and their strengths and possible shortcomings. In addition to enabling more effective bargaining, purchasing groups are expected to provide information on the quality of care provided by various health plans, to enable health plan enrollees to make informed choices among plans based on trade-offs between quality and price. The other two chapters in this section provide more in-depth analyses of the degree to which purchasing groups have been able to serve in this capacity. In Chapter Four, Helen Schauffler and Tracy Rodriguez describe the experience of the Pacific Business Group on Health (PBGH) in developing and implementing a system to assess the comprehensiveness of the preventive health services provided by different health plans. In Chapter Five, Andrew Bindman describes some of the conceptual and operational complexities of the health care "report cards" now used to communicate information on quality.

These three chapters illustrate a number of different types of market failure and the mainly private sector initiatives to overcome them. The most obvious market failure stems from the lack of demand-side market power; this has been quite successfully dealt with by purchasing coalitions. These chapters also touch on a number of other types of market failure, both those stemming from informational problems and those due to externalities. Purchasing coalitions are attempting to use their bargaining clout not only to get competitive prices but also to force the collection of information about quality of care. Although the PBGH is requiring such information specifically for the benefit of its member firms' employees, there should be a "spillover" benefit to all potential enrollees of these health plans. Despite such private sector efforts, we can see that our ability to measure and monitor quality of care via such "report cards" is currently limited, primarily by lack of standardized clinical and enrollee data collection systems. As a result, quality assessment in competitive managed care markets might be substantially enhanced by public sector intervention to subsidize and encourage the development of a common system.

Supply-Side Challenges and Responses

Competitive managed care controls costs primarily by radically reducing the use of high-intensity, high-cost medical services. In effect, this reduces the demand for such services in the industry. Thus the transition to competitive managed care can be expected to have a tremendous impact on the demand for and work life of nearly all types of health care professionals. In Chapter Six, Edward O'Neil and Leonard Finocchio discuss opportunities for cost reductions in health care delivery and implications of managed care for job reengineering, changes in the scope of practice and professional education. They focus on medicine, nursing, and allied and public health professions, which are expected to be most severely affected by the expansion of managed care. Chapter Seven, by Howard Waitzkin and Jennifer Fishman, focuses on how the structure and incentives of managed care affect the quality of the patient-physician relationship from the perspective of a primary care physician.

Chapters Six and Seven also illustrate a number of different types of market failure. Chapter Six discusses the need to change licensure laws to allow less expensive providers greater "scope of practice." The authors highlight how past professional licensure laws severely reduced competition, thus contributing to higher-than-necessary costs. But professional licensure, particularly in the case of physicians, does serve as more than a way for providers to exert monopoly power. Given the inherent difficulty in obtaining information about medical care quality, it is essential to maintain some method of assessing professional competence to guide consumer choice. The informational disadvantage of the health care consumer is explored further in Chapter Seven. In an era of competitive managed care, the physician is increasingly perceived as having a financial incentive to deny necessary care under the guise of professional authority. As a result, patients' trust in their physicians may be seriously eroding, with ominous consequences for the future quality of care.

Chapter Three

Group Purchasing in the Managed Care Marketplace

Linda A. Bergthold, Loel Scott Solomon

Group purchasing is a rapidly evolving market phenomenon with potentially significant effects on the cost, quality, and organization of health care in the United States. Recent anecdotal evidence suggests that the collective actions of health care purchasers are altering the dynamics of local health care markets by checking the aggregate power of providers and elevating quality as a dimension of competition among health plans and providers.

A number of types of groups purchase health insurance, including business and health coalitions, health insurance purchasing cooperatives (HIPCS), and health alliances. These arrangements reflect a range of organizational structures and interventions intended to bring multiple buyers together to improve the quality and efficiency of health care. (Throughout this chapter we use *purchasing groups* as a general term to describe a variety of organizational arrangements.) Some groups are sponsored by public entities, although most are privately controlled. While the majority are organized by and for private employers, others extend membership to public employers, labor unions, and even health care providers. Despite their diversity, however, purchasing groups tend to share one fundamental premise: collective action is more likely to achieve their goals than fragmented, single-party efforts.

In this chapter, we describe the evolution of group purchasing and discuss the purchasing strategies with the greatest potential to influence the market. Our preliminary evaluation of these strategies indicates a mixed and incomplete record of accomplishment. On the matter of cost, while purchasing cooperatives have achieved some success at bringing down premiums for their own members, it is unclear whether these reductions have been achieved through increased efficiency, by shifting costs to other purchasers, or by shifting higher-risk patients from managed care to traditional indemnity plans. With respect to quality, purchasers are requiring plans and providers to evaluate their processes and outcomes of care or face the prospect of lost business. Nonetheless, the tools available for measuring quality remain quite limited, and the impact of these initiatives on the quality of care remains largely undocumented. Finally, while approaches to group purchasing that move beyond individual local markets are too new to assess, they suggest significant shifts in the way health care is bought and sold.

As these strategies evolve, they are likely to have a number of implications for key sectors of the health care system. Purchasers will have to decide whether the benefits of joint purchasing are worth the reduction in autonomy it entails and the extra effort it requires. Managed care plans and providers will have to find ways to be more responsive—in terms of both price and quality—or face being denied access to the growing number of consumers represented by these purchasers. And policymakers will have to recast existing laws and regulations in ways that allow purchasing groups to thrive, while ensuring that these groups do not become yet another vehicle for risk selection.

The Evolution of Health Care Purchasing Groups

When the cost of health benefits for employees was a relatively small proportion of the total compensation package, corporations paid little attention to its purchase or offerings. It was not until the early 1970s, when the cost of health insurance and its proportion of the total benefits package began to increase noticeably, that some business leaders realized they needed greater control over this element of compensation and began to discuss how best to achieve that control.

Business was called to action by a Republican administration, when President Nixon's secretary of health, education, and welfare, Robert H. Finch, said in 1969, "We will ask and challenge

American business to involve itself in the health care industry, including the creation of new and competitive forms of organization to deliver comprehensive health services on a large scale" (Faltermayer, 1970, p. 127). Business leaders were challenged by their own peers in the opening article in a 1970 *Fortune* magazine: "American medicine . . . stands now on the brink of chaos. The time has come for radical change. . . . The management of medical care has become too important to leave to doctors, who are, after all, not managers to begin with" ("It's Time to Operate," 1970, p. 79).

Although business leaders may have recognized the inefficiency of the medical care industry, group purchasing was not the first strategy to which they turned. Health care purchasing groups are a much more recent intervention, emerging from an earlier organizational form, the "community" or "business and health care" coalition. Business and health coalitions grew rapidly in the mid 1980s, from 25 in 1982 to 173 by 1985 (Bergthold, 1990, p. 51). Several forces contributed to this rapid growth: the failure of the federal government to control costs through regulation or voluntary means throughout the 1970s, the participation and interest of large corporations in local and state attempts to control costs, the promotion of the private health care sector by the Reagan administration, the rise of large corporations delivering health care in multiple locations, the penchant of Americans for the use of informal groups to solve what are perceived to be community problems, and, perhaps most visibly, the influx of between $15 and $20 million in support from the Robert Wood Johnson and other foundations for the development of coalitions around the country in the early 1980s (Jaeger, 1983; Brown and McLaughlin, 1988).

By the mid 1980s, business leaders may have hoped that almost two decades of activity had finally succeeded in controlling health care costs and that intense organizational intervention would no longer be required. Neither turned out to be true, and the 1990s have brought about another generation of multiparty organizations determined to bring down costs—and more so than the business and health coalitions that came before them. This new wave of group purchasing has developed in response to the inability of individual employers and the traditional business and health coalitions to negotiate effectively with large insurance companies and

managed care organizations and to compete against public purchasers such as Medicare and Medicaid.

By early 1996, the National Business Coalition on Health had a
membership of over ninety employer-led coalitions around the
country. NBCH staff estimate between 125 and 150 business coalitions currently operating in over thirty states, representing roughly
ten thousand employers of all size and more than thirty-five million
enrollees. Of the NBCH's estimated 150 business coalitions on
health in 1995, approximately one third are actively purchasing
health care insurance and services jointly (National Business Coalition on Health, 1995). While there are no reliable national data
on the types or sizes of firms that participate in these coalitions,
the most active members of state-based or local coalitions tend to
be larger firms with adequate personnel to devote to this type of
activity; manufacturing, banking, or public sector organizations;
and firms with a direct economic interest in health care production or supply (Bergthold, 1990, p. 121).

Group Purchasing Strategies in the 1990s

The mid 1990s–style purchasing group is different from earlier
approaches in a number of important ways. First, instead of emphasizing consensus building among key stakeholders, these new
groups tend to emphasize the prudent purchase of insurance
through joint purchasing or negotiating. As a consequence, relationships with hospitals, doctors, and health care plans are undertaken at arm's length. Second, their intervention is no longer
focused solely on cost containment; rather, they have broadened
their mandate to include an emphasis on quality monitoring and
improvement. Finally, the geographic reach and membership
of group purchasing are starting to expand. While the majority of
groups remain focused on local markets and are controlled by
businesses that are either based or have a large number of employees in those communities, the last few years have witnessed the rise
of the superalliance—purchasing groups whose reach extends
across multiple markets.

Although the Clinton administration's ill-fated Health Security Act of 1993 can be credited with bringing health alliances into
the popular vocabulary, the alliance as a prudent purchaser of

insurance has its roots in the theory of managed competition first put forward by Stanford economist Alain Enthoven and further refined with the assistance of University of California professor Richard Kronick (Enthoven and Kronick, 1989). The centerpiece of this proposal was the "public sponsor," an entity that would purchase insurance on behalf of small companies and individuals not connected to the workplace. By aggregating the purchasing power of these disparate and independent purchasers, the authors of managed competition believed alliances could serve as a counterweight to the power of insurers in the small and nongroup markets.

It is somewhat ironic, then, that the most prominent purchasing groups today are not small-employer alliances but those organized by and for larger employers. Of course there are notable exceptions. For example, the community health purchasing alliances (CHPAs) in Florida and the Health Insurance Plan of California (HIPC) are attracting increasing numbers of small businesses with access to affordable, comprehensive benefits and the type of plan choice that small employers find it difficult to offer their employees.

Purchasing Groups as Negotiating Agents

Today's purchasing cooperatives undertake a wide range of activities related to negotiating with health plans and providers on behalf of group members. As pictured in Figure 3.1, these activities can be arrayed along a continuum based on

- The power and legal authority of the purchasing group to contract with plans or providers on its members' behalf.
- The degree of benefits standardization among policies offered by members of the group.
- The degree of risk sharing, or "community rating," across the participating entities.

On one side of the continuum are groups whose major function is merely to provide information on the price and quality of health plans. Members of these groups design their own benefit packages and retain contracting authority; they also assume the financial risk

Figure 3.1. Continuum of Group Purchasing Strategies.

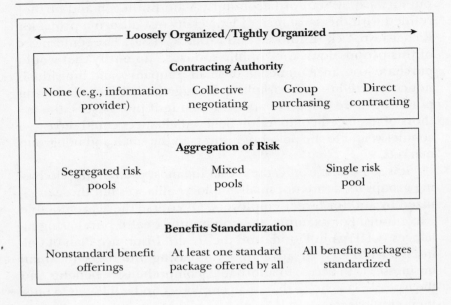

────── Loosely Organized/Tightly Organized ──────

Contracting Authority

None (e.g., information provider)   Collective negotiating   Group purchasing   Direct contracting

Aggregation of Risk

Segregated risk pools   Mixed pools   Single risk pool

Benefits Standardization

Nonstandard benefit offerings   At least one standard package offered by all   All benefits packages standardized

for health costs generated by their own employees. On the other side are purchasing groups that directly contract with provider networks, design plan benefits, and provide—directly or through contract—utilization review, managed pharmacy plans, and other cost-containment services. Most purchasing groups are clustered in the middle of this spectrum, however, as either *collective negotiators* or *group purchasers.*

The nature of the contracting relationship tends to be associated with other aspects of the group's purchasing strategy. For instance, individual entities engaged in group purchasing activities are more likely to offer at least one common benefit package and to share risk for that product than are entities engaged only in collective negotiation. By contrast, businesses that come together for the purpose of collective negotiation are more likely to pursue their goals through negotiated fee schedules or other cost-control strategies that allow segregated risk pools and considerable flexibility in benefit design. In order to conduct collective negotiations, coalitions need not necessarily be tightly organized along the dimensions in Figure 3.1.

The Pacific Business Group on Health (PBGH) is typical of the collective-negotiation model of joint purchasing. PBGH is the largest business and health coalition in California and the first private coalition in that state to negotiate collectively on behalf of its member companies. The group does not actually contract with plans on its members' behalf; the contracts are written directly between the health plans and PBGH's members. PBGH does, however, serve as a negotiating agent for eleven of its member companies, which represent four hundred thousand people and $400 million a year in premiums. In that role, PBGH negotiates the premiums for the HMOs that will serve the eleven companies. Each company decides which HMOs to offer, but all HMO plans must offer the same standardized benefit package to the group (Robinson, 1995; Lewin-VHI, 1995).

All PBGH members are large, self-insured firms—a factor that contributes to individual members' need for autonomy within the purchasing arrangement. PBGH's negotiating strategy is similar to that employed by several other alliances. After reviewing the operations of eleven different public and private cooperatives, the U.S. General Accounting Office found that while negotiating styles differ, most purchasing groups that engage in such activities share a common strategy. Most rely on "informed discussions" with health plans to review and debate premium increases. And while all require plans to submit data to the purchasing group to examine whether such rates are actuarially justified, some also use actuaries to develop target premiums for the plans (General Accounting Office, 1994a, p. 49). Many private groups of this type offer considerable choice to member companies, while individuals in those companies must join only those HMOs selected by the company.

Another California purchasing group, the California Public Employees' Retirement System, or CalPERS, serves as a good illustration of the group purchasing model on a statewide scale. Today, CalPERS has over nine hundred public employers, a million enrollees, and $1.6 billion in insurance spending. In contrast to PBGH, CalPERS has the authority to negotiate on behalf of all of its members and to decide unilaterally which plans will be offered to its members and under what terms. CalPERS standardized its

HMO benefits package in 1992, and each employee of CalPERS' members in the same geographic region has the same choice of plans, whether that individual works for a small city, an independent water district, or the state of California. The model of group purchasing provides maximum choice for employees, while organizational members have less choice because they must offer all HMOs selected by CalPERS.

A third model of group purchasing—direct contracting—is being forged by the Buyers Health Care Action Group (BHCAG) of Minneapolis–St. Paul, Minnesota. In 1991, BHCAG's focus shifted to collective purchasing. In 1993 the coalition began to offer its own health plan. One year later the group had ninety thousand employees and dependents of twenty companies enrolled in the plan—called Choice Plus—which is administered by a consortium called HealthPartners (General Accounting Office, 1994a).

Because of BHCAG's national visibility, the purchasing group made headlines in July 1995, when it announced that it would start directly negotiating contracts with small groups of hospitals and physician networks called "care systems," using HealthPartners to administer the contracts. HMOs will still have a role to play in this new scheme, as contractors providing marketing and data management services to the provider groups. Nonetheless, these new roles represent a dramatic flip in the balance of power between HMOs and providers in the Twin Cities marketplace. According to BHCAG officials, the intention behind this purchasing strategy was to bypass the administrative costs borne by HMOs and to inject meaningful competition into a market dominated by three major health plans (Meyer and others, 1996; Winslow, 1995; "Powerful Minn. Employer Coalition . . . ," 1995). While direct contracting is the central feature of this initiative, it is important to point out that the plan also represents a step back from direct employer control over workers' health benefits in one important respect. The direct contracting initiative also calls for broader employee choice under a voucher-based system in which employees select among a large number of care systems certified by BHCAG. Employees will pay the difference between the cost of the plan they pick and the voucher amount—a concept very close to the original concept of managed competition, which brought the term *purchasing cooperative* into the public vocabulary.

It is important to note that direct employer contracting is not a new strategy. Many individual employers adopted a similar strategy over the last two decades when they moved away from traditional health insurance in favor of self-insured arrangements. This earlier form of direct contracting, managed by third-party administrators and consultants, was driven by a number of different factors, including employers' dissatisfaction over traditional insurance carriers' inability to control costs, inadequate local networks, and the desire to avoid costly benefits mandated by state governments. (The growing prevalence of self-insurance is well documented elsewhere. See General Accounting Office, 1995.)

While the prevalence of self-insurance has continued to grow over the last five to seven years, particularly among smaller firms, this trend has coexisted with the even more rapid penetration of managed care—a trend that appears to have addressed employers' concerns about costs with some degree of success. BHCAG's plans to leapfrog over HMOs through direct provider contracting therefore signals an important change in current managed care practice, particularly with respect to control over the premium dollar.

Leveraging Local Markets Through Regional Purchasing

For many years, conventional wisdom has held that all health care markets—like all politics—are local. Unlike other goods and services, which can be shipped in from out of state or delivered over phone lines and computer cables, health care services are seen as an indigenous product, delivered to consumers by community hospitals and doctors. Local markets are traditionally viewed as the product of unique dynamics—namely, the particular disease patterns and health care needs of the population, the population's preference for one style of medicine over another, regional practice patterns, the shortage or excess of doctors and other health care professionals in the area, and special institutional relationships among doctors, hospitals, and the purchasers of health care.

Some of the nation's purchasing groups are challenging this notion by negotiating with plans on behalf of regional or national employers for multiple-market contracts. In contrast to market-by-market negotiations, these purchasing groups are seeking to maximize their members' regional clout by striking agreements with managed care plans that can deliver care across a wide geographic area. In the West, for instance, PBGH now negotiates with statewide HMOs for employers such as Pacific Telesis and Wells Fargo Bank that have employees across the state. The recent addition of firms in Washington and Oregon to PBGH's membership roster indicates that the group has extended the negotiation process beyond California (Robinson, 1995, p. 127).

Perhaps the most striking example of this movement toward multimarket contracting, however, is the so-called super-HMO initiative, or National Health Care Purchasing Alliance, rolled out in 1995. In that effort, ten of the nation's largest companies, including American Express, Merrill Lynch, IBM, and Marriott Corporation, announced that they were jointly releasing a request for proposals to HMOs to provide coverage to 240,000 employees in twenty-seven different health care markets in which they had some employee concentration (Freudenheim, 1995). A major reason for this unprecedented national strategy was the fact that this group of purchasers had noted the substantial inconsistency of quality and coverage across markets, even within the same managed care plan. In implementing their national purchasing strategy, the alliance discovered that there was even more local variation than they had anticipated. Instead of trying to select one or even a small number of HMOs to serve their employees across markets, the national alliance focused on selecting the highest-quality plan within each region, even when that plan was not necessarily the lowest-cost plan. According to Dr. Lonny Reisman, the physician consultant who helped devise the strategy, the purchasers agreed on a single plan design, asked for bids, and then gave equal weight to quality and cost in the first screen. Some of the lowest-cost plans did not meet quality screens and were dropped in second-round negotiations (L. Reisman, telephone interview, April 16, 1996). The result was not a single or super HMO, however, but a regional purchasing strategy implemented by multistate employers.

Continued sensitivity to how "national" HMO products differ region to region is realistic, given mounting evidence that there is significant variation in relative performance across the markets in which many national HMO plans are active. Moreover, employers have reported that regional plans with smaller networks are more successful at overseeing provider quality than larger, national plans (Mahar, 1996).

The Drive for Quality

Monitoring and improving quality have become major activities for a growing number of cooperatives. This development has been spurred by the understanding that value is a function of both price *and* quality. This view is reflected in the National Business Coalition on Health's definition of quality—"the right care from the right source at the right time" (1995, p. 1)—and its assertion that quality is now viewed by most coalitions as the best way to achieve sustainable cost control and maintain a healthy workforce. Purchasing coalitions are well suited to drive health care markets toward improved quality, for a number of reasons. First, their accumulated purchasing clout allows them to demand account-ability from providers and plans that are reluctant to compete on this new plane and may feel threatened about the prospect of doing so. Purchasing groups also have the ability to bring more financial and technical resources to bear on these initiatives than any individual member. Finally, groups can help bring about the standardization of quality information merely by acting in a concerted fashion. Standardization is important because it improves the usefulness of quality data (allowing apples-to-apples comparisons) and substantially reduces the cost of generating that data.

Quality initiatives undertaken by purchasing groups have var-ied considerably, in terms of both scope and sophistication. A recent assessment of group purchasing initiatives by Jack Meyer and his colleagues found that choice of quality initiative is often a function of the size and resources of the group, the interest and level of involvement of individual member companies, the rela-tionships between the group and the provider community, and the nature of the contracting arrangement. Perhaps the most common activity is the design and dissemination of consumer "report cards." While the specific elements of these report cards differ, most emphasize surveys of enrollees and plans on items ranging from customer satisfaction to waiting times to enrollees' opinions on the quality of care received. A growing number of report cards also in-clude HEDIS indicators—uniform measures of HMO performance developed by the National Committee for Quality Assurance and supported by the employer community (General Accounting Office, 1994b).

In addition to developing report cards, purchasing groups have required providers to buy and implement computer systems that collect and analyze detailed clinical information. Because these systems adjust for patient risk and uncover a finer level of clinical detail than either HEDIS or consumer surveys, purchasers and providers often find them more useful in pinpointing quality problems and designing strategies to address them (General Accounting Office, 1994c). Two cooperatives that have emphasized such systems in their quality improvement programs include Health Care 2000, a coalition representing eighty-two employers in Grand Rapids, Michigan, and the Central Florida Health Care Coalition, which represents six hundred thousand enrollees. Health Care 2000's quality initiative is built around an inpatient monitoring system developed by MEDSTAT that generates reports on a number of measures—including hospital charges, average length of stay, and mortality—and adjusts those measures for severity of illness prior to admission. The Central Florida Purchasing Cooperative has used a similar system developed by MediQual, another private health information systems vendor. In addition to requiring local hospitals to purchase and implement MediQual, the Central Florida coalition is developing outpatient monitoring initiatives for the top twenty-five major diagnostic categories as well as a patient survey designed to collect postintervention outcomes information for patients with hip and knee replacement surgery (Lewin-VHI, internal client memo, 1995).

Purchasing groups have also explicitly incorporated quality requirements into health plan contracts through network selection criteria and provisions of requests for proposals, as well as through contract provisions that establish financial incentives for providers to deliver high-quality care. In the first approach, quality is used as a screen to increase the likelihood that the purchasing group will contract with high-quality plans and providers. Contracts can also be drafted to require those entities to generate data, such as that described above, that can be used to monitor provider performance over the contract period. Incentive-based approaches represent an even more significant step in the evolution of value-based purchasing. One of the more innovative approaches in this area is that of the Colorado Health Care Purchasing Alliance—a Denver-based group that represents one hundred thousand enrollees

(Rybowski, 1994). In a program that began last year, the alliance puts 2 percent of health plan premiums into a bonus pool, which is paid out to the plans at the end of the year if the plans meet established performance targets. Plans are encouraged to set high standards for themselves, because those targets are made public in information given to employees prior to open enrollment.

In an increasing number of cases, quality improvement initiatives have been undertaken in collaboration with providers, often in stark contrast to the arm's-length approach typical of other group purchasing strategies. Emblematic of this approach is the creation of task forces and quality councils representing purchasers, clinicians, and, at times, consumers to address specific clinical and administrative issues. The goal is to assess current practices (usually on the basis of cost or utilization data), review best practices, and devise consensus-based practice guidelines and other action plans to move the community toward best practices (Lewin-VHI, internal client memo, 1995; Meyer and others, 1996, p. 15).

For example, as part of its national strategy, the National Health Care Purchasing Alliance is creating a partnership between the power of purchasers and the clinical expertise of consultants and outside experts. The alliance intends to use a panel of nationally recognized physician experts to consult with local plan physicians on complex cases, creating a dialogue between best national practices and actual physician interventions. While this approach is fully controlled by purchasers, it acknowledges the critical place of clinical knowledge in the purchasing decision. Collaborative strategies such as this have emerged because purchasers have found that they have neither the expertise nor the information necessary to bring about meaningful, concrete changes in clinical practice on their own. In large measure this reflects the simple fact that health care providers and health service researchers are vital partners in understanding the clinical practice of medicine and the implications of practice change on patient outcomes.

Consequences of Group Purchasing Strategies

What impact have these group purchasing strategies had on the marketplace? Have they reduced costs, improved quality in any measurable way, or had an impact beyond the local market?

Impact on Costs

Much of the evidence for the success of group purchasing initiatives at reducing cost comes from California. In 1994 PBGH achieved an average reduction in HMO premiums of just over 9 percent—a reduction attributed at least in part to collective negotiations (Robinson, 1995, p. 126). Over a similar period, CalPERS negotiated a 0.4 percent decrease for its HMO premium prices. In an environment where individual corporations had been bragging about limiting increases to single digits, the idea of an actual reduction was novel. Even CalPERS itself had seen HMO rate increases in 1991 and 1992 of 11 percent and 6 percent, respectively. On February 16, 1995, CalPERS announced that it had negotiated an overall 3.8 percent rate reduction in medical premiums for all of its plans for the 1995–1996 plan year (Lewin-VHI, 1995, p. B-3). These overall reductions represented 5.2 percent reductions for the HMO premiums and 2.3 percent increases for the preferred provider organization and self-funded plans. Meyer's review of purchasing coalitions in Madison, Wisconsin; the Twin Cities; and Edison, New Jersey, also provides evidence of savings for member companies, from 15 percent off charges (Madison) to 11 percent off comparable products offered in the market (Twin Cities) (Meyer and others, 1996).

Despite the success of CalPERS, PBGH, and other purchasing groups in reducing premiums for their members, a major unresolved issue is whether premium reductions reflect cost shifting or improved efficiency, which benefits the larger community. If group purchasing merely results in shifting costs to smaller, less organized purchasers, as many critics of purchasing groups contend, then collective purchasing may do more harm than good. For instance, cost shifting may contribute to the cost of insurance in the small-group and individual markets, leading to concomitant increases in premiums in those markets. Such a strategy may also imperil the financial security of safety net providers such as public hospitals, which provide the bulk of charity care and care to vulnerable populations. Moreover, as providers wring inefficiency from the health care system in response to increased demands from large employers and other buyers of health care and as public payers start to impose further limits on their payments (for example, through Medicaid managed care), there may be significant limits to the amount of additional cost reductions that can be brought about through strategies that depend on cost shifting rather than cost savings.

If, on the other hand, negotiations with providers and managed care plans result in new ways of controlling costs rather than merely shifting them, one can be more optimistic about the potential for continued savings. Cost controls with more promise for a lasting effect include changes in clinical practice patterns brought about through the development and adoption of practice guidelines, more efficient use of technology through technology assessment, provider education and centers of excellence, and programs emphasizing healthy behaviors, self-care, and greater consumer consciousness of the cost of medical care.

Empirical evidence of cost savings at the community level is scarce. One large-scale evaluation was the Robert Wood Johnson Foundation report on its $15 million project to promote affordable health care programs in sixteen communities in the mid 1980s (Brown and McLaughlin, 1990). After reviewing hospital spending per capita, admission rates per thousand, length of stay, trends in outpatient surgery, and prepaid group practice enrollment in the metropolitan areas where coalitions supported by the foundation were located, this study failed to produce hard evidence of cost containment at the community level—the level where the coalitions had hoped to achieve an impact. Their data yielded no evidence of hospital cost-containment outcomes that could be plausibly attributed to the existence of the programs for affordable health care in the sixteen communities.

The evaluators concluded that the variables that determine costs are not generally within a community's control. Many causes of health care inflation originate outside the local level, at the state or national level. They also found that there was not sufficient concentration of power in the hands of most local purchasers to force change and that the local purchaser leadership was not willing to make the hard decisions required to confront its providers.

Impact on Quality

Quality measurement and improvement activities initiated by purchasing alliances hold some promise for improving the health outcomes of group members and of the community as a whole. This is particularly true if these initiatives bring about changes in over-all practice patterns through the provision of new information and better communication and coordination among providers or through the creation of a competitive dynamic that rewards high-quality performance with larger numbers of enrollees. Hard evidence of such changes are sparse, but anecdotes abound. In central Florida the implementation of an inpatient performance monitoring system flagged abnormally high surgical wound infection rates following gall bladder operations. A change in the procedure (making a smaller incision) reportedly resulted in a fall in the infection rate as well as in the average length of stay and average cost of the operation. In Chicago, the Employers Purchasing Initiative for Quality (EPIQual)—an affiliate of the Midwest Business Group on Health—sponsored the development of a critical pathway for coronary artery bypass graft (CABG) surgery. An interim assessment indicated that the pathway helped reduce lengths of stay, readmission rates, and returns to surgery for all patients in four area hospitals (Rother, 1995; Rybowski, 1994). And in the Twin Cities, an organization established jointly by BHCAG and provider groups has developed no fewer than forty-one different practice guidelines, which are in the process of being implemented by twenty participating clinics that collectively serve between 85 and 90 percent of BHCAG's enrollees (Meyer and others, 1996, p. 15).

The Achilles' heel of most quality-improvement efforts, however, is the limited power of existing quality-monitoring systems to monitor outcomes and attribute findings to purchasers' interventions. For instance, many groups rely on private vendors such as MEDSTAT and MediQual to turn raw health care data into quality measures and to provide comparative benchmarks for assessing providers' performance. Reliance on these systems has a number of major limitations. First, with the exception of mortality and some limited measures of morbidity, the indicators focus on measures of resource use (for example, hospital charges, average length of stay, and utilization rates); data on whether patients actually got well or achieved improved physical functioning are largely unavailable from such systems. Second, quality improvement efforts based on these systems are typically limited to inpatient indicators, providing little information on outpatient services. Finally, the benchmarks they use are based on data from vendors' existing client bases or from the Medicare population (or both) rather than reflecting the best achievable practice (Lewin-VHI, internal client memo, 1995).

It is easy, however, to overemphasize the limitations of these monitoring initiatives; the value of these important first steps should also be acknowledged. At a minimum, group purchasers' demands for accountability have played an important role in the development of a new industry to support the collection and analysis of performance data. These demands have also forced providers to critically examine the way they practice medicine and, in some cases, to work together to see if their practice patterns can be improved to deliver higher-quality care in a more efficient manner. Evidence of these changes augurs well for the impact of purchaser-driven quality initiatives, even if there is little hard evidence to date of the actual impact of such initiatives.

Impact on Local Markets

While the implications of the move from local purchasing to trans-market purchasing are substantial for both group purchasers and local health care markets, the trend is also too new to fully assess. Consequently, this strategy prompts more questions than answers. One question concerns the nature of the good that is being purchased. Is managed care a product that is essentially local? What are the limits of regional purchasing? From how far away can you effectively manage clinical decisions? How much can you standardize care across markets? The "super HMO" alliance suggests that there are significant limits to standardization.

Another unanswered question is how this strategy will affect local providers and locally based managed care organizations (MCOs). One important effect of this strategy, confirmed in part by the "super HMO" initiative, may be that regional or national purchasing programs implicitly favor large MCOs and other health care systems that have broad, multimarket coverage. Group purchasers implementing a regional or national purchasing strategy may prefer to do business with only a few networks, because it is much easier to manage a handful of contracts, and the volume that purchasers are able to aggregate across markets offers leverage that they can use against these plans—leverage that is lost for MCOs that operate in only a handful of markets. The end result may be that smaller, homegrown MCOs, including the emerging provider-sponsored networks, may ultimately be disadvantaged by such strategies, unless they are able to develop multisite affiliations.

Other Implications of Group Purchasing

As the phenomenon of group purchasing expands, a number of implications are prompted by our discussion of where purchasing groups have been, the strategies applied by purchasing groups in today's managed care market, and what we know about the success of those strategies.

Implications for Coalition Members and Other Purchasers

Multiparty coalitions may not work if purchasing is their main goal. Buyers can and should form their own organization; the sellers should be involved in the discussions, particularly to the extent that quality is a major focus of the coalition's activity, but they need not be full-fledged members of the purchasing group.

A second implication purchasers should bear in mind is that, as purchasing groups grow, purchasers will face a moment of decision regarding their participation in those efforts. They will have to weigh the benefits of membership against the costs (namely, loss of autonomy and inability to use tailored benefits packages as recruiting or retention tools). Those that do not join, however, may face significant costs, such as higher premiums resulting from costs shifted from more organized purchasers. Individual purchasers' decisions not to join cooperatives will also have important implications for those that do join; some may end up getting a free ride, as the investment of purchasing groups results in beneficial change all around (for example, through changes in practice patterns) that become unfunded public goods.

A third implication for purchasers is that good data about the performance of health care systems are critical to the improvement of quality, but such data are difficult to collect and sometimes even more difficult to interpret. Development of such data can require substantial investments over a long period of time—something that the pooled resources of purchasers are well suited to support. Purchasers who are serious about quality improvement also need to engage local providers and other stakeholders in collaborative initiatives that build trust, draw on their expertise, and recognize providers' sense of professionalism. Purchasers must be ready to act decisively to reward high-quality providers with their business (for example, through selective contracting), but they must also be willing to develop partnerships that give plans and providers time and incentives to make the necessary investments and to develop the candor critical to accurately measuring and improving the quality of care.

A final implication for purchasers is that all of them must work together to achieve success. There have been many examples in this century of successful efforts by labor or management to enhance health and control costs. More efforts need to be made to bring labor and management together as purchasers with common interests. One encouraging effort in this regard is a joint initiative being undertaken by General Motors and the United Automobile Workers union in a number of communities with a large number of GM workers. The goal is to assess the performance of the health care system at the community level and to build support for systemwide change that can lower costs and improve quality for all members of the community. Both labor unions and employers are also participating in the Foundation for Accountability, or FAACT, an organization that is developing new outcomes-based standards for quality measurement that move beyond the process-based measures emphasized by HEDIS.

Implications for MCOs and Practitioners

Arguably the most significant implication of group purchasing for MCOs and providers is the need to meet new demands for accountability from highly organized, relatively sophisticated purchasers that are serious about evaluating the quality of the plans they select. Although business coalitions have been demanding quality data and the right to conduct quality audits for years, many health care plans have either not been able to deliver that data in a comprehensible format or have not taken such demands seriously. In order to be viable in this emerging market, providers will need to make investments in the data systems necessary to support quality-monitoring and quality-improvement activities. Second, although competition may begin with price, purchasers want to go beyond price to outcomes measurement. Offering the lowest price may allow a health plan entry into the market, but it will not keep it there if its quality and outcomes are not up to standards. A final implication for MCOs and providers concerns multimarket purchasing. To the extent that regional and national group purchasers control an increasing number of enrollees in local health care markets, locally based MCOs and provider networks may need to join forces with plans and networks in other areas. Such affiliations may provide these groups with the geographic coverage and one-stop shopping that multimarket purchasers demand.

Implications for Local Health Care Markets

Purchasing groups have a number of immediate implications for local markets. First, prevailing practice patterns are likely to change as a consequence of both quality-improvement initiatives and price pressures. To the extent that these activities result in greater efficiencies and higher-quality care, they are likely to spill over to the community at large. For example, a number of published studies examining the impact on hospital spending of managed care penetration within a given market indicate that HMOs appear to slow cost growth by inducing changes in the way hospitals and doctors treat *all* their patients—not just HMO enrollees but also fee-for-service and other non-HMO patients (Stapleton, 1995; Welch, 1994; Robinson, 1991). Evidence that coalitions have the potential to influence communitywide practice patterns in a similar way includes the adoption of the CABG pathway described above by five competing hospitals in the Chicago area (Meyer and others, 1996, p. 16). Through such spillover effects, coalitions can serve as engines of marketwide reform.

Local markets face a more tumultuous future if local providers respond to price pressure generated by purchasing groups by shifting costs rather than by managing those costs. Cost shifting from organized purchasers to unorganized purchasers is likely to increase the price of insurance for small employers and policyholders in the nongroup market, eventually resulting in higher numbers of uninsured people and more bad debt and charity care loads, bringing about additional cost pressure on unorganized purchasers. While it is difficult to predict whether providers will respond to cost pressure by shifting costs or by looking for new and better ways to practice medicine, characteristics of the markets themselves may influence their decision. For instance, cost shifting is likely to be more prevalent in markets with a relatively large number of small and unorganized purchasers. Markets where relatively easy changes in clinical practice have already been realized may also be prime targets for accelerated cost shifting as purchasing groups continue to flex their market muscle. Importantly, however, purchasing groups may also be able to influence this outcome by using their purchasing clout to seek changes in practice patterns rather than being satisfied with discounts on ever-increasing charges.

Finally, it is still unclear how local markets will respond to the increasing presence of unified buyers. On the one hand, the accumulation of purchasing clout represented by group purchasing may be a necessary correction to the increasing aggregation of market power on the supply side of the market. Organized purchasing may allow purchasers to exercise the "countervailing power" necessary to restore equilibrium between buyers and sellers in local health care markets. On the other hand, increasing buying power represents a further move away from a chief condition required for efficient markets—namely, the presence of multiple buyers and multiple sellers. For the time being, few markets appear to exhibit the significant aggregation of buying power that might represent monopsonistic buying.

Implications for Public Policy

Policymakers must find ways to ensure that purchasing groups can deliver value to their members in ways that are not detrimental to the community as a whole. Perhaps the biggest policy challenge in this regard concerns the establishment of meaningful community-rating laws that allow purchasing groups to negotiate premiums on behalf of small employers. Over the last several years, a number of states have passed some type of community-rating law to prevent insurance companies from skimming the good risks while avoiding the bad ones. The impact of these efforts may be eroded if small employers with healthy risks are allowed to opt out of the community rate by joining a purchasing group that either self-insures or negotiates special rates with insurance companies. Unfortunately, policymakers will have few good options at their disposal if cooperatives are allowed to remain unregulated. Options include implementation of risk-adjustment systems that compensate the community-rated pool for the better-than-average risk profile of coop members, application of guaranteed issue laws to purchasing groups, and strict prohibitions on selective marketing.

There also remains a critical role for policymakers in addressing the unresolved issues of access and coverage for those that remain outside the insurance system. Even the best private purchasing groups cannot be expected to address the inefficiencies and poor health outcomes that result from inadequate access to care for this population. Indeed, as the proportion of uninsured Americans grows, purchasing groups are likely to fight harder to avoid the cost shifting brought about by the bad debt and charity care associated with these individuals.

Conclusion

Group purchasing is a critical factor in the reform of the health care system. For the business sector, the central question is whether purchasing groups can succeed in their goals of reducing costs and improving quality for their members. Success in these endeavors is tied to a number of closely related factors, including the historic reluctance of one segment of the business community to challenge another; the ability of buyers to sustain their effort, particularly given that purchasers are typically in the business of something other than buying health care, whereas health care *is* the business of the supply side of the market; and whether purchasers have the fortitude to confront providers, particularly in markets where hospitals and other institutional providers are major contributors to the community's employment base.

For communities at large, the key questions for the future are somewhat different—namely, to what extent do purchasing group activities generate community benefit, and to what degree do those benefits accrue to group members at the expense of the entire community? The ultimate promise of group purchasing is that such organizations can improve the quality of care and make insurance more affordable to businesses that do not presently offer health insurance. The risk is that purchasing groups will segment the market, leaving the uninsured and less well-organized employers with an even more fragmented health care system.

References

Bergthold, L. *Purchasing Power in Health: Business, the State and Health Care Politics.* New Brunswick, N.J.: Rutgers University Press, 1990.

Brown, L., and McLaughlin, C. "'May the Third Force Be With You': Community Programs for Affordable Health Care." In R. M. Scheffler and L. F. Rossiter (eds.), *Advances in Health Economics and Health Services Research.* Vol. 9: *Private Sector Involvement in Health Care: Implications for Access, Cost, Quality.* Greenwich, Conn.: JAI Press, 1988.

Brown, L., and McLaughlin, C. "Constraining Costs at the Community Level." *Health Affairs,* 1990, *9*(4), 5–29.

Enthoven, A., and Kronick R. "A Consumer-Choice Health Plan for the 1990s." *New England Journal of Medicine,* 1989, *320*(1), 29–37; *320*(2), 94–101.

Faltermayer, E. "Better Care at Less Cost Without Miracles." *Fortune,* Jan. 1970, pp. 80–83, 126–132.

Freudenheim, M. "10 Companies Join in Effort to Lower Bids by H.M.O.s." *The New York Times,* May 23, 1995, p. D2.

General Accounting Office. *Access to Health Insurance: Public and Private Employers' Experience with Purchasing Cooperatives.* GAO/HEHS-94–142. Washington, D.C.: General Accounting Office, May 1994a.

General Accounting Office. *Health Care Reform: "Report Cards" Are Useful, but Significant Issues Need to Be Addressed.* GAO/HEHS-94–219. Washington, D.C.: General Accounting Office, September 1994b.

General Accounting Office. *Employers Urge Hospitals to Battle Costs Using Performance Data Systems.* GAO/HEHS-95–1. Washington, D.C.: General Accounting Office, October 1994c.

General Accounting Office. *Employer-Based Health Plans: Issues, Trends and Challenges Posed by ERISA.* GAO/HEHS-95–167. Washington, D.C.: General Accounting Office, July 1995.

"It's Time to Operate." *Fortune,* Jan. 1970, p. 79.

Jaeger, J. (ed.). *Private Sector Coalitions: A Fourth Party in Health Care?* Durham, N.C.: Duke University Press, 1983.

Lewin-VHI, Inc. "A Report on the State of Health Care in California." Paper prepared for the California Business Roundtable, San Francisco, June 1995.

Mahar, M. "Time for a Check-Up: HMOs Must Now Prove That They Are Providing Quality Care." *Barrons,* March 4, 1996, pp. 29–35.

Meyer, J., and others. *Employer Coalition Initiatives in Health Care Purchasing.* Vol. 1. Washington, D.C.: Economic and Social Research Institute, February 1996.

National Business Coalition on Health. *Health Care Data & Quality: The Role of the Business Coalition.* Washington, D.C.: National Business Coalition on Health, 1995.

"Powerful Minn. Employer Coalition Leads Market to Increased Direct Contracting with Providers." *State Health Notes* (Minn.), September 1995.

Robinson, J. C. "HMO Market Penetration and Hospital Cost Inflation in California." *Journal of the American Medical Association,* 1991, *266*(19), 2719–2723.

Robinson, J. C. "Health Care Purchasing and Market Changes in California." *Health Affairs,* 1995, *14*(4), 117–130.

Rother, L. "Employers in Orlando Create an Envied Model." *The New York Times,* June 30, 1995, p. C18.

Rybowski, L. *How Employers Are Reforming the Market for Health Care.* Washington, D.C.: National Business Coalition on Health, July 1994.

Stapleton, D. *The Impact of Managed Care on Health Care Spending Growth.* Fairfax, Va.: Lewin-VHI, 1995.

Welch, W. P. "HMO Market Share and Its Effect on Local Medicare Costs." In H. Luft (ed.), *HMOs and the Elderly.* Ann Arbor, Mich.: Health Administration Press, 1994.

Winslow, R. "Employer Group Rethinks Commitment to Big HMOs." *The Wall Street Journal,* July 21, 1995, pp. B1–B4.

Chapter Four

Exercising Purchasing Power for Prevention

Helen Halpin Schauffler, Tracy M. Rodriguez

Health plan purchasing alliances have the power to redefine the goal of health care reform from managing care to managing health. Increasingly, large purchasers of health care are seeking value for their health care dollars, and they are defining value in terms of disease prevention and improved overall health. Purchasing alliances offer an opportunity to improve Americans' health by combining economic incentives and systems of accountability to achieve public health goals and objectives.

In this chapter we report on the efforts of one of the nation's largest private employer purchasing groups—the Pacific Business Group on Health (PBGH)—to include health promotion and disease prevention in its definition of value, to pay health plans based on their performance in providing appropriate preventive care, and to encourage employers and employees to choose health plans that excel in promoting health and preventing disease.

Genesis of PBGH

In 1989 executives from the Bank of America and Wells Fargo Bank, frustrated by their inability to control the double-digit inflation

An earlier version of this chapter ("Exercising Purchasing Power for Preventive Care") was published in *Health Affairs*, 1996, *15*(1), 73–85.

of their companies' health care costs, formed the nonprofit Bay Area Business Group on Health. The coalition initially represented ten of the largest corporations headquartered in the San Francisco Bay area.

In the seven years it has been in existence, the coalition has changed in function, size, and name. In 1994 the coalition created a purchasing alliance that began negotiating health care benefits on behalf of eleven member companies, achieving premium reductions of 8 to 10 percent from many of the largest health maintenance organizations (HMOs) in California and saving participating employers more than $36 million. In 1995 the alliance negotiated another 4 percent reduction from HMOs for seventeen of its member companies. That same year the coalition changed its name to the Pacific Business Group on Health to reflect its growing membership of very large employers (those with more than two thousand employees) headquartered in California and its strategic alliances with other coalitions in the western United States. As of December 1995, PBGH membership had grown to thirty-two companies, representing more than 2.5 million Californians and more than $3 billion in annual health care spending.

In 1990, in its first strategic planning effort, PBGH identified disease prevention as a top priority. Its initial efforts focused on work site health promotion programs. The coalition developed and disseminated to its member companies comprehensive strategies to reduce stress, improve fitness, prevent back injuries, and in general enhance employees' health. Many of these strategies were implemented by PBGH companies.

By 1991, however, PBGH had begun directing most of its prevention efforts toward the health plans, encouraging them to provide comprehensive preventive care to all of their enrollees. This plan-based approach took advantage of PBGH's power as a major purchaser of health care. This approach also increased the provision of preventive services for all persons covered by participating employers, including many who often are not reached by work site wellness programs, such as employees in small work sites or remote regions, dependents, and retirees. Finally, this strategy has the potential to improve the health of the fifteen million Californians enrolled in the major health plans targeted by PBGH, not just the employees of PBGH companies.

In the past several years PBGH has adopted standard guidelines, benefits, and performance measures for preventive care, and through its negotiations with health plans it has established economic incentives to improve the provision of comprehensive preventive care to all health plan enrollees. Health plans in California that want a share of PBGH's health care dollars understand that they will be paid for performance that is consistent with the recommendations of the U.S. Preventive Services Task Force's (USPSTF) *Guide to Clinical Preventive Services* (1989) and that achieves or exceeds the health objectives for the nation set forth by the U.S. Public Health Service in *Healthy People 2000* (1990).

First Step: Adopting Guidelines

On January 30, 1992, PBGH convened the first meeting of the California Task Force on Preventive Services (CATFPS), which included the medical directors of major California health plans, the benefit managers of PBGH companies, and an academic research consultant. Its purpose was to discuss ways that health plans and employers could work together to ensure that employees and their families receive appropriate levels of preventive care and to encourage health plans and providers to assume more responsibility for that care (Rodriguez and Schauffler, 1993). The results of PBGH's 1991 employee survey, the Health Plan Value Check (HPVC), showed that although many plans offered health promotion programs to their members, few enrollees participated in them. The HPVC also found that physicians were not routinely discussing health promotion issues with their patients.

That same year PBGH also surveyed member companies on their work site wellness programs and polled health plans on their provision of preventive services. The employer survey found that although most companies offered health promotion programs, few of these programs extended to employees working in small sites and remote locations or to dependents and retirees. In addition, the survey of health plans found that many of the plans followed outdated guidelines for preventive care or used no guidelines at all, and most failed to collect data on their members' use of preventive services. These three surveys—of employees, member companies, and health plans—suggested that neither the employers nor the health plans were providing comprehensive preventive care and that data to assess the performance of health plans and employers on health promotion and disease prevention simply were not available.

Guidelines for Preventive Care

To remedy these problems, CATFPS decided to adopt uniform guidelines and core data elements for preventive care. The task force reviewed a number of preventive care guidelines and ultimately chose those of USPSTF, for the following reasons:

- The guidelines were developed by a national panel of experts rather than a single interest or professional group.
- They are grounded in a rigorous review of the scientific evidence on efficacy and effectiveness.
- They cover all age groups.
- They address more than one hundred interventions to prevent sixty illnesses and medical conditions.

By June 1992 CATFPS had agreed to adopt the preventive care guidelines for screening and immunizations that were recommended for healthy adults by USPSTF.

Guidelines for Counseling

Reaching agreement on guidelines for counseling on prevention was more difficult. The health plans and member companies were not as familiar with the research base behind USPSTF's recommendations for preventive counseling on such topics as smoking cessation, nutrition, exercise, motor vehicle injuries, household and environmental injuries, human immunodeficiency virus infection and other sexually transmitted diseases, unintended pregnancy, dental disease, and alcohol and drug abuse. They questioned the cost and cost-effectiveness of counseling; argued over who should provide the counseling, how often it should be provided, and how it should be done; and expressed concerns over plans' ability to measure their provision of counseling services.

In September 1992, after much debate, CATFPS reached final agreement on the precise wording of recommendations for appropriate preventive counseling. The task force also agreed that the recommended counseling services should be provided to all enrollees of all health plans at least once every three years. Working from a set of national guidelines, CATFPS had taken nine months to reach agreement on comprehensive preventive services recommendations. Next, CATFPS began to discuss ways to measure care against these guidelines. The task force developed a core data set for preventive care, which included standard definitions and suggested methods for measuring the provision of many of the recommended screening tests and counseling services.

Agreement with Health Plans

The chief executive officer of each health plan was then asked to sign an agreement indicating that his or her health plan "is dedicated to improving the health of its enrollees and agrees to encourage appropriate utilization of preventive services in California." The agreement stated that the health plan would

- Adopt the USPSTF *Guide to Clinical Preventive Services* for adult screening and immunizations.
- Adopt the counseling guidelines as defined by CATFPS, which are based on the USPSTF recommendations.
- Collect core data on the provision, use, and outcomes of preventive services for California enrollees.
- Collect and submit to PBGH the core preventive care data defined by CATFPS.

Data collection was to begin in 1993 with the submission of data on the proportion of continuously enrolled women aged fifty to sixty-five in California who had had a mammogram in the past two years, and the proportion of continuously enrolled women aged eighteen to sixty-five who had had a Pap smear at least once in the past three years.

CATFPS then made plans to distribute its *Preventive Care Guidelines for Healthy Adults* to the more than thirty thousand primary care physicians practicing in California (Rodriguez and Schauffler, 1993). PBGH implemented a media campaign in April 1993 to publicize its landmark agreement with sixteen of the major health plans and seventeen of the largest employers in California.[1] Using the same process, CATFPS completed its review and reached consensus on its *Preventive Care Guidelines for Healthy Children and Adolescents* in December 1993. These, too, were subsequently mailed to all family physicians and pediatricians practicing in California and released to the media.

Problems

Despite the commitments made to the agreement, full adherence to the guidelines has not yet been achieved. Some health plans, in an attempt to reach consensus with physicians and other health care professionals within their organizations, have interpreted the PBGH screening guidelines as minimum guidelines. Their internal guidelines, for example, may extend mammography to low-risk women between the ages of thirty-five and fifty or promote prostate screening for low-risk men over age fifty. On the other hand, a number of plans regularly communicate the guidelines to both physicians and enrollees, and a few have helped physicians implement reminder systems and other ways to improve use of the guidelines.

Most plans, however, have taken only minimal steps to promote the counseling guidelines. Some of the plans' medical directors question the original agreement—they argue that routine discussion of these topics with healthy persons is unnecessary. Others question the need for face-to-face communication and wonder whether newsletters, videotapes, and other materials would suffice. Clearly there is a need for USPSTF to better define what is appropriate counseling.

Incorporating the Guidelines into a Model Benefit

In 1993 PBGH began evaluating the feasibility of group negotiating for its member companies and of incorporating its preventive services guidelines into such negotiations. By the spring of 1993 PBGH employers had reached consensus on a model benefit plan for HMOs that incorporated the preventive care guidelines adopted

by CATFPS by requiring coverage for all preventive services recommended for healthy adults, adolescents, and children.

The initial model benefit plan proposed zero copayments for
preventive care to remove all financial barriers to preventive services (Schauffler and Rodriguez, 1993). Copayments for most
other outpatient services were set at five dollars. California HMOs
were asked for preliminary bids on the model benefit plan. The
majority indicated that they could not implement different copayments for preventive and acute care. Based on this feedback,
PBGH increased the preventive care copayments in its model benefit plan to five dollars.

The PBGH model benefit plan, which incorporates the recommendations of USPSTF, has been adopted by all of the employers participating in the PBGH negotiating alliance, by many PBGH
employers that have not participated in the alliance, and by a number of other employers and coalitions across the country.

Collecting Data on Health Plan Performance

Nearly all of the health plans provided the requested Pap smear
and mammography data to PBGH by 1993, as they had agreed to
do. Unfortunately, the quality of the data they provided was poor
(reported screening rates ranged from less than 5 percent to more
than 95 percent). PBGH quickly learned that simply requiring
health plans to provide data does not ensure that the data will be
comparable or reliable. Also, none of the plans provided all of the
data elements originally defined by CATFPS. Shortly before the
PBGH deadline for plan data, the National Committee for Quality Assurance (1993) released its *Health Plan Employer Data and
Information Set (HEDIS), Version 2.0.* The HEDIS 2.0 indicators
included childhood immunizations by the second birthday, cholesterol screening in the past five years for adults aged forty to sixty-
four, mammography screening in the past two years for women
aged fifty-two to sixty-four, Pap smears in the past three years for
women aged twenty-one to sixty-four, low-birthweight rates, prenatal care in the first trimester of pregnancy, asthma admissions,
eye examinations in the past year for persons with diabetes (to prevent blindness due to retinopathy), and outpatient follow-up after
admission for a major affective disorder. Following its release, the

health plans became reluctant to provide any data beyond the HEDIS measures, and PBGH employers agreed to forgo the other CATFPS-defined data elements that were not in HEDIS, including several that measured counseling.

Because the health plans had not provided PBGH with data it could use to assess and compare plans' performance on preventive care, PBGH began to collect its own data on use of preventive services, plan by plan. Given the limitations of most health plans in producing reliable data, other purchasing alliances may find themselves in a similar situation. PBGH began by including specific questions in its 1993 HPVC on the screening and counseling that employees received from their health plans. Every year a sample of employees randomly selected by health plan and employer is surveyed. Employees are asked about their satisfaction with their plan and their physician, if they received specific screening tests appropriate to their age and sex, and if a physician or other health care professional discussed smoking, exercise, nutrition, and other health promotion topics with them in the past three years.

Another PBGH effort to improve information on health plan performance in preventive care has been the development of the California Cooperative HEDIS Reporting Initiative (CCHRI). This is a collaborative, statewide effort that uniformly collects, audits, analyzes, and reports HEDIS data. Although the CCHRI is governed by purchasers, health plans, and providers, it is managed by PBGH. Each year between twenty and twenty-five plans participate in the effort. The initiative's major advantage is that all of the data are either collected or verified by a single, independent, third-party auditor. This method reduces the burden of data collection on medical care providers (whose records are reviewed only once for all participating health plans) and produces rates that are more comparable across plans. However, the CCHRI had difficulty obtaining charts from providers in both its first and second years. Overall, the CCHRI was unable to obtain nearly 20 percent of the sampled records. The number of unavailable charts varied by plan. Because HEDIS specifications require that unreviewed records be counted as negative and assume that services in such records have not been provided, plans with a large proportion of unreviewed records have lower rates of providing recommended services. In addition, the CCHRI identified differences in rates among the three collection methods HEDIS permits: from medical records, from administrative data, and from a combination of the two. Thus, comparisons of performance on HEDIS measures across health plans were fraught with difficulties. But despite these problems, the CCHRI is now in its third year of data collection.

Updating Guidelines and Benefits

CATFPS formally changed its name to the Health Services Advisory Committee (HSAC) in January 1994, to reflect the group's intention to address a wide variety of health care topics in addition to preventive care. For example, HSAC is defining benefits for mental health and fertility services. HSAC also continues to meet to develop additional preventive care guidelines to incorporate into the model benefit plan. Since January 1994 HSAC has adopted preventive guidelines for healthy adults over age sixty-five, as well as guidelines on preventive services that are not universally recommended for healthy adults under and over age sixty-five or for healthy children and adolescents. Next, HSAC will try to develop consensus on preventive care guidelines for pregnant women and high-risk persons, such as those with a family history of disease or with a chronic condition.

Through the work of HSAC, an ongoing mechanism has been established for PBGH to reach agreement with the major health plans and employers in the state on appropriate health care. This is then translated into benefit packages requested by employers and offered by HMOs. PBGH also has coordinated its work on preventive services with that of other groups, including the California Department of Health Services, which has developed preventive care guidelines and defined preventive services benefits for Medicaid managed care contracts. In addition, PBGH is working with other large employers and purchasers in California, including the California Public Employees Retirement System, which is a member of PBGH.

Second Step: Rewarding Health Plans' Prevention Efforts

PBGH has incorporated its preventive services guidelines into many aspects of its negotiations. During its first year of group negotiating, PBGH asked participating HMOs to make 2 percent of their premiums contingent on their performance on selected measures in three areas: customer service, quality, and provision of data. Where possible, the 1996 measures are defined by national standards, such as HEDIS.

PBGH meets with each HMO to negotiate targets and the dollar amounts at risk for each measure. Targets are negotiated based on a health plan's current performance, its performance relative to competing HMOs, and its ability to change its performance. Plans with lower performance measures are encouraged to undertake significant efforts to improve their rates. Plans with better performance measures are allowed to set targets that will maintain or only slightly improve their performance. In addition, PBGH employers ask health plans to accept greater financial risks in areas needing the most improvement.

The amount of money at risk in the 1995 benefit year was nearly $7 million, approximately 30 percent of which, or $2.2 million, was allocated to prevention performance measures. Health plans will receive approximately $500,000 if they meet targets for Pap smears and mammograms. They will receive more than $1.7 million if they provide data on smoking cessation, childhood immunizations, and other HEDIS quality indicators.

If a health plan has reason to question the availability or reliability of its data on a particular measure, the measure is moved to the provision-of-data category. In this category, health plans are financially rewarded if they submit accurate data by the date requested. Once a health plan demonstrates that it is able to collect the required data, the measure is moved to the customer-service or quality category, where performance targets are set and financial incentives negotiated.

New preventive care quality measures for 1996 include three additional HEDIS indicators—prenatal care, diabetic retinal exam, and cholesterol screening—and a new provision-of-data measure, on the extent to which plans have informed members of the availability of wellness programs. In 1996 these measures will be used with point-of-service plans as well as HMOs. In addition, a number of employers that are not part of the PBGH negotiating alliance have adopted these measures.

Third Step: Influencing Market Share

Health plans can also be encouraged to improve their performance with the prospect of additional enrollees. PBGH shares report card information with purchasers and seeks to identify the kind of information that consumers desire and that is most useful.

Publishing Performance Data

PBGH also influences health plans' provision of appropriate preventive care by publishing health plan performance data on prevention, to influence employers' and consumers' choice of plans. One source of information on plan performance in preventive care is PBGH's HPVC survey. PBGH uses the results of its annual consumer survey to rank plans according to their provision of preventive screenings and preventive counseling (Pacific Business Group on Health, 1995). In general, screening rates are relatively high, averaging 80 percent, while counseling rates are low, averaging 20 percent.

The rankings are shared with health plans and purchasers in an annual report card. PBGH encourages purchasers to use the report cards to choose plans that excel in preventive care and to work with plans to improve screening and counseling rates. CCHRI released its first public report card based on its first year of data collection in February 1995. This report card graded twenty-one HMOs that collectively provide health care services to more than 95 percent of all HMO members in California on the provision of the preventive care screening measures included in HEDIS. CCHRI also released a lengthier, more detailed report to participating health plans and employers that provided actual rates for each of the performance measures. Because of problems resulting from variations in the availability of medical charts across health plans, CCHRI decided not to produce a public report card for its second year but will produce a report card for its third year.

Finding Out What Consumers Need

PBGH sponsors focus groups to identify the types of information consumers want and need to choose a health plan and to determine how that information should be presented. The questions asked of recent focus groups and their responses are summarized below.

1.   *What information would you like to have to help you choose among health plans with the same coverage, prices, doctors, and hospitals?* Consumers had difficulty answering this question, despite significant probing. Many participants mentioned that they would discuss their choice with family and friends. Information about enrollee satisfaction was mentioned only once. Quality of care was never mentioned.

2.   *Would you like to receive information on health plans' rates of preventive care to help you choose a plan?* Consumers were asked to use a scale of 1 to 10 to indicate how much they would like to receive information on plan performance on each HEDIS preventive care measure (a 10 indicated that they would really like to obtain the information). Nearly all of the HEDIS indicators received a score of 8 or higher. Participants rated prenatal care and childhood immunizations the highest and diabetic retinal exams the lowest. Although some participants questioned health plans' role in influencing rates of preventive care, others responded that health plans could improve these rates by sending out reminders to patients. In general, consumers highly valued health plan information on prevention.

3.   *How would you like this information to be presented?* Participants were shown a variety of formats. In general, consumers preferred simpler formats. They preferred letter grades (A, B, or C) to the *Consumer Reports* format ("above average," "average," or "below average"), and they preferred either of those formats over actual rates, such as 80 percent or 85 percent. In addition, consumers made fewer mistakes interpreting the results when they were shown grades than when they were shown other formats. Consumers reported that numbers took too much time to decipher and that they had difficulty reading charts with bars and graphs, interpreting information about confidence intervals, and understanding population targets, such as those defined in *Healthy People 2000.*

4.   *Would you use this information?* Most consumers indicated that in choosing a new health plan they would use the information on the report cards, along with other information, such as suggestions from family, friends, and coworkers.

5.   *Would you change health plans based on this information?* Consumers indicated that they would not change their health plan

based on this information alone. If, however, they were unhappy with their health plan, a poor performance on its report card might provide the impetus to change plans.

The findings from the PBGH consumer focus groups suggest that although people do not think of using information on quality of care or preventive care to choose health plans, they value this information and would use it if it were available. PBGH encourages its member companies to use the findings from the HPVC report cards in their open enrollment materials to influence employees' selection of a health plan. The focus group findings suggest that employees will use this information, particularly if they are unhappy with their plan and contemplating a change.

Several PBGH employers have begun to incorporate the results from the HPVC survey into their open enrollment materials for their employees. For example, in 1995 Chevron, Stanford University, the Fireman's Fund, Lockheed, and Union Bank included scores or grades for health plan satisfaction; and Stanford, Lockheed, and Union Bank also included scores or grades on preventive care.

Defining a Health Behavior Measure for Smoking

Of all of its performance measures, PBGH has had the most difficulty obtaining consensus on a measure related to smoking cessation. There are well-established, validated instruments—such as the Centers for Disease Control and Prevention's Behavioral Risk Factor Surveillance System—that ask about individual smoking behavior. The difficulty lies in the uncertainty over how and how much health plans can be expected to affect their members' smoking rates and the possible perverse incentives that might be introduced if health plans were held accountable for their members' health-related behavior.

Measuring actual smoking rates or changes in smoking rates could induce health plans to avoid enrolling smokers as members. Relying on quit rates, while encouraging health plans to focus on the preferred outcome, may place a plan with a higher proportion of members who are heavy smokers at a disadvantage and would not address the problem of recidivism, which may be as high as 90 percent. Also, any action that health plans and providers take to discourage smoking is likely to be only one of many factors contributing to smoking behavior, many of which are outside plans' and providers' control.

To avoid these problems, PBGH initially elected to hold health plans responsible only for providing appropriate smoking cessation counseling to their members. The smoking performance measure in 1994 was the percentage of smokers who had discussed smoking cessation with a health professional in their health plan at least once in the last three years. This measure encouraged health plans to identify smokers (most plans are unable to do so at this time) and encouraged providers to discuss smoking cessation with their patients.

However, the measure for smoking cessation counseling also was problematic because it did not assess the content, length, or quality of the counseling. Thus, a high rate of counseling could mean that health plan providers are simply asking patients if they smoke or not, or it could mean that providers are helping smokers to set a quit date, offering them prescriptions for nicotine patches, and referring them to smoking cessation programs. In addition, since providers do not routinely record provision of preventive counseling in the patient record, these rates have to be obtained from patient reports that cannot be easily validated.

The PBGH performance measure for smoking cessation was changed in 1995 to measure what health plans are doing to reduce smoking, rather than relying on patients' reports of what providers are doing. The new measure requires health plans to

- Provide an action plan for the identification of the smoking population
- Indicate what they are doing to help smokers quit
- Describe how they influence providers to make smoking cessation counseling a routine part of patient care

This measure will not provide PBGH with information on how many smokers were helped or how many have quit, however.

The problems that PBGH has had in identifying a measure for smoking cessation are likely to be repeated as it develops measures for changes in other health-related behaviors. However, USPSTF concluded that "the most promising role for prevention in current medical practice may lie in changing the personal health behaviors of patients" (U.S. Preventive Services Task Force, 1989). Thus, the development of performance measures addressing health behavior is critical if health plans' practices are to be aligned with goals to improve public health.

Funding Research on Preventive Care

PBGH employers established a quality improvement fund in 1994 to support the HPVC and the CCHRI, as well as health services research, including research on preventive care. PBGH has funded research to learn if health plan performance on prevention influences employees' satisfaction with their health plan. The research found that employees who reported that they were offered or used their plan's health promotion programs are more likely to be satisfied with their health plan, are more likely to recommend their plan to family and friends, and are less likely to switch to another plan in the future (Schauffler and Rodriguez, 1994). In addition, employees who reported that their health care professional discussed health education topics with them in the past three years are more likely to be satisfied with their physician (Schauffler, Rodriguez, and Milstein, 1996). These findings suggest that health plans that provide and encourage the use of prevention programs may increase member satisfaction and be in a better position to maintain or even increase their market share.

Conclusion

The experience of PBGH suggests that many strategies are available to purchasing alliances to improve access to and quality of health promotion and disease prevention services. PBGH's efforts to influence health promotion and disease prevention for its member companies have focused on creating systems of accountability, combined with the imposition of economic incentives, to influence health plan provision of clinical preventive services, particularly screening and immunizations. The definition of guidelines, benefits, and performance measures for preventive counseling and other health promotion activities has been more difficult.

The implications of the widespread adoption of the PBGH model among large-group purchasers are enormous. Since 1993 the growth of health plan purchasing groups has been remarkable. More than twenty states now have health plan purchasing groups. Ten states have government-run groups, seventeen states have small-business purchasing groups, and there are estimated to be at least forty large-employer groups. Six states (California, Kentucky, Florida, Minnesota, New Mexico, and Washington) have both government and private employer purchasing groups. These groups have the potential to build accountability and economic incentives into their contracts with health plans and providers that can fundamentally shift the priorities of the health care delivery system.

To the extent that these groups define value for their health care dollar in terms of measurable improvements in health status and disease prevention, their efforts may contribute significantly to achieving public health goals and objectives. In 1990 the U.S. Public Health Service released *Healthy People 2000,* a document laying out the federal government's strategy for health promotion and disease prevention for the decade. The document built upon "the strong foundation of federalism that undergirds the American public health system by involving both private and public sectors at all levels," in the words of James O. Mason, who was then assistant secretary for health in the Department of Health and Human Services (Mason, 1990, p. 23). The approach taken by PBGH, to expressly include health promotion and disease prevention in its definition of value, is a model for how the private sector can take seriously this mandate to improve the health of the general population. Both public and private purchasers can use their purchasing power to shift the priorities of the health care system from managing the delivery of medical services to improving health.

However, a major barrier to holding health plans accountable for their enrollees' health status is the limited role medical care plays in determining health behavior and health status (Schauffler and Rodriguez, 1994). To the extent that purchasers push to define value as health improvement (measured by health status), they eventually will force health plans to look outside the confines of the clinical encounter and beyond the actions of physicians to identify others in the community with whom they can work collaboratively to influence the real determinants of health—the health-related behaviors of individuals and the social, environmental, economic, and political health of our communities.

Notes
1.   A copy of the PBGH preventive care guidelines may be obtained from the authors at the University of California, Berkeley, School of Public Health, 406 Warren Hall, Berkeley, California 94720–7360.

References

Mason, J. "A Prevention Policy Framework for the Nation." *Health Affairs,* 1990, *9*(2), 22–29.

National Committee for Quality Assurance. *Health Plan Employer Data and Information Set (HEDIS), Version 2.0.* Washington, D.C.: National Committee for Quality Assurance, October 1993.

Pacific Business Group on Health. "PBGH a Key Player in Development of Breakthrough HMO Quality Report." *Pacific Currents,* 1995, *1*(1), 3.

Rodriguez, T., and Schauffler, H. "Measuring Quality of Preventive Services." *Business and Health,* 1993, *11*(5), 65–70.

Schauffler, H., and Rodriguez, T. "Managed Care for Preventive Services: A Review of Policy Options." *Medical Care Review,* 1993, *50*(2), 153–198.

Schauffler, H., and Rodriguez, T. "Availability and Utilization of Health Promotion and Disease Prevention Programs and Satisfaction with Health Plan." *Medical Care,* 1994, *32*(12), 1182–1196.

Schauffler, H., Rodriguez, T., and Milstein, A. "Health Education and Patient Satisfaction with Physicians." *Journal of Family Practice,* Jan. 1996, pp. 62–68.

U.S. Preventive Services Task Force. *Guide to Clinical Preventive Services: An Assessment of the Effectiveness of 169 Interventions.* Baltimore, Md.: Williams and Wilkins, 1989.

U.S. Public Health Service. *Healthy People 2000: National Health Promotion and Disease Prevention Objectives.* Department of Health and Human Services pub. no. (PHS)91–50212. Washington, D.C.: U.S. Department of Health and Human Services, 1990.

Chapter Five

The Challenge of Measuring and Monitoring Quality

Andrew B. Bindman

Throughout most of the twentieth century, the quality of health care has been defined by the medical profession, and little information on quality has been publicly available. The public is now demanding greater accountability from its health care system, however, and it is no longer satisfied to leave judgments about quality to physicians. Although the desire for information about health care quality is high, few data are available.

Publicly reported health care quality "report cards" emerged in the 1980s. While the notion of report cards is readily understood by the public, the term has negative connotations for those being evaluated, and there is a growing movement to instead refer to these quality evaluations as quality indicators or performance measures. Most of the initial activity in reporting performance measures emerged from government agencies and focused on hospitals (Brinkley, 1986); however, private organizations are increasingly developing performance measures for health plans and physicians. This shift appears to be directly attributable to the increased competition among health plans and health care providers.

Different participants in the health care marketplace are likely to have different uses for performance measures. Employers, as purchasers of health care services, are interested in identifying the differences in quality among health plans of varied cost. Patients, who increasingly are enrolled in managed care plans that limit their choice of physicians, want to know about the quality of different health plans and their providers. Physicians might use performance measures to determine if they want to be associated with a particular health plan. Health plans would like to incorporate performance measures into their marketing strategies. Both health plans and providers want to use performance measures to stimulate quality improvement projects. Public health agencies can use performance measures to monitor progress toward public health goals.

While performance measures hold much promise, several important questions should be answered before they are embraced by participants in the health care marketplace. First, who should be evaluated—hospitals? health plans? individual physicians? Second, what should be measured, and is it a valid indicator of health care quality? Third, are performance measures reliable, available in a timely manner, and sensitive to differences in the types of patients a plan covers or a provider sees? Finally, how should performance measures be disseminated and used?

Who Should Be Evaluated?

Indicators of performance are typically activities or outcomes that can be used to compare the providers at a given level in the health care delivery system (for example, health plans, hospitals, or physicians). Ideally, all levels should be evaluated, because legitimate questions can be raised about the performance of each one. To a large extent, however, what can be measured at a given level is determined by the availability of data. For example, a physician's performance with particular types of patients generally cannot be evaluated, as most physicians' activities are highly diversified, and no single activity is performed often enough for performance to be estimated reliably. When events occur at relatively low rates, random error can create a false impression of the quality of the performance. For example, in 1992 the New York State Department of Health began to report physician-specific mortality rates for cardiac surgery procedures. The low rate at which many surgeons performed certain procedures resulted in low year-to-year agreement of quality rankings (the correlation equaled 0.22, but in fact 46 percent of the surgeons moved from one half of the ranked list to the other during a one-year period; Green and Wintfeld, 1995). In a statistical demonstration of the pitfalls of using mortality rates to assess physician performance, Luft and Hunt (1986) showed that if the expected death rate for a condition were 1 percent, it would take more than five deaths among two hundred patients to conclude at a probability of less than 0.1 that the outcome was worse than could be expected by chance. In this example, it is statistically impossible to demonstrate a better-than-expected outcome with mortality rates.

In some cases, broadening the time frame for evaluation will sufficiently increase the number of observable events. Another approach to this statistical problem is to broaden the unit of analysis from an individual physician to a group of physicians. Medical care in a group practice may not be uniform, however, and therefore it may not be legitimate to judge the performance of an individual physician based on how the others in his or her group care for similar patients. Based on the number of observable events, health plan data are currently the most amenable to statistical analysis.

Performance Measures: Selection and Validity

Stimulated by large employers' desire for data on the quality of health plans of varied price, the National Committee for Quality Assurance (NCQA) (1993) proposed a standardized set of performance measures for health plans: the Health Plan Employer Data and Information Set (HEDIS). HEDIS is the most widely accepted set of performance measures, and a growing number of health plans has agreed to share their results on several of the HEDIS measures. There are five main categories of HEDIS measures: quality, access and satisfaction, utilization, plan management, and finance. The majority of the HEDIS indicators measure structures or processes of care.

While HEDIS has galvanized health plans to collect and report similar types of data, the validity of these and other proposed measures as indicators of health care quality and access has rarely been scrutinized. Bindman and his colleagues (1995) examined the validity of one HEDIS indicator—asthma admission rates—to determine if it was in fact a measure of access to primary care.

Comparisons were made between community residents' reports of access to care and the community's admission rates for asthma, chronic obstructive pulmonary disease, congestive heart failure, diabetes, and hypertension. At the community level, 50 percent of the variation in hospitalization rates across areas could be explained by differences in self-rated access to care: the greater the difficulty in obtaining access to care, the higher the hospitalization rate. The strength of the association between self-rated access to care and preventable hospitalization rates suggested that admission rates for conditions such as asthma are indeed a valid indicator of health care access.

The growing enthusiasm of many health plans for HEDIS as a basis for equitable comparisons of quality suggests that consensus on performance measures can eventually be reached. Nevertheless, health plans still differ more than they agree in the quality-assessment data they collect. Validating indicators of quality remains a critical step in building confidence within the health care marketplace that the measurement process is legitimate and worthwhile.

Measures of physician performance, contained in "physician profiles," are even less standardized than health plan performance reports; most are used internally within health care organizations and are not publicly available. Increasingly, physician profiles are being developed to stimulate continuous quality improvement projects in various clinical settings. In general, when physicians participate in defining quality standards and receive feedback on how their care processes differ from those of other providers in a reference group, differences in how care is delivered tend to diminish over time. Although profiling techniques can lead to statistically impressive reductions in such variability, the fact remains that in most cases the care processes that lead to the best health outcomes are not known. While it is hoped and assumed that physicians who work together to decrease variation in their practice styles are developing standards that will result in the best outcomes, that is not necessarily the case. Group practices that are more uniform in their care processes do not necessarily provide better quality care.

Some institutions and health plans are also using physician profiles to make decisions about credentialing, hiring, and firing. The legality of firing physicians from a health plan on the basis of their statistical deviation from other providers on quality measures has been challenged by physicians who argue that the profiling methodology is often cryptic and flawed (Boschert, 1996). Moreover, physicians confronted with poor performance evaluations legitimately raise the point that their performance might have appeared better had their patients complied with all of their recommendations. No published report to date has demonstrated the validity of any quality indicator used for physician profiling (General Accounting Office, 1994).

Additional Methodological Concerns

If performance measures are to become a useful tool for evaluating and improving health care delivery, they must also be reliable, be reported in a timely fashion, and be adequately adjusted for confounding variables.

Missing, inaccurate, and miscoded data can lead to false impressions of a physician's performance, and data collection practices vary considerably across health plans and providers. Although groups such as NCQA are trying to standardize data collection methods, there is no mandated auditing process, and health plans retain control over what score is reported on their own plan. If users of performance measures are to have confidence in the results, some method of rigorous external auditing must be established.

The development and use of performance measures has been facilitated by the availability of computerized administrative and clinical databases that provide relatively easy and inexpensive access to the information. However, data entry and verification typically create time delays that can limit the usefulness of the findings. For example, California hospital discharge data are typically eighteen to twenty-four months old before they are released to investigators, and data analysis may require an additional year or more. Rapid changes in the structure of health care delivery, including closures and mergers of hospitals, may make reports based on such data obsolete even before they are published. Although computerization throughout the health care delivery system should diminish these time delays, some time lag will inevitably persist, potentially threatening the usefulness of the data.

The greatest challenge to the interpretation of performance measures is controlling for demographic and other differences in the patients cared for by different providers and plans. The best variables for case-mix adjustment of performance measures are not known, and different variables are probably needed for different clinical indicators. Moreover, case-mix adjustment methods vary enormously in complexity and cost, and agreement among them is often poor (Iezzoni and others, 1995). With few objective data about the validity and reliability of case-mix adjustment approaches, government and private organizations attempting to evaluate health care quality are either choosing very different approaches or ignoring case-mix adjustment altogether (Kerr and others, 1995).

Inadequate case-mix adjustment is problematic even when quality is assessed using validated performance measures. For example, in the above-mentioned validation study of preventable hospitalization rates as a measure of access to care, race, education, and income also affected the admission rates (see Figure 5.1). Making judgments about the quality of health plans on the basis of preventable hospitalization rates without considering these confounders could lead to faulty conclusions. A preventable hospitalization rate of sixty-five hospitalizations per ten thousand individuals might reflect the best possible access to care or only moderately good access, depending upon the demographic makeup of the patient population.

Not only is the proper case-mix adjustment methodology complex, but in many cases variables that are likely to be important are not available for consideration. For example, race is strongly associated with health service utilization patterns and health outcomes, but civil rights protections often preclude the systematic collection of this information by health plans. Even when data on race are available, a question can be raised about whether they should in fact be used as an adjustment variable, since adjusting for race could mask important variations in the quality of care delivered to individuals from different racial groups.

Case-mix adjustment methods that explain more of the variation are generally considered better than those that explain less. Salem-Schatz, Moore, Rucker, and Pearson (1994) showed that variations in the patterns of referral by primary care physicians to

Figure 5.1. Preventable Hospitalization as a Function of Self-Rated Access in Different Populations.

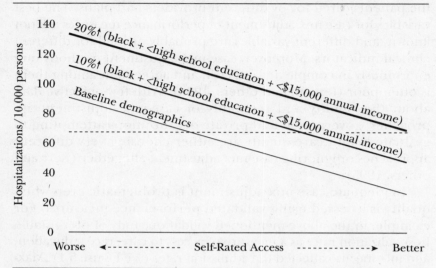

Hospitalization rates and self-rated access in urban California among individuals aged eighteen through sixty-four. Preventable hospitalizations indicate cumulative admission rates for asthma, chronic obstructive pulmonary disease, congestive heart failure, diabetes, and hypertension per ten thousand individuals in a community. The line labeled "Baseline demographics" is derived from a multivariate model including self-rated access, age, gender, race, education, income, and health insurance status to predict preventable hospitalization rates (adjusted R^2 = .84). The lines labeled 10 percent and 20 percent "black, + <high school education + <$15,000 annual income" are derived from the same model showing 10 and 20 percent absolute increases in the percentage of black individuals who have less than a high school education and individuals who have an annual household income of less than $15,000.

specialists were greater when diagnostic information was used in addition to patients' age and gender as a case-mix adjustment variable. While these results might suggest that age and sex are less satisfactory than age, sex, and diagnostic information as case-mix adjustment variables, Welch, Black, and Fisher (1995) have warned of the potential for overadjustment when diagnosis is used as an adjustment variable. Patients might need to see a specialist because they truly have more diagnostic problems, in which case-mix adjusting for diagnoses would be appropriate. If specialists tend to respond to the consultation by making additional diagnoses, however, then adjusting referral rates for the number of diagnoses may lead to an underestimate of primary care physicians who refer excessively.

The problem of overadjusting is the result of using databases that do not reveal the order of events and using variables to adjust outcomes that are themselves potential indicators of quality. For example, a hospital's mortality rate may be an indicator of the quality of care it provides. Since the number of cases of myocardial infarctions that the hospital cares for may be associated with its overall mortality rate, it might be reasonable to adjust its overall mortality rate for the number of individuals it cares for with a myocardial infarction. However, since the number of myocardial infarctions events recorded at a hospital is related both to the number of patients who present with this condition and to the number of patients who acquire this condition in the hospital as a result of poor care, using the myocardial infarction rate as an adjuster could conceal a quality problem.

The fundamental question that remains regarding case-mix adjustment is whether it can adequately correct for nonrandom differences in the distribution of demographic and other characteristics of patients seen by different health plans and providers. Case-mix adjustment can explain significant amounts of variation in the utilization patterns and health of groups of similar patients but only small amounts of such variation in an individual patient. Because many health events are unpredictable, it is unrealistic to expect that case-mix adjustment could explain all of the variation in utilization or health. Therefore, the test of acceptability of a case-mix adjustment method is its ability to explain the predictable aspects of health care utilization and health outcomes. Newhouse, Sloss, Manning, and Keeler (1993) explored the ability of various case-mix adjustment models to explain variations in health care expenditures on children. Using subjective and objective measures of health status and prior utilization, these authors were able to explain prospectively 65 to 70 percent of the variation in medical care use. However, even this high rate of prediction was not sufficient to protect against the possibility of health plans' appearing to provide better or worse care purely on the basis of their patient population.

Disseminating Performance Scores

Even if the methodological difficulties of defining and collecting accurate performance measures are resolved, important issues will remain about the best way to report the information. Moreover, although some performance measures have already been made available to the health care marketplace, the criteria for interpreting them have not been established. If performance measures are to become a guide for assessing the quality of health care, then users will need a clear and uniform understanding of what constitutes better and worse scores. For example, is the health plan with the highest percentage of eligible women receiving mammograms necessarily the highest-quality plan? A woman concerned about breast cancer might consider this an attractive feature, but a high rate of mammography screening is likely to consume resources that could otherwise be used for other health care services. Therefore, if breast cancer is not a matter of great concern, a plan that scores highly on screening for breast cancer might be a poor choice.

Although it is reasonable to assume that health plans would desire the best scores on all performance measures as a means of attracting patients, financial incentives might make it more likely that health plans would actively work toward *poor* performances on some indicators. For example, because treating patients with AIDS or mental illness is costly, some plans might aim for lower scores in those areas in the hopes that those patients would choose other health plans.

Who should receive performance scores and how they should be made available are open questions. Hospitals and physician groups have fought (generally in vain) against publishing performance scores in the media for fear that the information will create negative impressions of health care delivery (Vibbert, 1991). Publications in the lay press reach a broad audience, but their content must be simplified. In addition, information disseminated in the lay press is not necessarily available when it is needed by consumers. Cataloging the results in reference guides may be useful for those who have the luxury of ample time to make decisions about health care, but reference materials are not useful in emergencies—a person having a heart attack cannot be expected to research the best available heart specialist, even over the Internet.

Little is known about the public's understanding of or response to published reports on the performance of hospitals and individual providers (Donaldson and Lohr, 1994, pp. 93–94), but public disclosure of such information has apparently resulted in measurable changes in hospital and physician performance. For example, health department officials in New York State have attributed decreases over time in case-mix-adjusted mortality rates after heart surgery to the introduction of the Cardiac Surgery Reporting System (Hannan and others, 1994). Supporting this assertion is the report from one New York hospital that its providers used the publicly released data to identify quality problems and to improve its mortality rate over time (Dziuban, McIlduff, Miller, and Dal Col, 1994). However, the improved outcome could also reflect a decreased willingness among cardiac surgeons to operate on extremely ill patients (Omoiguia and others, 1996). Furthermore, Green and Wintfeld (1995) project that 41 percent of the apparent reduction in mortality rates after heart surgery is attributable to more aggressive coding of mortality risk factors and an artificial inflation of the predicted mortality rate. Between 1989 and 1991, coding of renal failure and congestive heart failure in patients undergoing cardiac surgery increased 600 percent and 350 percent, respectively. These increases probably reflect changes in coding practices rather than a change in the prevalence of these risk factors.

Although they were among the first to demand data on the quality of health plans, employers acknowledge that their choice of health plans is still based largely on cost. As yet, there is no established method for translating differences in performance measures into monetary values. The Pacific Business Group on Health (PBGH), which negotiates managed care contracts for approximately 2.5 million employees in thirty-two San Francisco Bay Area businesses, is leading attempts to develop a strategy to link health insurance premiums to quality. PBGH has negotiated commitments with its contracted health plans to withhold 2 percent of premiums, totaling approximately $8 million; these monies will ultimately either be paid to the health plans or returned to the employers, depending on how the plans perform on twelve agreed-upon measures (Pacific Business Group on Health, 1995).

Supporters of competition in the health care marketplace hope that it will create incentives for improving care processes. On the other hand, detractors argue that competition could adversely affect providers' willingness to share knowledge and shift their focus from fighting disease to battling one another (Berwick, 1995).

Conclusion

The systematic collection and public reporting of performance measures are still in their infancy, but it is likely that progress will be made on many of the methodological issues that limit the usefulness of these indicators today. The most vexing methodological issue that remains is the need to develop a cost-efficient case-mix-adjustment method that clinicians can accept as legitimate. Indeed, there is a growing skepticism that this can ever be done (Newhouse, 1994).

In view of the fact that it may take a long time to resolve all of the methodological shortcomings of performance measures, the question arises as to when these indicators should be considered a tool that can be used to produce more good than harm. Some argue that the health care marketplace is so dominated by cost data that even poor-quality data on performance measures merit public release, to stimulate improvements in quality assessment. On the other hand, early experiences with public reporting of performance measures suggest that health plans and providers may respond to an externally generated poor-performance score by shifting away from severely ill patients rather than by seeking to improve care. In such cases, the performance scores might appear to indicate high-quality care but would actually reflect a low-risk population. Thus, the premature introduction of performance measures could lead to financial windfalls for health plans and providers without stimulating an improvement in the quality of health care. In addition, if the health care marketplace rewards plans and providers on the basis of an inadequate case-mix adjustment of performance measures, the efforts of health plans and providers to attract low-risk patients are likely to result in greater access barriers for high-risk, high-cost patients.

Despite opposition by many in the health care industry, increased public reporting of performance measures appears to be inevitable in the near future. The medical profession, which already has suffered some loss of public trust, will best be served by being willing to participate in the search for accurate measures of health care quality. In exchange for their participation, health care providers should demand that the methods used to rate their performance be explicit and scientifically valid (Kassirer, 1994).

In the long run, the usefulness of performance measures will be judged on the basis of whether collecting and analyzing the data lead to improved health care delivery. Initial efforts to estimate the direct and indirect costs to health plans of collecting data on performance measures are just getting under way. Data collection activities are likely to be costly, and the focus on performance measures that can be compared across plans will probably consume resources that might be better used for quality-improvement projects that are potentially more relevant for a particular plan's patients.

Competition in the health care marketplace has created an unprecedented demand for performance measures, as quality has become another facet of health care delivery that can potentially be differentiated and marketed. However, the competition for patients may have a more significant impact on health care quality than performance measures ever will. Ironically, the most important role for accurate performance measures of quality may be to monitor the impact of competition itself—on the quality of the health care system and on the health of the population.

References

Berwick, D. "Quality Comes Home." *Quality Connection,* 1995, *4,* 1.

Bindman, A., and others. "Preventable Hospitalizations and Access to Health Care." *Journal of the American Medical Association,* 1995, *274,* 305–311.

Boschert, S. "Deselection Battle Heats Up, Heads to Courts." *Internal Medicine News,* March 1, 1996.

Brinkley, J. "U.S. Releasing Lists of Hospitals with Abnormal Mortality Rates." *New York Times,* March 12, 1986, p. 1.

Donaldson, M. S., and Lohr, K. N. (eds.). *Health Data in the Information Age: Use, Disclosure, and Privacy.* Washington, D.C.: National Academy Press, 1994.

Dziuban, S. W., McIlduff, J. B., Miller, S. J., and Dal Col, R. H. "How a New York Cardiac Surgery Program Uses Outcomes Data." *Annals of Thoracic Surgery,* 1994, *58,* 1871–1876.

General Accounting Office. *"Report Cards" Are Useful, but Significant Issues Need to Be Addressed.* GAO/HEHS-94-219. Washington, D.C.: U.S. General Accounting Office, September 1994.

Green, J., and Wintfeld, N. "Report Cards on Cardiac Surgeons: Assessing New York State's Approach." *New England Journal of Medicine*, 1995, *332*, 1229–1232.

Hannan, H., and others. "Improving the Outcomes of Coronary Artery Bypass Surgery in New York State." *Journal of the American Medical Association*, 1994, *271*, 761–766.

Iezzoni, L. I., and others. "Predicting Who Dies Depends on How Severity Is Measured: Implications for Evaluating Patient Outcomes." *Annals of Internal Medicine*, 1995, *123*, 763–770.

Kassirer, J. "The Use and Abuse of Practice Profiles." *New England Journal of Medicine*, 1994, *330*, 634–636.

Kerr, E. A., and others. "Managed Care and Capitation in California: How Do Physicians at Financial Risk Control Their Own Utilization?" *Annals of Internal Medicine*, 1995, *123*, 500–504.

Luft, H., and Hunt, S. "Evaluating Individual Hospital Quality Through Outcome Statistics." *Journal of the American Medical Association*, 1986, *225*, 2780–2784.

National Committee for Quality Assurance. *HEDIS: The Health Plan Employer Data and Information Set*. Washington, D.C.: National Committee for Quality Assurance, 1993.

Newhouse, J. "Patients at Risk: Health Reform and Risk Adjustment." *Health Affairs*, 1994, *1*, 132–146.

Newhouse, J., Sloss, E., Manning, W., Jr., and Keeler, E. "Risk Adjustment for a Children's Capitation Rate." *Health Care Financing Review*, 1993, *15*, 39–54.

New York State Department of Health. *Coronary Artery Bypass Graft Surgery in New York State, 1989–1991*. Albany: New York State Department of Health, 1992.

Omoiguia, N. A., and others. "Outmigration for Coronary Bypass Surgery in an Era of Public Dissemination of Clinical Outcomes." *Circulation*, 1996, *93*, 27–33.

Pacific Business Group on Health. *Pacific Currents*. San Francisco: Pacific Business Group on Health, 1995.

Salem-Schatz, S., Moore, G., Rucker, M., and Pearson, S. "The Case for Case-Mix Adjustment in Practice Profiling." *Journal of the American Medical Association*, 1994, *272*, 871–874.

Vibbert, S. "Judge Orders New York to Release Physician-Specific Death Rates." *Medical Utilization Review*, 1991, *19*, 1.

Welch, H. G., Black, W. C., and Fisher, E. S. "Case-Mix Adjustment: Making Bad Apples Look Good." *Journal of the American Medical Association*, 1995, *273*, 772–773.

Chapter Six

The Future of the Health Professions Under Managed Care

Edward O'Neil, Leonard J. Finocchio

As the other chapters in this book argue, the U.S. health care system is changing dynamically. While there are many factors contributing to the changes, the single most important factor remains the overall cost or level of resources allocated to health care. What is different now than in earlier efforts to reform the system is that these changes are being driven by an emerging health care market that, to be best understood, should be thought of as three interrelated markets—health care purchasers, insurers, and providers.

Purchasers of care, both private and public, are increasingly organized to demand both lower costs and improved performance in terms of both health care outcomes and patient satisfaction. The demands of this first market have pressured most insurers to offer diversified products that lower costs and enhance outcomes (or at least claim to), however these elements are measured. This interaction between purchasers and insurers has driven one of the most dramatic changes in the health care infrastructure—the consolidation of providers, both hospitals and professional practices, into large integrated systems of care.

At each level of these market-driven changes there is an orientation toward more carefully "managing" the resources associated with care. Purchasers manage their expenses by negotiating a fixed fee per member, per month and demanding and receiving real performance data from the health plans and providers that deliver care. Health plans bargain with providers for lower fees or shift the financial risk to providers through fixed payments for all needed services (capitation). There is now some balance among providers between making a profit and managing the health of the enrolled population. Providers that participate in fully capitated plans have strong incentives to deliver care in innovative ways that can lower costs and improve quality. Because health care is labor-intensive, such dramatic changes cannot help but significantly impact the work of all health care professionals.

These changes are of course occurring at different rates and in different ways across the many and varied health care markets in the United States, but there is growing evidence that they will eventually play out in all markets, regardless of their current condition. For the purposes of understanding health workforce and education issues in the context of these developments, three stages in the evolution of managed care markets seem to be particularly important—assembly, integration, and management.

The first stage is the *assembly* of the basic elements. During this phase, purchasers begin to combine their bargaining strength, particularly by combining the negotiating power of the public and private sectors. Insurance companies begin to assemble modified plans that offer to better manage the insurance obligations of purchasers. The insurance plans also begin to develop their networks of providers, both hospitals and physicians. The providers themselves recognize these changes and begin to move toward organized yet loose affiliations. In this phase health care professionals are primarily affected by negotiated fee reductions and the growing use of prospective and retroactive management techniques such as prior approval and utilization review.

The second stage in the evolution toward intensively managed systems of care might be called *integration*. In this phase, there is more consolidation of purchasers and clearer articulation of expected performance standards, principally in terms of price but also with a growing concern for quality. As a consequence, insurers (which are more appropriately called "organizers" of care) pay more attention to the costs of providing care, which translates into negotiated cuts in payments to health care providers and an increased focus on enrollee satisfaction.

Providers' experience at this stage is marked by movement into tightly organized relationships with other providers, creating larger integrated systems. These systems need not be *financially* integrated, but individual providers and provider groups will find it increasingly difficult to work outside the primary system with which they are affiliated. This phase is also marked by increased competition between systems and a reduction of excess capacity in the general health care delivery system, particularly in acute care hospital beds and specialty physician services.

The third and final stage is best called *management.* This period will hopefully provide some payoff for the painful experiences of the assembly and integration periods, in which resources and capacity were reduced and new and often awkward relationships were created among purchasers, insurers, and providers. In the management phase there are no more gains to be had by reducing capacity or taking resources out of the system. Lowered prices must reflect increased value, however, in terms of enhanced consumer satisfaction and improved quality. Accomplishing this requires no less than a redesign of the health care delivery process. Purchasers are likely to see an advantage in becoming active partners with health care providers in this reengineering effort.

The organizers of care (that is, insurers) will find this period precarious, unless they can use their access to information systems, their special expertise in organizing care, and their capacity for managing change to add value to the overall health care system. If they cannot compete in these arenas, their traditional role as marketers is likely to lose out to direct contracting between purchasers and providers, eliminating them as nonproductive middlemen.

Implications of Managed Care for the Health Professions

The future system of care will not replace the existing system entirely but will alter it with new values, institutions, patterns of practice, and policies. These structural changes are already dramatically increasing managed care enrollments and forcing more cost constraints and greater accountability on providers. These transformations are also bringing an increased emphasis on primary care, prevention, population-based practice, interdisciplinary teamwork, and clinical effectiveness research. The success of the future U.S. health care system will depend upon the willingness of health care professionals to acquire the new knowledge and skills needed to adapt to this changing system.

The system that is emerging will be integrated through the delivery of primary care, because it is less expensive, more comprehensive, and of higher quality (Starfield, 1992; Stewart and others, 1989; Greenfield and others, 1992). This will mean that all health care practitioners—generalists and specialists—must be able to understand the values and functions of coordinated, comprehensive, and continuous care and direct their practices to support such goals. The delivery of primary care will not be dominated by physicians, as it is today, because there is growing evidence that nurse practitioners, nurse midwives, and primary care physician assistants deliver care that is of high quality and is responsive to patient needs for access and satisfaction.

The complexity and acuity of care needs will require health care professionals to work effectively as team members in organized settings that emphasize the integration of all services. As these integrated systems of care become the dominant means of health care delivery, health care professionals must learn how to ensure the highest levels of quality through interdisciplinary and interinstitutional work. This will entail practicing more effectively within multiple care delivery settings and coordinating treatment and complementary services with interdisciplinary team members and with other social and academic organizations.

For example, one important emphasis of the emerging paradigm is ambulatory care. There is growing attention to care delivered outside traditional institutional settings, in the community or at patients' homes. This broader perspective will require different sets of skills and entail the integration of a range of services across professional, disciplinary, and institutional boundaries to promote, protect, and improve health.

One potential positive result of a more integrated system of care—especially if it holds provider organizations financially responsible for patient outcomes—is the new value that will be placed on the active prevention of disease. The existing system's focus on treating acute conditions has proven very expensive because it waits until patients' needs are most extreme. Public health advocates have long known that a predominance of such "downstream" expenditures is not in the best interests of society or of individual patients. But until now there has been no organization, outside of public health institutions, with a vested interest in health promotion and disease prevention.

Clearly the emerging system is pushing for a greater balance between treatment and prevention. To accomplish this balance, practitioners must be able to help individuals, families, and communities maintain and promote healthy behaviors. To contribute to this goal, all health care providers must be able to understand when and how to use primary and secondary preventive strategies. Future practitioners will have to possess a broad understanding of all the determinants of health, such as the patient's physical environment, socioeconomic status, behavioral health care (that is, mental health), and genetic background.

Practitioners must be able to help patients and their families actively participate in health care decisions. The most pressing concerns facing the health care system are fundamental issues—how social resources are spent, how decisions are made, how individuals take responsibility for their own health, and what role society plays in insuring people against risk. To provide appropriate care, practitioners must appreciate the growing diversity of the population and understand the effects of different cultural values on patients' health status and care. Practitioners of the future must be able to frame their work in ethically sensitive ways and provide education and counseling to patients, families, and communities when ethical issues arise.

The combination of increased competition among providers and increased demands from purchasers and consumers will continue to force health care systems and practitioners to continually assess quality. Demands for quality measures, both for internal benchmarking and for external review, have been driven in part by the large volumes of information on quality held by government and insurance entities. To remain a vital part of a complex, managed, information-driven system, health care professionals must be able to manage and use large volumes of scientific, technological, clinical outcomes, and patient information in a way that helps them deliver effective clinical care that meets the needs both of the community and of the overall health care system. Traditional quality improvement and continuous quality improvement—which promote efficiency and effectiveness—as well as the newer "best practices" programs are being utilized to a greater extent in a variety of settings.

In order to participate in the system evolving today, professionals must be responsive to increasing levels of public, governmental, health system, and health plan scrutiny. Individual practitioners must be held accountable to provide cost-effective, high-quality, appropriate care. This does not mean making cost the paramount value in health care, but it does mean that the provider must work to achieve price and cost reductions; health professionals can either participate in this process or abdicate their authority to nonclinicians. Such an abdication would not be in the interest of the nation's health. The practitioner of the future must be able to understand and apply increasingly complex technologies in an appropriate and cost-effective manner. This will mean balancing clinical and system demands.

This transformation of health care in the United States from a professionally governed, fee-for service enterprise of independent professionals and hospitals to a publicly and privately governed, managed system with large networks of providers will clearly bring about considerable dislocation. Nothing will be as significant as the changes in how the professional health care workforce is regulated, how it carries out its work, its overall size, and the skills and competencies its members must have to be competitive. These four challenges—reengineering the health care process, reregulating professional practice, rightsizing the health care profession, and restructuring health education—will come to dominate health care reform in the next decade.

Reengineering and the Health Care Workforce

In many ways reengineering the workforce is already part of the health care landscape. Whether forced upon the profession by hospitals, health plans, or other outside entities, the process of redesigning or reengineering the processes by which care is delivered and health promoted is already well afoot. In its best manifestation, reengineering establishes a set of desired outcomes or standards for the overall health care system, for sets of health care institutions, for individual health care organizations, for single practices, and even for elements of diagnostic or therapeutic technologies. The goal of such reengineering is to achieve better quality of care, improved outcomes, and reduced costs by altering the inputs to the care delivery process, based on empirical evidence.

For the health care professional, reengineering care delivery processes and organizations poses this challenge: can their work be improved, as measured by outcomes and costs, by altering some pattern of their practice, such as how they involve and utilize other health care professionals or paraprofessionals? Reengineering will inevitably raise the issue of the substitution of one health care provider for another whenever one can potentially produce an equivalent or better outcome at a lower cost. This active experimentation will continue in health care systems as they pursue the challenge of lowering costs and improving quality. The challenge to health care professionals will be to take this dislocating task on as a process that they will lead.

Reregulating Professional Practice

The rules and laws that currently govern professional practice in health care are the vestiges of regulations established in the late nineteenth century, an age that did not have the influential educational institutions and hospitals that guide and direct professional practice today. Moreover, even the regulatory modifications of the past fifty years were established without the presence of integrated systems of care or the information resources of a managed care system. All of these developments point to the need to realign the goals and processes of professional regulation (Finocchio and others, 1995). While there are many goals that such a reform could address, three issues will be particularly important over the next decade.

First, reform efforts will pressure regulations to more effectively and efficiently protect and promote the public's health. Historically, professional regulation has served only to protect the public from harm, but in a transforming system, all regulatory mechanisms should serve to promote good health outcomes. This can be accomplished prospectively by ensuring professional competence through the initial and continuing licensure processes. Current requirements for continuing education are feeble attempts at guaranteeing ongoing professional competence. In a retrospective manner, the public would be better protected from substandard providers by more aggressively identifying professional practices that lie outside of acceptable standards for practice and clinical outcomes.

Second, an improved regulatory system must permit more flexibility in the scope of practice of professionals working to meet the changing needs of a transforming system of care. This flexibility must not come at the expense of the public's safety or the subordination of professional standards to institutional licensure but should allow all professionals to provide services to the fullest extent of their current knowledge, training, experience, and skills. Scopes of practice should be based on demonstrated initial and continuing competence, and those of different professionals should be allowed and expected to overlap.

Finally, regulation must reflect the interdisciplinary and public accountability demands of the changing health care delivery system. Health care professionals' regulatory boards are typically composed of members of single professions. Only recently have public members been allowed to sit on boards, and experience indicates that those members must be trained and supported to be effective. Rarely if ever do members of one profession sit on the boards of the other professions, despite the obvious need for interdisciplinary exchange of information and innovations for the developing care systems that use teams of health providers to deliver care. In this respect, some of the professional autonomy that has been protected by current regulatory law will have to be lost.

Rightsizing the Health Care Workforce

As the U.S. health care system grew from 6 percent of the nation's gross domestic product in 1960 to its current size of over 15 percent, it also engendered considerable growth in the size of the professions and in the length of time required to matriculate into professional practice. One major difference in comparing U.S.

health care expenses to other nations' is the labor-intensive nature of our system of health care delivery. Even without the significant transformation to systems of managed care, the 1990s would have experienced a growing oversupply of many health professionals. As managed care takes hold in this decade, the attendant workplace redesign will highlight the significant oversupply of some professional groups.

One of the unfortunate dimensions of these changes is that much good has been accomplished through the growth of the professional education system. But this is increasingly more than the nation can afford, as the resources consumed by professional education take away from other areas. In the long run this will only erode the strength of the professions purportedly being served.

The challenge over the next decade will be to downsize the number and size of education and training programs in a manner that recognizes excellence but ensures real progress toward reducing the size of some of the professions. A more difficult task will be for the professions to reconsider the length of time required for education and training programs. The professions, which will ultimately have to respond to market demands for efficiency, should use the opportunity to lead with solutions rather than merely respond to external mandates.

Restructuring Health Professions Education

While changing the size and length of education and training programs are certainly relevant challenges in the overall reform of health care, there are additional issues to which the education establishment must respond. Three seem to be particularly important. First, the health care professions will find themselves challenged to broaden their curriculum beyond the biomedical core currently regarded as the basic science of health care. A changing epidemiology, a new system of care, and a better understanding of the relationship between mind and body will necessitate a more complex core curriculum that addresses the psychological, social, and behavioral aspects of health care in addition to the biomedical aspects. Second, the health care system itself will demand more of a population-based approach to care. Included in such competencies will be clinical epidemiology, clinical prevention, health education, and more effective use of resources. Finally, the increased complexity of patient needs and sophistication of the emerging system will demand a better integration of skills across the professions and effective team competencies.

As the health care system changes over the next decade, these three issues will be the principal challenges to the health professions and their educational institutions. Many professional groups and schools will fight these changes, seeing them as a direct attack on their professional prerogatives and privileges. Others will see the challenges as dislocating but will also recognize the enormous opportunity that is presented as the health care system in the United States changes so dramatically.

Implications of Managed Care for Specific Professions

This chapter now turns its focus to four professions—nursing, medicine, allied health, and public health—with some observations about how they will likely be affected over the next decade.

Nursing

The largest of all the health care professions, nursing enters the next decade with the advantage of being in virtually every health care setting from the surgical suite to the home health agency. This advantage, coupled with nursing's professional orientation toward care and its intellectual basis in both the biomedical and the psycho-social-behavioral sciences, positions the profession well for the transition to more integrated systems of managed care.

There are some realities of the nursing profession that must be addressed if it is to take full advantage of this emerging opportunity. First, two thirds of the nation's 1,853,000 employed registered nurses (RN) work in hospital settings (Moses, 1994, p. 46). Of all health care institutions, it will be hospitals that will undergo the most significant transformations over the next ten years. Estimates vary but consistently point to an oversupply of hospitals and hospital beds, ranging from 25 to 60 percent. If these beds and hospitals close, it will have a dramatic impact on the employment prospects of hospital-based RNs. A conservative estimate of a 30 percent reduction in hospital beds over the next decade would easily reduce the 1.2 million RNs employed in hospitals in 1992 by a corresponding 20 to 30 percent. Such a situation would mean a loss of 240,000 to 360,000 hospital nursing positions. Undoubtedly there will be opportunities for nurses in ambulatory settings as care moves out of hospitals, but these positions will also be sought by allied health care workers and physicians.

The second big challenge to nursing will be the need to differentiate between nursing practice and education. The available pathways to becoming an RN include hospital-based diploma programs, two-year associate degree programs, and four-year university programs leading to a baccalaureate degree in nursing. The current nursing population was prepared in roughly even measure from each of these three programs; but the associate degree programs now dominate the production process, producing 64 percent of RNs in 1991 (Aiken, 1995). The challenge lies not in the varied pathways into nursing but in the fact that these pathways involve different amounts of time and differently oriented curricula, yet they all produce individuals eligible to become RNs and to be employed in the same capacity in health care organizations. In order to take full advantage of the changes in the system, the nursing profession must develop a clear and meaningful differentiation between its educational structures and patterns of practice.

For instance, education in a diploma program might prepare an RN for service limited to an acute care hospital setting. The associate degree might include hospital care and also provide more background for a somewhat more independent practice in a long-term care facility. A baccalaureate course of study would provide preparation for any of these settings and also include the more independent work associated with home and community practice.

Related to the issue of RN training is confusion in the current health care system about advanced-practice nursing. On the one hand, certificate- and master's-prepared clinical nurse specialists will have an expanded opportunity in hospital settings as medical training programs decline and the complexity of patients' needs increases. On the other hand, the demand for independent nurse practitioners in a variety of settings, including hospitals, will grow as the health care system seeks practitioners that have flexibility and a different set of skills and are less expensive than physicians. However, the same confusion that exists for the RN now exists for the advanced-practice nurse. The profession needs to develop clear national standards for their preparation and practice if advanced-practice nurses are to take advantage of the opportunities in the evolving system.

The nursing profession is well established through practice-defining legislation (known as practice-acts) enacted in every state of the nation. These acts have done much to help define the professionalism of nursing and move it into its enviable role of service and professional prominence. The first response by the profession to recent changes in care has been to use these laws and the strength of nursing professional associations to defend the profession from all efforts by managed care to change the workplaces in which nurses practice. This strategy seems destined to fail. Though the claimed concern behind these efforts is a desire to protect the public's health, the growing pressure on hospital closings will increasingly make the nursing profession's political position look to be what it truly is—an effort to save the status quo of nursing employment.

What the profession should embrace is the opportunity to position itself as the key workforce component of the new system. This will occur only with a willingness to give up on the traditional patterns of professional action and focus on creating practice laws that creatively place nurses in a variety of inpatient and outpatient settings with a growing level of independence. Nursing should welcome the opportunity to move out of the many narrow duties that have kept it from reaching its fullest potential.

Finally, nursing must build on its already strong commitment to patient care management, providing nursing students with a thorough experience of the demands of patient care in managed care settings. As the new system emerges, it will look for clinicians that can both provide care and comprehensively manage care and resources at the point of service delivery. Because of their number and the nature of their education, nurses are particularly well suited to balancing these two needs, but the profession must focus some of its research attention on this topic, and educational programs must embrace the demands of managed care.

The challenges facing nursing are great, but so is the opportunity afforded by a health care system in transition. Over the next ten years, nursing must better rationalize the education and practice continuum for RNs. Nurses' training should reflect real differences in nursing practice, and nursing practice and education should provide an easy ladder for all nurses to advance their skills and credentials.

Nursing should reduce the number of training programs by 20 to 25 percent. These reductions must come from the diploma and associate degree programs, because they represent a type of preparation that will be in declining demand. Furthermore, nursing should aggressively redefine the profession's intellectual grounding in a manner that embraces the management needs of integrated systems of care. All nursing curricula, from those directed at preparing nurses for clinical work in hospitals to those covering leadership positions in large health care organizations, must incorporate these qualities.

Medicine

Because of its historical position of dominance in the health care system, medicine has far and away the greatest amount to lose in the coming transformation. Each of the four major issues discussed earlier—reengineering, reregulating, rightsizing, and restructuring in education—will have a profound impact on medicine. Medicine, in turn, will remain in a leadership position as it comprehends these changes and makes accommodations to seize upon the opportunities, but it will not be able to do this without giving up some of the ways in which education and practice are organized and carried out.

By almost any measure there is a growing oversupply of physicians in the United States (Weiner, 1994; Council on Graduate Medical Education, 1995). This does not mean there are not many underserved areas of the nation; they remain, but given the existing evidence it seems obvious that continued expansion of the physician supply has not and will not address this problem. In fact, oversupply now threatens the viability of the profession. As health care moves into a market-dominated system, all of its professional resource inputs may become commodities, and any oversupplied commodity loses much of its value.

The oversupply of physicians is derived from two sources: an increase in the average size of graduating classes in U.S. medical schools and the growth in the number of international medical school graduates that come to the United States for training, 80 percent of whom have historically remained here to practice (Gamliel, Politzer, Rivo, and Mullan, 1995). This oversupply would have existed even without the advent of managed care, but with managed care's push for more efficient use of resources, it will become dramatic over the next ten years. Of over 650,000 practicing physicians, the oversupply is likely to be as great as 100,000 to 150,000, all of them in medical subspecialties (Finocchio and others, 1995). This excess represents an even greater percentage of employed professionals than will be experienced by nursing.

The growth in the size of medical training is easy to understand. Opportunities for new physicians seemed endless during the past five decades as more and more money went into health care and as the incomes of physicians relative to other professions grew. Federal and state education subsidies—either direct, through the educational capitation program of the 1970s, or indirect, through research grants, indirect cost recovery, and government support for graduate medical education—also contributed to the expanding physician workforce. The private sector also contributed by allowing generous billing by academic health centers and faculty practices. The first challenge to medicine over the next decade will be to gain some measure of control over the size and growth rate of the procession.

With this growth in the number of physicians, the medical profession has become increasingly oriented toward specialized knowledge and care. This orientation has become so pervasive that it has come to determine compensation levels for all physicians, their status within and outside of the profession, the nature and orientation of publicly sponsored research, and the length of medical training, all of which favor the specialists. This is not to say that specialized knowledge is not needed—clearly it is, but it must be understood within the context of fixed resources. Within these limits, such an overwhelming orientation toward specialization does harm to other approaches to the organization and delivery of care, particularly primary care (Starfield, 1992). This then is the second challenge to medicine—how to reorient or reengineer the profession so that specialty knowledge and practice might be better fitted into the generalist orientation of the primary care physician.

This means a great deal more than just adjusting the relative number of training programs so that there is a balance between generalist and specialist tracks. For fifty years the U.S. health care system has been understood from the perspective of the specialist. The emerging system values specialists and what their perspective can bring to managing patients' health, but it is increasingly turning to primary care physicians to provide care that integrates all of the system's resources with the needs of the patient. Ample and growing evidence indicates that such an orientation is better (or at least neutral) for patient care outcomes, and it saves money (Stewart and others, 1989; Greenfield and others, 1992). As the nation's health care system turns more and more to primary care for a host of answers, it is essential that medicine reaffirm its commitment to this approach to care delivery. Other providers will happily fill any void left by medicine. This will require the profession to affirm its commitment to and understanding of primary care. It will also mean that the incipient fights between specialists and generalists must be recognized as what they are—self-defeating efforts that will not help the profession or enhance the nation's health. This agenda for change has implications for education, practice regulation, and professional governance.

The Allied Health Professions

The allied health professions represent over 60 percent of the total health care workforce. Invisible for many years, they have now emerged as over two hundred distinct professions (O'Neil, 1993, p. 35). They are often associated with a particular clinical technique or type of medical technology, yet many have developed distinct bodies of knowledge that require specialized graduate training. They are by no means limited to hospital practice, yet much of their employment is in this sector.

Because of the cost basis for hospital care, the allied professions will be the focus of many efforts to change the way care is delivered in hospitals. This will create a corresponding demand for changes in the way allied health professionals are regulated and how they carry out their practice. Independent professions have been allowed to proliferate in each state because there were few reasons for reigning in such growth. States continue to feel pressures to change the processes for regulating these professions.

Education has followed practice with a panoply of programs to fit each of the narrow specializations in hospitals. The growing accreditation and degree requirements of these programs now tax the resources of two- and four- year colleges, and educational leaders have spent the past decade looking for some relief from this growing burden. They have had little help from the professions themselves (O'Neil, 1994). Of the four great challenges that face the health care professions, only downsizing does not seem to loom as great for the allied professions, in part because these programs are generally small and flexible compared to nursing or medicine.

To meet the challenges presented by managed care over the next decade, the allied health professions must develop and sustain three fundamental changes, in how they are trained, how they are organized, and how they practice. If they meet these challenges they will be well positioned to take advantage of the turbulence of the next ten years. Without such changes they will find themselves and their practices defined by other professions and the growing strength of consolidated delivery organizations.

The first challenge to the allied professions is to create a professionally determined pathway to multiskilled practice. Much has been written about such schemes to cross-train and develop multiple skills (O'Neil, 1992; Bergman, 1994; Boston and Vestal, 1994; Bard, 1994). In general, such proposals have been greeted coolly by the allied health professions, or they have been rejected out-of-hand. It would seem that most of this reaction is born from these professions' using the old standards of professionalism and complying with the now aging economics of fee-for-service practice. In this model, professional groups advanced and gained more prestige, greater workplace control, and better pay by limiting the ability of others to carry out their work tasks and by increasing the education required for licensing. While serving the interests of the professions, this has tended to balkanize the delivery of care, splintering it into far too many subsets to be effectively managed to meet the goals of systemwide cost reduction and quality improvement.

The independence of all the professions threatens the capacity of the emerging integrated system of care to deliver on these goals. The emerging system will not value professional independence; it will value the ability to collaborate toward achieving system-defined goals. Because the allied health professions are so numerous in hospitals, the arena that will see these changes come first, they are in an excellent position to reinvent themselves to serve this emerging requirement. This will not be easy, of course.

The organization of the professions may seem an unlikely place to begin, but it is the one area where the professions maintain the most discretion for action. Not all allied health professionals will need to be cross-trained for all other roles. They each possess unique skills and varying abilities to meet specific patient and system needs, and these should determine which professions work with which other professions and in what capacity.

Work done as part of the National Health Care Skill Standards Project grouped allied health occupations into four clusters based on their primary focus: therapy, diagnosis, information services, or environmental services (Far West Laboratories, 1994). For example, the therapy cluster includes case managers, dentists, dieticians, home health professionals, physicians, nurses, pharmacists, physical therapists, and respiratory care providers, among others. The diagnosis cluster includes cardiologists, diagnostic imaging specialists, medical laboratory technicians, and radiography specialists, among others. The information services cluster includes medical records managers, unit coordinators, and utilization reviewers, among others, and the environmental services cluster covers central supply, facility maintenance, food service, housekeeping, and other environmental support personnel.

Occupational and physical therapy, for example, are by far the most independent and distinctively rationalized professions among the allied health professions. But these professions will face growing demands for their services, particularly in outpatient settings, and these services will be more efficiently and perhaps better delivered if a single professional with the knowledge and skill base of both professions is able to provide care. This can be thought of as a threat to each of these separate professions—or, if it is embraced in a spirited manner, it could be regarded as an enormous opportunity for both to best position themselves for the changing health care environment. Such potential partnerships will present themselves across all the allied health professions over the next decade. Leadership in the professions will be needed to seize this chance.

The practice setting for allied health professionals will and is being redefined, with or without the support and involvement of the professions themselves. As noted, health care is a labor-intensive endeavor, and any effort to reengineer the processes by which care is delivered will of necessity bring about a restructuring of the health care workplace. Again, this redesign will happen first in hospitals, because that is where the need is greatest. Integrated health care systems, like the Henry Ford Health System and the Community Hospitals of Central California, are actively engaging the process of change to achieve a set of locally determined but nationally driven goals for reduced costs, enhanced patient satisfaction, and improved quality of care. These efforts are being carried out as experimental activities for which there are few givens about inputs, only about what will best achieve the desired performance. Here the leadership mantle has been taken from the professions; they are presented with a stark choice of either participating in the process or passively watching their workplace be redefined or perhaps disappear.

Although the professions could use educational programs to lead these changes, more likely the current trend is for employers to take the initiative in redefining the workplace and the knowledge and skills needed to be competitive. Or the professions may create new ways to organize themselves. But schools can help in this process by anticipating the new skills that their students will need, with or without redirecting their programs toward cross-training and the development of multiple skill areas. The first Pew Health Professions Commission report identified seventeen competencies that would enable all of the health professionals to be truly effective in the future (Shugars, O'Neil, and Bader, 1991):

- Care for the community's health.
- Expand access to effective care.
- Provide clinically competent care.
- Emphasize primary care.
- Participate in coordinated care.
- Ensure cost-effective and appropriate care.
- Practice prevention.
- Involve patients and families in the decision-making process.
- Promote healthy lifestyles.

- Assess and use technology appropriately.
- Improve the health care system.
- Manage information.
- Understand the role of the physical environment.
- Provide counseling on ethical issues.
- Accommodate expanded accountability.
- Participate in a racially and culturally diverse society.
- Continue to learn.

While all of these remain important for future success, two seem to be worthy of particular emphasis here. Participating in coordinated care means developing the skills and capacities to make effective use of the resources available in the health care system. Allied health professionals currently working at the point where care is delivered are in the best position to make the changes in practice that can produce the changes now being demanded by the system.

A related competency is key to this work. As information and computer technologies become more important resources in the realignment of health care, they will become essential parts of the allied practice of the future. They must be integrated into the work of faculty and into the curriculum in such a way that they are not seen as add-on activities but are integral to the delivery of allied health care.

Public Health

While the other three professional groups discussed here—nursing, medicine, and allied health—may be uncomfortable both with the changes managed care is likely to bring and with this discussion of their likely impact, public health professionals may celebrate the new emphasis managed care places on many of the principles they have long espoused. They may also find that the next decade brings some new and unfamiliar allies to address many of the problems that have long been the exclusive concern of public health advocates (O'Neil, 1995).

One way of understanding the changes brought by market-driven reform is that a force very alien to public health (profit) is now driving the system to recognize something essential to the traditional values of public health—managing the health of a population. As managed care plans take more financial risk and responsibility for the care of enrolled populations, there will be, perhaps for the first time, a powerful entity that has an immediate stake in successfully managing the health of enrolled populations. This means that the system will feel significant pressure to utilize what are known to be effective strategies and programs for preventing the onset of both chronic and acute disease, by changing the behavior of patients, organizing health care resources in a manner that derives the maximum benefit for the lowest costs, changing the environment to reduce health hazards, and lobbying for public laws to prevent or reduce the severity of accidents or disease. Such a dynamic has rarely existed in this country.

These changes will produce a new demand for the knowledge and skills of the public health professional, despite the fact that those who will be asking for these changes (managed care organizations) will seem unlikely political bedfellows for public health officials. Public health professionals may reject a profit-driven orientation for health care, but they should not. Rather than refusing to participate in the new dynamics of health care, public health professionals should capture the strengths of the system and work with them to achieve their larger goals. As a social driver, the market is a powerful resource, but it must be understood and mastered if it is to serve both the private purposes of investors and the broader health needs of the public.

To do this will require a shaping of and commitment to population-based goals for the new system and a new regulatory framework that will permit the market to work yet serve these broader social purposes. Again, there simply is no better professional group to understand both of these dynamics than the public health community.

To address these challenges will mean significant restructuring by schools of public health. The master's of public health (MPH) degree remains the principal avenue for training public health practitioners. This degree will require a bit of reconsideration and perhaps redesign to meet the job requirements of large systems of integrated care. The profession should reconsider both the core courses and concentration options currently offered by MPH programs.

In addition, schools of public health should take the lead now to forge broad partnerships with integrated systems of care. These partnerships should be used not only to understand and develop their educational programs but also as the basis for new research programs and student practicums. In much the same way that U.S. medical schools prospered during the postwar years with the changing fortunes of hospitals, schools of public health should now forge a fundamental link with integrated systems of care and grow with them as they expand.

Conclusion

While most of the suggestions for these four professions are germane only to the individual professions, several themes cut across and are essential components for these and all health professions that face the challenge of responding to the movement to managed care. The first is that whatever the health professions do in the future—in practice or in education—it must be directed toward adding value to health care dollars, enhancing patient satisfaction, and improving health care outcomes.

Second, these contributions must be demonstrated by empirically based, scientifically valid data. The movement to an evidence-based health care system may be obscured by all of the frenzy around the consolidation of providers, but it will remain as an essential component of the health care system in the next century.

A third issue that all health care professions must address aggressively is the incorporation of information and communications technology in the delivery of care. In the past, health care knowledge was locked inside the head of the health care professional, and the organization and financing of health care centered around developing, accessing, and utilizing that knowledge. Today this knowledge is increasingly digitized and transported around the country; health care professionals cannot afford to miss this revolution.

The changes proposed here concerning how professionals practice and are educated are rather overwhelming. Individual professionals and their associations have limited ability and resources to fully respond to this broad set of changes. To be strategically successful in the future, professionals must seek out partnerships to leverage the strengths needed to build a new health care reality. These may be with managed care firms, pharmaceutical companies, purchasers of care, or information management companies. The exact nature of the partnership will vary from group to group and location to location. It is the partnership that will be essential.

Finally, health care professionals will be successful in this brave new world if they approach the future creatively. Little will be given to health care professionals in the new health care system. Those professions, practices, associations, and schools that can spend less time defending the past and bemoaning its loss and more time understanding (if not embracing) the future and the opportunities it will bring will eventually look back on the coming decade as the beginning of their golden age.

References

Aiken, L. "Medicare Funding for Nurse Education: The Case for Reform." *Journal of the American Medical Association,* 1995, *272*(19), 1528–1531.

Bard, M. "Reinventing Health Care Delivery." *Hospitals and Health Services Administration,* 1994, *39,* 397–402.

Bergman, R. "Reengineering Health Care." *Hospitals and Health Care Networks,* February 5, 1994, pp. 28–35.

Boston, C., and Vestal, K. "Work Transformation." *Hospitals and Health Care Networks,* April 5, 1994, pp. 50–54.

Council on Graduate Medical Education. *Fourth Report: Recommendations to Improve Access to Health Care Through Physician Workforce Reform.* Rockville, Md.: U.S. Public Health Service, 1995.

Far West Laboratories. *Health Care Skill Standards.* San Francisco: Far West Laboratories, 1994.

Finocchio, L. J., and others. *Reforming Health Care Workforce Regulation: Policy Considerations for the 21st Century.* San Francisco: Pew Health Professions Commission, December 1995.

Gamliel, S., Politzer, R. M., Rivo, M., and Mullan, F. "Managed Care on the March: Will Physicians Meet the Challenge?" *Health Affairs,* Summer 1995, pp. 135–138.

Greenfield, S., and others. "Variations in Resource Utilization Among Medical Specialties and Systems of Care: Results from the Medical Outcomes Study." *Journal of the American Medical Association,* 1992, *267*(12), 1624–1630.

Moses, E. B. *The Registered Nurse Population: Findings from the National Sample Survey of Registered Nurses, 1992.* Rockville, Md.: United States

Department of Health and Human Services, Public Health Service, Health Resources and Services Administration, 1994.

O'Neil, E. H. "Multiskilled Health Practitioners and the Changing Environment of Health Care: Challenges for the Future." In W. K. Kellog Foundation, *Healing Hands: Customizing Your Health Team for Institutional Survival.* Battle Creek, Mich.: W. K. Kellog Foundation, 1992.

O'Neil, E. H. *Health Professions Education for the Future: Schools in Service to the Nation.* San Francisco: Pew Health Professions Commission, 1993.

O'Neil, E. H. "Critical Issues Facing Allied Health Accreditation." *Journal of Allied Health,* 1994, *23,* 15–19.

O'Neil, E. H. "Health Care Reform and the Future of Public Health." *American Journal of Preventive Medicine,* 1995, *11*(31), pp. 11–12.

Pew Health Professions Commission. *Critical Challenges: Revitalizing the Health Professions for the 21st Century.* San Francisco: University of California, San Francisco, Center for the Health Professions, December 1995.

Shugars, D. A., O'Neil, E. H., and Bader, J. D. (eds.). *Healthy America: Practitioners for 2005: An Agenda for Action for U.S. Health Professions Schools.* Durham, N.C.: Pew Health Professions Commission, 1991.

Starfield, B. *Primary Care: Concept, Evaluation and Policy.* New York: Oxford University Press, 1992.

Stewart, A. L., and others. "Functional Status and Well-Being of Patients with Chronic Conditions: Results from the Medical Outcomes Study." *Journal of the American Medical Association,* 1989, *262*(18), 907–913.

Weiner, J. "Forecasting the Effects of Health Care Reform on U.S. Physician Workforce Requirements: Evidence from HMO Staffing Patterns." *Journal of the American Medical Association,* 1994, *272*(3), 222–230.

Chapter Seven	

Inside the System

The Patient-Physician Relationship in the Era of Managed Care

Howard Waitzkin, Jennifer Fishman

We begin our discussion of the impact of managed care on the relationship between patient and doctor with two case descriptions. These encounters illustrate some generic issues that will increasingly play themselves out as managed care proliferates.

The first patient was a fifty-eight-year-old male engineering professor, insured by UC Care, the University of California's new self-insured managed care program. This patient developed severe substernal chest pain at 1:00 A.M. one morning during a Thanksgiving holiday weekend. The patient called the on-call primary care internist to approve a visit to an emergency room, as he had been instructed to do when he signed up for the plan. The doctor, who was a little hard of hearing (and was sleeping soundly when the call came, since he had covered more than thirty patients on the inpatient wards, in the intensive care units, and by phone the prior day for his colleagues), didn't hear the phone until a half hour later, when the answering service tried again to reach him. By that time the patient had left for the emergency room because of continuing pain. The physician then called the emergency room to approve the visit. As soon as the patient arrived, his electrocardiogram revealed a huge myocardial infarction involving the anterior wall of the left ventricle. If the patient had waited for approval, as he was supposed to do, he would have arrived too late for treatment with streptokinase to help lyse the clot in his coronary artery, which was the standard of care for a patient with this type of heart attack.

The second patient, a twenty-five-year-old, Spanish-speaking woman who worked as a hospital maintenance worker, was insured by Health Net, the health maintenance organization that workers for the University of California can join for the cheapest rate. She presented to the emergency room during her shift at 3:00 A.M. with a sore throat and a fever of 101 degrees. Because she had not realized that she was supposed to call the on-call physician for permission, the emergency room staff called the physician and woke him up. Groggy and mad at being awoken solely for this bureaucratic reason, he asked to speak with the patient (fortunately, he could speak Spanish). He realized that the problem could wait until daytime and did not approve the emergency room visit. The patient complained that it would be difficult to come during the day because of child care responsibilities, but she could not persuade the doctor to approve the emergency room visit, since he had been instructed not to approve such visits for minor outpatient problems.

In dealing with these cases, the doctor experienced several feelings:

- Guilt that he had not heard or responded quickly to the initial phone call from the patient having a heart attack.
- Anger that the nature of managed care led to a critical delay in this patient's evaluation and treatment.
- Sympathy for the patient whose visit he refused to approve because a later visit would prove inconvenient and because she hadn't understood the rules.
- Annoyance that he had to perform mainly a gatekeeping role in both cases, using essentially none of his clinical skills.
- Awareness that financial considerations underlay all these decisions:

    He and his colleagues would receive a bonus at the end of the year if they could hold down emergency room utilization.

    The paltry $7 per month that two of his colleagues received to cover all outpatient care for each of these patients would decrease even further if utilization became much higher.

    His own motivation to provide services subtly decreased with such managed care patients, since doing more work was not associated with more income.

He also thought of Health Net's chief executive officer at the time, Roger Greaves, who reportedly received a salary of almost $3 million, plus bonuses and stock options, in 1994 and who seemed the main beneficiary of doctors' good work as gatekeepers (Coyle and Hostetter, 1996).

- Frustration that all these emotions deviated enormously from those he had expected to have in medicine, a career he selected with the assumption that he would mainly have the opportunity to serve those in need and to receive an adequate salary for doing so, not compensation linked to patients' ability to pay or insurance coverage.

- Most of all, awareness that his communication with managed care patients was becoming distorted by the structural nature of these payment arrangements and that the openness and honesty he valued were becoming ever more tenuous.

As managed care has proliferated in the United States and spread from here to other countries, it has transformed the nature of the patient-doctor relationship in very fundamental ways. This transformation has occurred rapidly, with little accompanying preparation on the part of either clinicians or patients. In any assessment of managed care's impact, its effects on patient-doctor relationships deserve attention. The debate so far has raised many potential problems, few of which have received serious enough analysis to exert an impact on health care policy, either within or outside the managed care industry.

Gatekeeper or Double Agent?

The reader may already have guessed that the above situations were actually experienced by one of us (Howard Waitzkin); without doubt, many readers who are clinicians have had similar experiences. That is why some clinicians have been struggling for suitable policies that would not require such very conflictual activities.

Advocates of managed care often claim that this method of organizing services can and should actually improve the patient-doctor relationship. For instance, since managed care organizations generally assign patients to a single primary care physician, that person presumably can provide continuity and can help improve the coordination of services. The primary care provider can communicate with patients about preventive services and encourage their utilization. Since managed care services are mostly paid for in advance through capitation, the predictability of copayments required for each outpatient visit may also reduce financial barriers to access for some patients.

To our knowledge, however, not a single research project has conclusively demonstrated improved patient-doctor communication processes or patient satisfaction in managed care systems. The limited studies comparing communication and satisfaction in managed care versus fee-for-service plans have found either no difference or observations disfavoring managed care (Davies and others, 1986; "Health Care in Crisis . . . ," 1992; Rubin and others, 1993). The adverse impact of managed care on communication processes and the patient-doctor relationship has also received attention in several influential editorials and position papers (Angell, 1993; Emanuel and Dubler, 1995; Balint and Shelton, 1996). Further, the claimed advantages of managed care in the arenas of communication and interpersonal relationships have not been assessed in detail for growing subgroups of enrollees, including minorities, the poor, non–English speakers, the elderly, and the chronically ill.

Meanwhile, managed care refers to primary care practitioners as "gatekeepers." That is, such doctors are supposed to keep the gate closed, as a cowboy might do against a corral of wild stallions trying to break out with great energy. Or, given the notable political apathy of the U.S. public (only 55 percent of eligible voters cast ballots in the 1992 presidential election, for instance [Pear, 1992]), might a better metaphor be that primary care doctors are shepherds, keeping the barnyard closed for their sheep? That is, such doctors tend the gate, keeping it closed for expensive procedures or referrals to specialists or emergency visits, and open the gate only when it is absolutely necessary for the preservation of life or limb. The reason for tending the gate carefully is very clear: that's how doctors and their bosses keep enough of patients' capitation payments to break even or maybe come out a little ahead.

Double agent, as Marcia Angell (1993) and others have pointed out, has probably become a more cogent metaphor for doctors' role under managed care. In essence, while continuing to masquerade as patient advocates, doctors are actually acting as double agents, working both for their patients and for managed care organizations. Unfortunately, the latter's interests are often diametrically opposed to the former's.

"Masquerade" may not be totally accurate. One of the authors of this chapter recently spent nearly an entire day advocating for a single patient, a fifty-eight-year-old psychologist with a displaced fracture of her elbow, before various Health Net bureaucrats in order to convince them that she really did need an orthopedic appointment that day rather than in three weeks and that she also really needed surgery in three days rather than possibly in the indefinite future. Many clinician colleagues are burning out at the energy such maneuvering takes, with such little apparent benefit for either the patients or the gatekeepers. At the very least, doctors find that such activities lead to "rationing by inconvenience" (Grumet, 1989). That is, when obtaining services for patients entails such inconvenience, an incentive arises not to pursue the matter vigorously, thus decreasing the probability that the patient will receive the services, even though they are needed.

More often, clinicians feel an inherent conflict—either ethical or financial or both—between patients' interests and those of the managed care systems they represent as gatekeepers. This is the essence of doctors' work as double agents. Clinicians experience this conflict even when they supposedly benefit financially by keeping the gate closed. In light of such occupational conflicts and the meager earnings generated, it becomes less astounding to realize that many colleagues are leaving medicine entirely for greener pastures—such as the furniture business (a major semiretirement career for southern California physicians) or telephone marketing of household appliances (which appears to be an emerging career path for burned-out primary care practitioners in southern Florida).

Of course, these structural constraints also affect patients' experience, with medicine in general and with managed care in particular. The two patients in the above case summaries directly confronted the limitations managed care imposes on individual discretion. In the first case, the patient—though knowledgeable about the rule that emergency room visits must be preapproved to be paid for by the managed care plan—overrode that constraint through a judgment about the urgency of his symptoms. As it later became clear, his sophistication as a scientist and educator contributed to his choice to take action without the gatekeeper's permission—a decision that may have saved his life. The second patient acted from a position of ignorance about the structural constraints of the plan in which she had enrolled and could not present a convincing enough argument to accomplish her own preferences to be seen sooner rather than later. In neither case did the structural constraints imposed by managed care's gatekeeping principle conform with a close and trusting patient-physician encounter, in which the patient's preferences could guide the course of care in a predictable way.

Also from the patient's viewpoint, the structure of managed care constrains the very nature of the communicative process. Here, instead of exploring possible options with full participation by patients in decision making, the patient must make a case strong enough to be accepted by the gatekeeping physician. Financial interests reinforce the physician's skeptical appraisal. Under these conditions, especially as patients become more aware of these financial relationships, patients' trust of their physicians may seriously erode.

Further, the communicative process increasingly occurs under constraints of time. The on-call doctor, unpaid for time spent on the phone in the middle of the night, is not disposed to lengthy and supportive conversation, especially with a patient who is a stranger. For more routine encounters during daylight hours, additional constraints on communication arise, as the productivity expectations of managed care organizations create standards that require physicians to see greater numbers of patients per unit of time. From the organizational viewpoint, the fixed capitation received per patient exerts pressure to maximize the number of patients seen by each salaried practitioner in each patient-care session. Since managed care organizations strive to fill doctors' schedules, patients may have to see practitioners other than their own, including physician substitutes like nurse practitioners and physician assistants. (Managed care organizations frequently employ midlevel practitioners to handle overflow from physicians' full schedules.) Physicians employed by managed care organizations therefore enjoy little discretion in determining how much time to spend with each patient.

On the other hand, we also want to make clear our position that structural constraints in the patient-doctor relationship did not begin with managed care. Under the fee-for-service system, communication between patients and doctors suffered from a variety of problems, some tied to the financial underpinnings of that particular form of reimbursement (Waitzkin, 1984, 1991; Roter and Hall, 1992). For instance, encounters between primary care practitioners and patients tended to be hurried, and little time was spent communicating information. Interruptions and dominance gestures by physicians commonly cut off patients' concerns. Further, exploration of issues in the social context of medical encounters, which patients experienced as important components of their lived experience of illness, tended to become marginalized in patient-doctor encounters.

The financial structure of fee-for-service medicine created an incentive to maximize patients seen per unit of time and to decrease the time devoted to in-depth exploration of patients' concerns. In contrast to managed care, this productivity constraint usually permitted practitioners substantial discretion in choosing how much time to spend with a given patient. Patients' dissatisfaction with communication under the fee-for-service system ranked among the most frequently voiced complaints about U.S. medical practice (Waitzkin, 1984). In recent years, even before the advent of managed care, many calls for improvements in physicians' communicative practices came to the surface (Roter and Hall, 1992; Lipkin, Putnam, and Lazare, 1995; Smith, 1996)

It therefore would be an error to see the fee-for-service structure as necessarily more conducive to favorable communication and relationships than managed care. The financial incentives of fee-for-service medicine have created their own adverse effects. Yet the structure of managed care does little to improve those earlier problems and, in addition, introduces a new set of constraints that may prove even more contradictory and discouraging for patient-doctor relationships.

Legal and Ethical Implications of Managed Care

In this litigious society, when doctors act as double agents one can expect trouble—and trouble is what is going to happen. Some beneficial results will probably come from this trouble, at least for patients and for those doctors who vaguely remember why they went into health care in the first place.

For several years now, legal sharks who work the malpractice circuit have been turning to managed care because of its lucrative potential for big settlements. The reason is precisely the financial conflict of interest imposed upon practitioners by managed care. If doctors screw up (or if it can be alleged that they have screwed up), it is very easy to make a case that they screwed up because a financial conflict of interest caused them to limit care to the injured patient. A current malpractice case in southern California is seeking big money from a managed care organization whose practitioners refused to approve a gastroenterology consultation for vague abdominal pain in a thirty-six-year-old woman who later died from metastatic colon cancer (Olmos and Roan, 1996). Similar malpractice cases are pending against other managed care groups for limitations on needed services due to financial conflicts of interest. Such conflicts of interest are completely changing the fabric of patient-doctor communication and relationships.

Previous Barriers to Information Sharing

During the last two decades, even before the growth of managed care, several researchers have documented many barriers to communication between patients and physicians. These barriers derive from differences in social class, education, gender, ethnicity, cultural background, language, and age. In particular, physicians have performed very poorly in responding to patients' desire for information about their medical problems, diagnostic testing, treatments, and other aspects of care (Roter and Hall, 1992).

Our own research from the early 1980s provides information on the nature of these problems (Waitzkin, 1984, 1985). One way that we looked at the transmittal of information was simply to measure the amount of time devoted to the process. We found that doctors spent very little time giving information to their patients.

In general we discovered that doctors spent very little time actually providing information during encounters with patients and vastly overestimated the amount of time they spent informing patients.

We tried to relate the way doctors provide information to their patients to patient characteristics that we thought might be important. We assessed both the time doctors spent providing information and the quality of the information they provided (in the sense that it both provided relevant technical details and was presented in a manner the patient could find useful). In particular, patients' education and social class (measured by occupation) were predictors of doctors' tendency to give them information. College-educated patients tended to receive more information than patients who did not go to college; patients from upper- or upper-middle-class backgrounds received more doctor time and better explanations than did patients from lower-middle-class or lower-class backgrounds. It is important to recognize that there was no difference between poorly educated, lower-class patients and better-educated, upper-class patients in their *desire* for information. However, doctors did not perceive this desire much more commonly for poorly educated or lower-class patients. This observation confirmed what other researchers had already observed: lower-class patients tend to be diffident; that is, they usually ask fewer questions. Partly as a result, doctors tend to miss these patients' desire for information and generally believe that they want or could use less information. This finding is clinically important; lower-class patients want more information than doctors may think, and their diffidence reinforces a structural barrier to communication in patient-doctor interactions.

In addition, various studies have revealed the importance of ethnicity and language as barriers to the communication of information (Castillo, Waitzkin, Villaseñor, and Escobar, 1995). Regarding verbal communication, interpreting spoken language poses a challenge in primary care encounters. Lay interpreters who accompany monolingual patients are often family members or friends who lack formal training in interpretation techniques that help ensure accuracy. In addition to limited knowledge of medical terminology, lay interpreters may experience cultural inhibition or embarrassment in explaining patients' symptoms or in conveying requests for information. Because of these difficulties, the participation of trained, professional interpreters is highly desirable, though it frequently is not feasible in primary care settings (Putsch, 1985; Hardt, 1991; Haffner, 1992).

Such difficulties in communication may have begun to improve somewhat, partly as patients and doctors gain greater awareness of barriers to communicating information and the importance of information to ensuring quality care. We also believe that the changing gender and ethnic composition of the profession is contributing to these improvements (Roter, Lipkin, and Korsgaard, 1991; Hall and others, 1994).

Information Withholding

Beyond such barriers to communication under prior practice arrangements, a new barrier—information withholding—has arisen from the requirements of managed care. Doctors participating in managed care rarely, if ever, explain to patients that doctors' own financial earnings under capitated arrangements improve to the extent that they limit services such as diagnostic tests, expensive treatments, and specialty consultations. In other words, doctors tend not to reveal the financial conflict of interest inherent in managed care.

Of course, managed care organizations also do not communicate this conflict of interest to the people they seek to enroll. In fact, an increasing source of contention involves "gag rules" that many managed care organizations require their physician employees to follow. These rules prohibit physicians from disclosing a range of diagnostic or treatment options to patients when they are different from those approved by the administrators of the managed care organization (Woolhandler and Himmelstein, 1995; Olmos and Roan, 1996). The gag rules that restrict physicians in managed care from sharing information that they believe may prove important for patients' health and well-being create a basic conflict with doctors' responsibilities under the Hippocratic oath and current ethical norms, which call for placing the patient's welfare over all other concerns (American College of Physicians, 1993).

While physicians find themselves in an ethical bind over these gag rules, patients are caught in an even more precarious situation. Seen from the patients' viewpoint, contracts that forbid a physician to reveal the full range of treatment options or diagnostic techniques violate patients' rights, particularly the right to informed consent (Brennan, 1993; Rodwin, 1995). The legal doctrine of informed consent requires that physicians explain to patients the choices available, the risks and benefits of the proposed treatment, and any alternatives (Rodwin, 1995). Because a patient's access to this information is restricted as a result of managed care gag rules, informed consent is not achieved, and subsequently the patient is put at risk. Most patients are unaware that such gag rules exist and therefore falsely assume that they are receiving all relevant information to give informed consent for the procedure chosen. Not recognizing physicians' conflict of interest, they predictably assume that they can trust physicians' advice and recommendations because of the physician's ethical responsibility to act in his or her patients' best interests. Therefore, under a gag rule, not only can truly informed consent not be obtained, because the patient is in essence not given all the necessary information to make a consensual decision, but consent is actually obtained under false pretenses: the patient believes that the physician has given all necessary information because it is the physician's responsibility to do so.

These constraints lead to a strange and ethically difficult situation in which patients remain naive about the financial motivations that underlie many clinical decisions. In some ways, this naïveté is reminiscent of the ignorance and lack of information that physicians paternalistically used to maintain around patients who developed cancer or other fatal illnesses. Physicians in the United States used to assume that revealing their inability to cure a condition would prove deleterious to patients' morale, and so patients very often remained in the dark, even when they desperately wanted to know what was going on (Waitzkin and Stoeckle, 1972). That has changed in the United States over the last two decades, partly in response to the demands of the consumer movement and parallel struggles for full information within the women's movement and civil rights movement (Novack and others, 1979).

Nowadays, doctors, or the organizations for which they work, may assume that to reveal the true financial structure of managed care would lead to major problems in patients' morale (and certainly in their acquiescence to professionals' decisions to limit services). Therefore, physicians tend to withhold that critical piece of information. To maintain the advances of the last twenty years in patients' rights, there is an ethical obligation to allow patients to give truly informed consent by fully disclosing one's financial and ethical conflicts of interest within the managed care system. Furthermore, such disclosure should be a requirement not only for physicians but also for managed care organizations.

Recently a public interest law firm in Arizona asked one of us to consult on a monumental lawsuit based on the conflict of interest that causes doctors and managed care organizations to withhold the financial components of clinical decisions from patients. In recruiting patients and their employers, the managed care company that was being sued, like most managed care companies, promises comprehensive, easy to obtain services but provides no information about the financial structure of managed care. After several malpractice cases based on the ill effects of decisions to limit services, this law firm has initiated a class action suit against the managed care firm; a successful outcome, of course, could be used as a precedent in suits against other firms.

Some of the doctors working with this managed care company have responded to the suit with an interesting argument that creates a sense of déjà vu: if doctors told patients that they or their companies make more money when they limit tests and referrals, patients would lose morale and confidence in the patient-doctor relationship (Kilgore, personal communication, 1996). Paternalism thus has moved from maintaining the patient's ignorance about death and dying to maintaining the patient's ignorance about the financial motivations in restricting services to the living and otherwise healthy.

Structural constraints on communication may vary among different types of managed care organizations. For instance, different plans place different restrictions on time spent communicating with patients and on openness about the financial underpinnings of managed care. Nonprofit health maintenance organizations, where physicians work as members of a professional partnership (such as Kaiser-Permanente) might exert less pressure on physicians to shape their communication in certain ways than do for-profit staff-model HMOs (such as FHP, Aetna, and CIGNA). For-profit group-model HMOs (such as Foundation or Health Net) likely occupy an intermediate position in this spectrum of institu-tionalized control over information sharing.

However, we know of no research that has compared commu-nication policies, or actual communication, in different types of managed care organizations. Predictions that organizations with somewhat different financial structures have different patterns of communication remain almost entirely untested at this point. Fur-ther knowledge about such variability may come from research, though it will more likely come from a spate of litigation address-ing gag rules and other restrictions on communication in managed care organizations.

Social Problems in Medical Encounters

One of our research interests over the last few years has been the question of how patients and doctors deal with social problems in medical encounters (Waitzkin, 1991; Waitzkin, Britt, and Williams, 1994). The following encounter, which conveys an elderly woman's loss of home, community, and autonomy, illustrates this problem:

> An elderly woman visits her doctor for follow-up on her heart disease. During the encounter she expresses concerns about decreased vision, her ability to continue driving, lack of stamina and strength, weight loss and diet, and financial problems. She discusses her recent move to a new home and her relationships with family and friends. Her physician assures her that her health is improving; he recommends that she continue her current medical regimen and that she see an eye doctor.

> From the questionnaires that the patient and doctor completed after their interaction, some pertinent information is available: The patient is an eighty-year-old white high school graduate. She is Protestant, Scottish-American, and widowed, with five living children ranging in age from forty-five to fifty-nine; she describes her occupation as "homemaker." Her doctor is a forty-four-year-old white male and a general internist. The doctor has known the patient for about one year and believes that her primary diagnoses are atherosclerotic heart disease and prior congestive heart failure. The encounter takes place in a suburban private practice near Boston.

> The patient recently has moved from a home that she occupied for fifty-nine years. The reasons for giving up her home remain unclear, but they seem to involve a combination of financial factors and difficulties in maintaining it.

During silent periods in the physical examination of the patient's heart and lungs, the patient spontaneously communicates more details about her loss of possessions and relationships with previous neighbors, along with satisfaction about certain conveniences of her new living situation. Further, as the patient speaks, the doctor asks clarifying questions about the move and gives several pleasant fillers before he cuts off this discussion by helping the patient from the examination table:

P: Yeah . . . [moving around noises]. Well, I sold a lot of my stuff.

D: Yeah, how did the moving go, as long as [word]?

P: And y'know take forty-ni—fifty-nine years' accumulation. Boy, and I've got cartons in my closet it'll take me till doomsday to, ouch.

D: Gotcha.

P: But I've been kept out of mischief by doing it. But I've got a lot to do; I sold my rugs 'cause they wouldn't fit where I am. I just got a piece of plain cloth at home.

D: Mm hmm.

P: Sometimes I think I'm foolish at eighty-one. I don't know how long I'll live. Isn't much point in putting money into stuff, and then, why not enjoy a little bit of life?

D: Mm hmm [words].

P: And I've got to have draperies made.

D: Now, then, you're [words].

P: But that'll come. I'm not worrying. I got an awfully cute place. It's very very comfortable. All-electric kitchen. It's got a better bathroom than I ever had in my life.

D: Great. . . . Met any of your neighbors there yet?

P: Oh, I met two or three.

D: Mm hmm.

P: And my, some of my neighbors from Belmont here, there's Mrs. F— and her two sisters are up to see me, spent the afternoon with me day before yesterday. And all my neighbors, um, holler down the hall [words] . . . years ago. They're comin', so they say. So, I'm hopin' they will. I hated to move, cause I loved, um, I liked my neighbors very much.

D: Now, we'll let you down. You watch your step.

P: You're not gonna let me, uh, unrobed, disrobed today.

D: Don't have to, I think.
P: Well!
D: Your heart sounds good.
P: It does?
D: Yep.

After the doctor mentions briefly that the patient's heart "sounds good," he and the patient go on to other topics. The doctor's conversational cutoff, returning to a technical assessment of her cardiac function (he previously has treated her congestive heart failure) has the effect of marginalizing a contextual problem that involves loss of home and community.

From the patient's perspective, the move holds several meanings. First, in the realm of inanimate objects, her new living situation, an apartment, contains several physical features that she views as more convenient, or at least "cute." On the other hand, she apparently has sold many of her possessions, which carry the memories of fifty-nine years in the same house. Further, she feels the need to decorate her new home but doubts the wisdom of investing financial resources in such items as rugs and draperies at her advanced age.

Aside from physical objects, the patient confronts a loss of community. In response to the doctor's question about meeting new neighbors, the patient says that she has met "two or three." Yet she hated to move because of the affection she held for her prior neighbors. Describing this attachment, she first mentions that she "loved" them and then modulates her feelings by saying that she "liked them very much." Whatever the pain that this loss has created, the full impact remains unexplored, as the doctor cuts off the line of discussion by terminating the physical exam and returning to a technical comment about her heart.

Throughout these passages, the doctor supportively listens. He offers no specific suggestions to help the patient in these arenas, nor does he guide the dialogue toward a deeper exploration of her feelings. Despite his supportive demeanor, the doctor here functions within the traditional constraints of the medical role. When tension mounts with the patient's mourning a much-loved community, the doctor returns to the realm of medical technique.

Dealing with Social Context Under Managed Care

Even before managed care made its inroads into clinical practice, many practitioners felt reluctant to get involved in helping to improve the contextual problems that patients face—no matter how important such problems may be. Doctors may rationalize that there is not time or that intervening in social problems goes beyond the medical role. The answers have never been simple, but the productivity expectations and financial structure of managed care further discourage efforts to deal with such problems. Several years ago, a member of our research group and one of the authors worked out some preliminary criteria to guide practitioners in addressing contextual concerns.

These criteria try to address the question of to what extent physicians *should* intervene in the social context. The answer to this question depends partly on clarifying the practitioner's role, especially the degree to which intervention in the social context comes to be seen as appropriate and desirable. Practitioners may reasonably respond to this analysis by noting the time constraints of current practice arrangements, the need to deal with challenging technical problems, and the lack of support facilities and personnel to improve social conditions. How doctors should involve themselves in contextual difficulties, without increasing professional control in areas where doctors claim no special expertise, thus takes on a certain complexity.

On the other hand, our research suggests that the presence of social problems in medical encounters warrants more critical attention. Elsewhere, we and others have spelled out suggestions for improving medical discourse by dealing with contextual difficulties more directly (Mishler and others, 1989; Waitzkin, 1991). Briefly, on the most limited level, we have argued that doctors should let patients tell their stories with far fewer interruptions, cutoffs, and returns to technical matters. Patients should have the chance to present their narratives in an open-ended way. When patients refer to personal troubles that derive from contextual issues, doctors should try not to marginalize these connections by reverting to a technical track.

Although such suggestions encourage more "attentive patient care" (Mishler and others, 1989) and greater acknowledgment of patients' contextual stories (Smith, 1996), some preliminary criteria may also prove helpful for physicians in deciding when and under what circumstances they might initiate, extend, or limit discussions about contextual matters:

1.   *When patients initiate a discussion of contextual issues, physicians should pursue the discussion rather than marginalize it, and they should offer contextual interventions.* It is important to recognize that patients differ in their openness and their desire for contextual discussion; physicians should take their cues from the initiative patients take to raise contextual concerns. For instance, in the above encounter the patient introduces extensive contextual material concerning loss of home and community, social isolation, transportation problems, financial insecurity, and nutritional concerns. Rather than merely providing supportive listening, the physician might have responded more directly to these patient-initiated concerns with relatively simple contextual interventions: referring the patient to a seniors' organization in her new neighborhood; arranging for home-care services, including nursing and nutritional assistance; suggesting social work support to help with financial issues; providing information about transportation services; and making an effort to coordinate care with the patient's family members and friends.

2.   *When patients do not initiate discussion of contextual issues that are clearly present, physicians should inquire briefly if they wish to discuss these issues and take part in contextual interventions.* Physicians should remain sensitive to patients' differing desires and needs. Variations in patients' preferences should be recognized, as should their right to refuse discussion or interventions.

3.   *In making decisions about the time and costs to be devoted to contextual discussion, physicians and patients should consider evidence that contextual conditions affect outcomes of care such as prognosis, functional capacity, and satisfaction.* This point is of particular concern to managed care organizations. Regarding the above encounter, for instance, the geriatric literature provides extensive evidence that social isolation, lack of convenient transportation, financial insecurity, and inadequate nutritional support all worsen the functional capacity of older people (for example, Reuben and others, 1992). Current productivity standards in managed care are leading to

tighter scheduling and thus shorter appointments, which do not encourage the exploration of contextual concerns. When time and cost constraints require prioritization, existing evidence about the importance of specific contextual problems for health outcomes can help guide physicians and patients in targeting contextual issues for discussion and intervention. Likewise, a reasonable hypothesis for future research is that the marginalization of contextual issues may be inversely related to patient satisfaction, an important outcome of care (see Roter and Hall, 1992).

4.   *Practitioners should consider making referrals to social workers, psychologists, or psychiatrists in addition to the option of dealing with contextual issues in the primary care setting.* In managed care, the primary care practitioner usually initiates such referrals, but administrative reviewers, often through utilization review committees, must approve them for reimbursement. For some patients, experiences with mental health professionals prove unsatisfactory or financially prohibitive. In addition, mental health professionals' role in mediating socially caused distress has received criticism from both outside and inside the psychiatric profession (for example, see Laing and Esterson, 1970; Kupers, 1981; Davis, 1986, 1988). Because many patients do not feel comfortable seeking help from mental health professionals, primary care practitioners will probably continue to see the majority of patients with emotional problems who present to physicians for care (Depression Guideline Panel, 1993). While referrals to mental health professionals sometimes may prove necessary or appropriate, a broad mandate encouraging such care for people suffering from contextually based distress is not a solution.

5.   *Physicians should try to avoid "medicalizing" societal problems that require long-term reforms in social policy.* Medicalization requires further critical attention (Waitzkin, Britt, and Williams, 1994). At the individual level, medicalization can become a subtle process. For instance, there is a fine line between physicians' discussing contextual interventions and assuming professional control over broad areas of patients' lives. It is important that physicians not imply that the solution of contextual difficulties is ultimately the patient's own responsibility.

Even from the standpoint of utilization and cost, it can be argued that attention to contextual concerns can in many instances improve patients' functional status, decrease unnecessary utilization, and possibly reduce the costs of care, especially for at-risk people like the elderly and those affected by poverty. Aiming toward a more supportive and humanistic encounter, one that addresses contextual concerns rather than simply marginalizing them, may emerge as a goal that even some enlightened managed care organizations will support.

Clearly, it would be helpful if patients and doctors could turn to more sources of assistance outside the medical arena to help in solving social problems, but current conditions do not evoke optimism about broader changes in medicine's social context. Such changes will require time and financial resources (although not necessarily more than what is now consumed in inefficient conversations that marginalize contextual issues). From our study we are convinced that contextual problems warrant new social policies to address unmet needs. Of course, these suggestions are not new. Yet it is evident that meaningful improvements in discourse between doctors and patients will depend partly on such wider reforms, which go beyond the changes inherent in managed care.

Policy Efforts and the Contours of the Medico-Political Struggle

As managed care transforms the patient-doctor relationship, the questions of consent and acquiescence present themselves. Why have patients and doctors put up with such a fundamental shift in their relationship? Do patients see little space to resist a new system of care in which physicians—professionals with whom they previously had close and trusting (if sometimes flawed) relationships—have become double agents, gatekeepers who purportedly represent the interests of both patients and managed care corporations but whose remuneration depends in large part on restricting services? Have physicians' quest to maintain their livelihoods really become so desperate that they have become, as some have argued, like lemmings marching into the ocean of managed care?

Resistance among patients has mounted, although slowly. In many states, consumers' organizations have initiated major campaigns to resist some of the observed excesses of managed care. These efforts have led to state-level lobbying activities for protective legislation to prohibit unreasonable limitations and delays in services. Also, some advocacy groups have heavily criticized gag rules and similar restrictions that make physicians feel either formally or informally restrained from advising patients about the full range of diagnostic and therapeutic options available. As noted earlier, some of this advocacy work has culminated in class action lawsuits and similar legal actions that may lead to reforms in some of the constraining policies that managed care has imposed on the patient-doctor relationship.

Physicians' resistance is also gradually increasing, despite the surprising acquiescence they have shown so far in accepting administrative control and micromanagement of the everyday conditions of practice. State medical associations and the American Medical Association have supported legislative efforts to curb gag rules and other constraints on free communication between patients and doctors. Such efforts, however, have so far proven surprisingly mild, with little criticism of the underlying structural features of managed care (especially concerning its corporatization) that impinge on the patient-doctor relationship.

An important exception to this passivity involves an organization that has worked to achieve a national health program for the United States. Physicians for a National Health Program (PHNP), which has chapters in all fifty states, initiated a series of proposals between 1989 and 1994 calling for a national health policy based on a single-payer approach (Himmelstein and others, 1989; Grumbach and others, 1991; Harrington and others, 1991; Schiff, Bindman, and Brennan, 1994). Modeled on the Canadian system but advocating policies to correct problems that have arisen in Canada, PNHP's proposals led to the most widely supported alternative to the managed care–oriented proposal of the Clinton administration. Although legislative measures based on the single-payer model failed along with those of the Clinton plan, PHNP has continued to work actively at the national and state levels to maintain the vision of a well-organized national program as a viable policy option.

One component of PNHP's work since the failure of the Clinton proposal has been a continuing, sharp critique of managed care's impact on the patient-doctor relationship. PNHP leaders have called attention in many forums to the deleterious effects of gag rules and other restrictions on free communication between patients and doctors (Woolhandler and Himmelstein, 1995). These efforts have contributed to movement in state legislatures and (gradually) in Congress toward reforms that will modify such practices. Further, PNHP has called attention to the adverse impact of corporate policies on access to appropriate care.

A major part of this critical work has focused on administrative waste and the erroneous view that physicians' practice patterns account for much of the problem of high costs in health care. Although uncontrolled costs are a multifaceted problem, administrative waste deserves special emphasis from this viewpoint (Woolhandler and Himmelstein, 1991; Shulkin, Hillman, and Cooper, 1993). Administrators represent the fastest-growing sector of the health care labor force, expanding at three times the rate of physicians and other clinical personnel. Even before the latest proliferation of managed care, the United States spent more on administration than any other economically developed country; currently, administration consumes approximately 24 percent of U.S. health care spending. This figure compares unfavorably to all countries with national health programs, which spend between 6 and 14 percent of health care costs on administration. If the United States could reduce administrative spending to a proportion comparable to that of countries with national health programs, the savings (approximately 10 percent of $1 trillion, or about $100 billion) would be adequate to provide universal access to health services without additional government spending (General Accounting Office, 1991). Yet because managed care is administratively intensive, it will increase the proportion of health care expenditures devoted to administrative activities well beyond the current 24 percent figure.

A national health program in the United States could drastically reduce such wasteful administrative practices by eliminating the need for billing by hospitals and through other, related reforms. As in Canada and several European countries, hospitals could be funded through global annual budgets negotiated with the national health program, rather than being burdened by the present costly billing and utilization-review processes. Administrative practices that curtail services and constrain communication in the patient-doctor relationship under managed care are themselves costly. The evidence that these added administrative costs can be justified by appropriate reductions in clinical costs has been quite limited (Langwell, Staines, and Gordon, 1992; Gabel and Rice, 1993; Waitzkin, 1994).

Inappropriate physician practices account for a small part of this country's health care cost crisis compared to administrative waste (Woolhandler and Himmelstein, 1989, 1991, 1995). Overall expenditures on unnecessary procedures ordered or performed by physicians are currently unknown. Even generous estimates, however, put this figure at no more than about 10 percent of total spending on health care (National Leadership Commission on Health Care, 1989).

Table 7.1 shows the potential savings from reducing the volume of selected high-volume, high-cost medical and surgical procedures. A 5 percent reduction is used for these calculations because it represents a reasonable percentage of inappropriate procedures that might be eliminated in the application of practice guidelines (National Leadership Commission on Health Care, 1989, p. 127). As is evident from the estimates, the potential savings from a national health program that would reduce administrative waste are approximately 70 times larger, depending on the assumptions, than those from reducing "inappropriate" medical and surgical procedures. While it is difficult to reach completely precise estimates here, the differences in the order of magnitude between the expected savings from a national health program and those from more rationalized practice patterns are clear. Under the circumstances of managed care's unproven effects in improving efficacy or reducing overall costs, the micromanagement policies that restrict clinical decisions and physicians' open explanations of them deserve greater critical attention than they have received thus far.

Conclusion

To sum up: we have tried to spell out some of the troubling contradictions that managed care has created in day-to-day patient-doctor encounters and relationships. We have discussed practitioners as double agents and the financial structures that constrain open communication. Managed care has created enduring legal and

Table 7.1. Estimated Potential Savings from Reducing the Volume of Ten Selected Procedures by 5 Percent.

Procedures	Total savings per procedure ($ millions)
Hip replacement	66.9
Total knee replacement	100.7
Pacemaker insertion	73.5
Coronary artery bypass graft	245.1
Carotid endarterectomy	51.7
Upper GI endoscopy	8.4
Cholecystectomy	339.4
Transurethral resection of the prostate	65.6
Hysterectomy	195.9
Cesarean section	160.2
Total savings	1,307.4

Source: Used with permission from *For the Health of a Nation: A Shared Responsibility.* Report of the National Leadership Commission on Health Care. Chicago: Health Administration Press, 1989, p. 129.

ethical dilemmas in interpersonal relationships that warrant attention in health policy.

Toward that end, we have touched on the unresolved question of what kind of patient-doctor encounter we should be striving to create, and we have outlined some of the struggles that have and will continue to emerge as managed care flowers. The very future of the patient-doctor relationship as we have known it is at stake. The era that preceded managed care obviously was not free of problems in this regard, but the conflicts of interest and mixed loyalties inherent in managed care have further clouded patients' and health professionals' relationships with one another. A loss of trust and open communication will continue to generate conflict and policy debate. Without such conflict and debate, medicine will lose its most basic qualities—caring and compassion.

References

American College of Physicians. *Ethics Manual.* (3rd ed.) Philadelphia: The College, 1993.

Angell, M. "The Doctor as Double Agent." *Kennedy Institute for Ethics Journal,* 1993, *3,* 279–286.

Balint, J., and Shelton, W. "Regaining the Initiative: Forging a New Model of the Patient-Physician Relationship." *Journal of the American Medical Association,* 1996, *275*(11), 887–891.

Brennan, T. A. "An Ethical Perspective on Health Care Insurance Reform." *American Journal of Law and Medicine,* 1993, *19*(1–2), 37–74.

Castillo, R., Waitzkin, H., Villaseñor, Y., and Escobar, J. I. "Mental Health Disorders and Somatoform Symptoms Among Immigrants and Refugees Who Seek Primary Care Services. *Archives of Family Medicine,* 1995, *4,* 637–646.

Coyle, W., and Hostetter, G. "Kaiser Leader in Care Payout." *Fresno Bee,* February 13, 1996, p. E1.

Davies, A. R., and others. "Consumer Acceptance of Prepaid and Fee-for-Service Medical Care: Results from a Randomized Controlled Trial." *Health Services Research,* 1986, *21,* 429–452.

Davis, K. "The Process of Problem (Re)formulation in Psychotherapy." *Sociology of Health and Illness,* 1986, *8,* 44–74.

Davis, K. *Power Under the Microscope: Toward a Grounded Theory of Gender Relations in Medical Encounters.* Dordrecht, Holland: Foris, 1988.

Depression Guideline Panel. *Depression in Primary Care.* (AHCPR Publication No. 93–0550). Rockville, Md.: Agency for Health Care Policy and Research, 1993.

Emanuel, E. J., and Dubler, N. N. "Preserving the Physician-Patient Relationship in the Era of Managed Care." *Journal of the American Medical Association,* 1995, *273*(4), 323–329.

Gabel, J. R., and Rice, T. "Is Managed Competition a Field of Dreams?" *Journal of American Health Policy,* 1993, *3,* 19–24.

General Accounting Office. *Canadian Health Insurance: Lessons for the United States.* Washington, D.C.: General Accounting Office, 1991.

Grumbach, K., and others. "Liberal Benefits, Conservative Spending: The Physicians for a National Health Program Proposal." *Journal of the American Medical Association,* 1991, *265,* 2549–2554.

Grumet, G. W. "Health Care Rationing Through Inconvenience." *New England Journal of Medicine,* 1989, *321*(9), 607–611.

Haffner, L. "Translation Is Not Enough: Interpreting in a Medical Setting." *Western Journal of Medicine,* 1992, *157,* 255–259.

Hall, J. A., and others. "Satisfaction, Gender, and Communication in Medical Visits." *Medical Care,* 1994, *32*(12), 1216–1231.

Hardt, E. J. *The Bilingual Medical Interview.* Boston: Boston Department of Health and Hospitals and Boston Area Health Education Center, 1991.

Harrington, C., and others. "A National Long-term Care Program for the United States: A Caring Vision." *Journal of the American Medical Association,* 1991, *266,* 3023–3029.

"Health Care in Crisis: Are HMOs the Answer?" *Consumer Reports,* 1992, *57*(August), 519–531.

Himmelstein, D. U., and others. "A National Health Program for the United States: A Physicians' Proposal." *New England Journal of Medicine,* 1989, *320,* 102–108.

Kupers, T. A. *Public Therapy.* New York: Free Press, 1981.

Laing, R. D., and Esterson, A. *Sanity, Madness and the Family.* New York: Penguin Books, 1970.

Langwell, K. M., Staines, V. S., and Gordon, N. *The Effects of Managed Care on Use and Costs of Health Services.* Washington, D.C.: Congressional Budget Office, 1992.

Lipkin, M., Jr., Putnam, S. M., and Lazare, A. (eds.) *The Medical Interview: Clinical Care, Education, and Research.* New York: Springer, 1995.

Mishler, E. G., and others. "The Language of Attentive Patient Care: A Comparison of Two Medical Interviews." *Journal of General Internal Medicine,* 1989, *4,* 325–335.

National Leadership Commission on Health Care. *For the Health of a Nation.* Technical Appendix III. Washington, D.C.: National Leadership Commission on Health Care, 1989.

Novack, D. H., and others. "Changes in Physicians' Attitudes Toward Telling the Cancer Patient." *Journal of the American Medical Association,* 1979, *241,* 897–900.

Olmos, D. R., and Roan, S. "HMO Gag Clauses on Doctors Spur Protest." *Los Angeles Times,* April 14, 1996, p. A1.

Pear, R. "The 1992 Elections: Disappointment—The Turnout." *New York Times,* Nov. 5, 1992, p. B4.

Putsch, R. W. "Cross-Cultural Communication: The Special Case of Interpreters in Health Care." *Journal of the American Medical Association,* 1985, *254*(23), 3344–3348.

Reuben, D. B., and others. "The Use of Targeting Criteria in Hospitalized HMO Patients: Results from the Demonstration Phase of the Hospitalized Older Persons Evaluation (HOPE) Study." *Journal of the American Geriatrics Society,* 1992, *40,* 482–488.

Rodwin, M. A. "Conflicts in Managed Care." *The New England Journal of Medicine,* 1995, *332*(9), 604–605.

Roter, D. L., and Hall, J. A. *Doctors Talking with Patients/Patients Talking with Doctors.* Westport, Conn.: Auburn House, 1992.

Roter, D., Lipkin, M., Jr., and Korsgaard, A. "Sex Differences in Patients' and Physicians' Communication During Primary Care Visits." *Medical Care,* 1991, *29*(11), 1083–1093.

Rubin, H. R., and others. "Patients' Ratings of Outpatient Visits in Different Practice Settings." *Journal of the American Medical Association,* 1993, *270,* 835–840.

Schiff, G. D., Bindman, A. B., and Brennan, T. A. "A Better-Quality Alternative: Single-Payer National Health System Reform." *Journal of the American Medical Association,* 1994, *272,* 803–808.

Shulkin, D. J., Hillman, A. L., and Cooper, W. M. "Reasons for Increasing Administrative Costs in Hospitals." *Annals of Internal Medicine,* 1993, *119,* 74–78.

Smith, R. C. *The Patient's Story.* Boston: Little, Brown, 1996.

Waitzkin, H. "Doctor-Patient Communication: Clinical Implications of Social Scientific Research." *Journal of the American Medical Association,* 1984, *252,* 2441–2446.

Waitzkin, H. "Information Giving in Medical Care." *Journal of Health and Social Behavior,* 1985, *26,* 81–101.

Waitzkin, H. *The Politics of Medical Encounters: How Patients and Doctors Deal with Social Problems.* New Haven, Conn.: Yale University Press, 1991.

Waitzkin, H. "The Strange Career of Managed Competition: From Military Failure to Medical Success?" *American Journal of Public Health,* 1994, *84,* 482–489.

Waitzkin, H., Britt, T., and Williams, C. "Narratives of Aging and Social Problems in Medical Encounters with Older Persons." *Journal of Health and Social Behavior,* 1994, *35,* 322–348.

Waitzkin, H., and Stoeckle, J. D. "The Communication of Information about Illness: Clinical, Sociological, and Methodological Considerations." *Advances in Psychosomatic Medicine,* 1972, *8,* 180–215.

Woolhandler, S., and Himmelstein, D. U. "Resolving the Cost/Access Conflict: The Case for a National Health Care Program." *Journal of General Internal Medicine,* 1989, *4*(1), 54–60.

Woolhandler, S., and Himmelstein, D. U. "The Deteriorating Administrative Efficiency of the U.S. Health Care System." *New England Journal of Medicine,* 1991, *324*(18), 1253–1258.

Woolhandler, S., and Himmelstein, D. U. "Extreme Risk—The New Corporate Proposition for Physicians." *New England Journal of Medicine,* 1995, *333,* 1706–1708.

Part Three

Public Sector Initiatives and Responses

Intervention to Enhance Market Efficiency

The government may intervene in a variety of ways to enhance market efficiency in general and within the health care sector in particular. This section presents two very different examples of government interventions designed primarily to improve the competitive balance in the health insurance market—controlling the expansion of market power by health maintenance organizations (HMOs) and helping small purchasers develop their own countervailing bargaining power. In Chapter Eight, Ruth Given discusses the role of government antitrust regulators in curbing excessive market concentration. She illustrates this concept by describing the economic issues raised by a recent HMO merger case. In Chapter Nine, Thomas Buchmueller discusses government intervention to promote efficiency through the demand side of the market. Buchmueller evaluates the early experience of the Health Insurance Plan of California, a state-sponsored purchasing pool established to improve access to and affordability of insurance coverage for small employers.

The most obvious form of market failure immediately apparent in both of these chapters relates to the problem of reduced competition. Chapter Eight describes government's role in ensuring that markets that should be competitive actually remain so.

This is accomplished through evaluation and selective denial of mergers that raise concerns about anticompetitiveness. Chapter Nine also addresses the issue of reduced competition; it suggests that there is an important government role in helping small employer groups increase their bargaining power with insurers, just as large purchasing coalitions have been able to do. Another form of market failure addressed in Chapter Nine is adverse selection. In addition to providing bargaining clout for small groups, the HIPC also serves to pool risk for all participants, reducing the likelihood of adverse selection and making more comprehensive policies available and affordable for this population. However, other opportunities for adverse selection remain, due to the structure of the HIPC. Evidence of their severity and possible solutions are discussed.

Intervention to Address Equity Concerns

While a perfectly competitive market guarantees maximum efficiency, it may not result in a socially acceptable degree of equity in access to health care. In the end, the responsibility to ensure equity in the health care marketplace is left to government. Government health care programs for vulnerable populations, in particular Medicaid, are being profoundly affected by the market forces of competitive managed care. In Chapter Ten, Michael Sparer describes the nearly universal rush by the states to shift Medicaid recipients from fee-for-service to managed care. In Chapter Eleven, Kelly Devers provides an in-depth look at the experience of a single state, Colorado, in its recent attempt to devise and implement a managed care program for the special population of Medicaid recipients requiring mental health services.

As we have noted, even a perfectly competitive market cannot ensure that societal goals for equity will be met. As a result, government must reallocate resources in a fashion that the citizens find preferable to a free-market distribution. Although Chapters Ten and Eleven deal primarily with government's role in promoting equity, they also touch on a few issues related to market failure and market efficiency. One important current topic of public debate revolves around the relative efficiency and value to society of public and private nonprofit providers, as well as their prospects for survival in an increasingly price-competitive managed care marketplace. Advocates of nonprofit institutions claim that they fill a special niche, providing services to populations shunned by profit-oriented firms. Their detractors claim, however, that nonprofits are essentially indistinguishable in their behavior from for-profits, that they have unfair tax advantages, and that because of a past lack of market discipline, nonprofits have contributed to overall market inefficiency.

This debate is unlikely to be resolved soon, but it is particularly important because nonprofit and public institutions frequently serve as a safety net or as the providers of last resort for vulnerable populations whose care is subsidized by the government. The threat of cutbacks in state and federal funding, together with the growing unwillingness of private purchasers to cover the costs of uncompensated care, has created a funding crisis for many of these safety-net providers. A major policy-relevant area of research for the future is to determine whether these institutions are merely inefficient and should be allowed to fail or whether they serve a unique social purpose that profit-oriented firms cannot.

The Politics of Intervention

Government can promote market efficiency by acting to directly enhance competition, improve market information on price and quality, and introduce incentives (typically taxes and subsidies) to reduce negative externalities and increase positive ones. Government can also improve upon the outcomes of competitive markets through resource redistribution to address societal concerns about equity. However, government intervention is necessarily a political process. As a result, policy developed to deal with these market failure problems can reflect the personal and political agendas of policymakers as much as the prescriptions of disinterested policy analysts.

Chapter Twelve, by John Wilkerson, examines the recent proposal to introduce market competition into the Medicare program, to illustrate how politicians and policymakers are using popular rhetoric about free markets to promote far-reaching changes that have little to do with improving the efficiency of the system. Although these changes are being presented as a solution to one perceived and important source of market failure (health care consumer's moral hazard), it is also obvious that perhaps a more important rationale is to support the sponsoring politicians' own social agendas. Therefore the strength of the analytical rationale underlying policy proposals should always be carefully scrutinized, because the potential benefits of reducing market failures through government intervention must be balanced against the potential costs of government failure.

In Chapter Thirteen, Donald Light describes the recent British effort to inject competitive market forces into the National Health Service and draws out a number of lessons for U.S. policymakers. Light's description of the attempted reforms shows how political resistance in Britain ultimately severely limited any meaningful changes to the system. Moreover, evidence from the British experience suggests that a competitive approach to health care financing and delivery may not provide the best outcomes for society, even in a system that has already addressed the issue of equity through universal coverage.

Chapter Eight

Ensuring Competition in the Market for HMO Services

Ruth S. Given

Antitrust enforcement activity with respect to physicians and hospitals has become increasingly common since the mid 1970s (Lerner, 1984; Flynn, 1994). Health maintenance organization (HMO) merger activity, as well as other aspects of potentially anticompetitive behavior in the managed care industry, are just now beginning to attract attention and raise concerns among direct consumers and purchasers of care, providers, and government regulators (Klein, 1995; Kassirer, 1996; Johnsson, 1996). This chapter provides background on the economic rationale for current antitrust policy on corporate mergers as well as some of the special issues that arise when applying this policy to health insurers. The chapter focuses on a recent merger case involving the St. Louis, Missouri, subsidiaries of two national HMOs, United HealthCare and MetraHealth. This case illustrates how government intervention can, through merger evaluation and selective approval, improve efficiency in health care markets.

Antitrust Policy

Antitrust policy consists both of federal and state laws that make certain types of business practices illegal and of the interpretation and enforcement of those laws. The business practices prohibited or regulated by antitrust laws include price fixing, price discrimination, the use of tying clauses, exclusive contracting arrangements, and mergers among competitors. The purpose of antitrust policy is to ensure the competitiveness, and thus the efficiency, of economic markets. As Joseph Stiglitz, chairman of President Clinton's Council of Economic Advisors, has put it, "Antitrust laws exist to protect competition, which is central to the success of our market economy. It spurs producers to contain costs, to be responsive to consumer demands by offering innovative products and to deliver these products at low prices. In short, competition promotes efficiency and delivers the resulting benefits to consumers" (Stiglitz, 1995, p. A22).

Unlike government economic regulation of industries considered to be natural monopolies, antitrust policy applies to industries in markets that should be inherently competitive. However, firms in a competitive industry have an incentive, although not always the means, to act anticompetitively in the ways mentioned above. The major differences between the government's role in regulating natural monopolies and its role in enforcing antitrust laws can be illustrated by use of a medical metaphor, in which the market is the patient and the government is the provider (Scherer and Ross, 1990). An optimally healthy market would be characterized by perfect competition, which would produce a healthy (that is, efficient) allocation of resources. Industries described as natural monopolies might be considered chronically ill and in need of long-term care by government regulators to safeguard efficiency. This intervention takes the form of ongoing oversight and monitoring of production and pricing (for example, by requiring rate approval).

Industries in competitive (healthy) markets do not require such constant attention from government. However, these markets may occasionally become ill, requiring government intervention to treat—in accordance with the protocols of antitrust policy—acute attacks of anticompetitiveness. There are certain risk factors that increase the likelihood of such attacks. The most important is a reduction in the number of competitors, which leads to increased market concentration. In addition to treating acute problems as they surface, antitrust policy is also responsible for preventing the development of market conditions that raise the risk of anticompetitiveness, such as increased concentration.

This chapter focuses on an important form of preventive therapy that exists under antitrust policy—the evaluation of proposed horizontal mergers to deter any unnecessary increases in market concentration. Although popular opinion tends to focus on the negative (monopolistic) aspects of horizontal mergers, such mergers sometimes result in beneficial outcomes. The government, to safeguard the competitive health of the economic market, need not prevent or even challenge all proposed mergers. However, the key challenge for regulators is to distinguish between beneficial and detrimental mergers and respond appropriately.

Current Horizontal Merger Policy

Mergers can be either horizontal, vertical, or conglomerate. A horizontal merger combines firms that produce or sell the same good or service in the same geographic market; a vertical merger joins firms that are upstream or downstream in the production process for a particular product. Popular notions of conglomerate mergers from the 1960s are that they combine firms with nothing whatsoever in common. However, this category also includes mergers of firms that sell similar products but in different geographic markets (market extension mergers) and mergers of firms that sell different products but in the same geographic market (market expansion mergers).

This chapter will focus on the potential problems of horizontal mergers in which the firms in question share both product line and geographic market. Horizontal mergers potentially raise the most substantive antitrust concerns since they reduce the number of direct competitors in a market, giving the merged firm increased market power and possibly reducing market efficiency.

There are a number of reasons that firms pursue horizontal mergers. Motives with the most relevance for antitrust policy and merger evaluation are the desire to increase market power and the desire to increase efficiencies of operation. The first motivation clearly has negative consequences for market efficiency. Firms naturally want to increase their market power. Considered from a market-efficiency perspective, however, this can be detrimental, since a merger between direct rivals reduces competition. Firms also merge for reasons that have more positive social consequences, such as achieving economies of scale. In this case a merger would result in lower costs of production, increasing overall market efficiency. Hence, a merger need not be detrimental to the efficiency of a market as a whole.

Any particular merger may have positive or negative consequences or both. Williamson has described the trade-off between the societal loss from increased market power, which enables a firm to raise prices above its cost of production, and the savings from economies of scale that reduce the average cost per unit of output (Williamson, 1968). Figure 8.1 shows the consumer's downward sloping demand curve in a market for a particular good. The hypothetical merger portrayed here has contrasting and somewhat offsetting effects on market efficiency. On the one hand, the resulting increase in market concentration allows the newly merged firm to wield increased market power, allowing it to raise its price above its cost of production. This is the change from P1 to P2. The related negative effect appears in the area of triangle A, which represents the deadweight societal loss (that is, implicit cost) due to inefficiency, since the price for the product can now be raised above its cost of production. On the other hand, the merger reduces the cost of production, due to economies of scale. This is the change from AC1 to AC2. The related positive effect is reflected by the area of rectangle B. Horizontal mergers thus may have both cost-saving (that is, positive) aspects as well as market power–enhancing (that is, negative) aspects. Casual inspection of this example indicates that this should be considered, on net, a positive merger.

The preceding suggests that mergers that apparently result in a net cost savings are beneficial and should not be challenged by regulators. But there are a number of reasons for caution about this conclusion. First, despite the fanfare with which managers promote mergers to stockholders, the prospective cost savings of a merger are very hard to project and therefore to document. Second, this merger trade-off model implies that all of the benefits of the reductions in the cost of production accrue to the merging firms. Although this does, on net, increase overall societal benefits, distributional concerns may arise because the cost savings will not necessarily be passed along to consumers in the form of reduced prices; in this case the benefits would accrue only to the owners (stockholders) of the merged firm.

Figure 8.1. Merger Trade-Off Analysis.

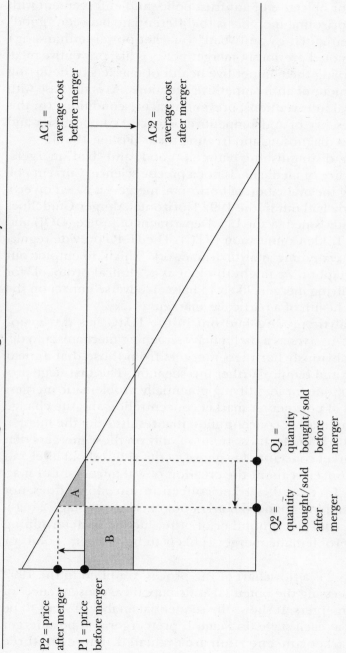

AC1 = average cost before merger

AC2 = average cost after merger

Q1 = quantity bought/sold before merger

Q2 = quantity bought/sold after merger

P2 = price after merger

P1 = price before merger

A = Deadweight loss to society due to monopoly pricing

B = Cost savings due to increased efficiency

The major objective of antitrust policy and enforcement with respect to horizontal mergers is to differentiate between "good" (efficiency-enhancing) and "bad" (market power–enhancing) mergers. As noted previously, merger policy is like preventive medicine, preserving the competitive health of markets by deterring the development of anticompetitive situations. As is the case with many medical interventions, preventing acute conditions (in this case, the presence of anticompetitive practices) can be easier and cheaper than diagnosing and treating them (Fisher, 1987).

However, distinguishing between "good" and "bad" mergers, like the practice of medicine, is not a precise science. Current policy regarding the evaluation of horizontal mergers is based on economic criteria laid out in the 1992 Horizontal Merger Guidelines (HMG), jointly issued by the U.S. Department of Justice (DOJ) and the Federal Trade Commission (FTC). The HMG provide regulators with an economic analytic framework, which, to employ our medical metaphor, we might think of as a "clinical protocol" for use in identifying mergers likely to have an adverse impact on the competitive health of a particular market.

The analytic process laid out in the HMG has two major stages. Stage 1 serves as a preliminary screening mechanism to differentiate obviously harmless mergers from those that appear problematic and require further investigation. This first stage provides a technique for identifying potentially problematic mergers on the basis of postmerger market concentration and the change in the level of market concentration that results from the merger. Stage 2 of the HMG focuses attention only on those mergers that increase market concentration above a critical threshold level and thus raise concerns about the creation or enhancement of market power. Increased market concentration alone does not inevitably lead to enhanced market power. Thus, in Stage 2 regulators must consider a number of other factors in determining whether a problematic merger is likely to be, on net, "good" or "bad."

Figure 8.2 is a flowchart of the process outlined in the 1992 HMG for assessing the potential anticompetitive consequences of horizontal mergers. It shows the sequential analytical steps to be considered at each stage. In Stage 1, premerger and postmerger levels of market concentration are evaluated. There are three steps underlying this task. The first step (1a) is to define the

Figure 8.2. The 1992 DOJ-FTC Horizontal Merger Guidelines.

Stage 1

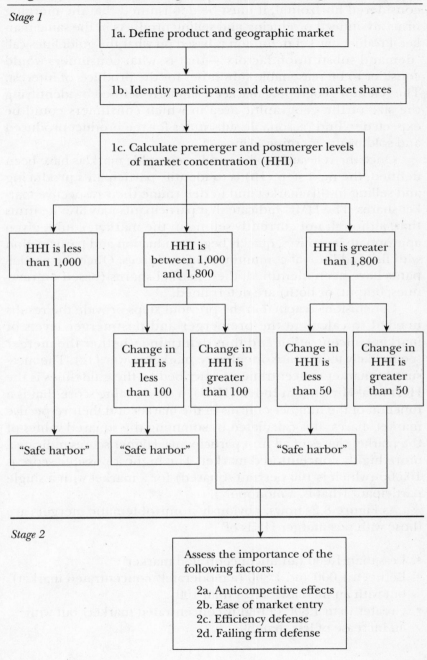

1a. Define product and geographic market

1b. Identity participants and determine market shares

1c. Calculate premerger and postmerger levels of market concentration (HHI)

HHI is less than 1,000

HHI is between 1,000 and 1,800

HHI is greater than 1,800

Change in HHI is less than 100

Change in HHI is greater than 100

Change in HHI is less than 50

Change in HHI is greater than 50

"Safe harbor"

"Safe harbor"

"Safe harbor"

Stage 2

Assess the importance of the following factors:

2a. Anticompetitive effects
2b. Ease of market entry
2c. Efficiency defense
2d. Failing firm defense

appropriate product and geographic market. For a merger to be considered horizontal, it must be determined that the merging firms are indeed producing and selling products in the same market. Product market definition is based on what the guidelines call "demand substitution factors"—that is, what consumers would consider to be reasonable substitutes for the products of interest. The relevant geographic market is similarly defined by identifying the size of the geographic area in which consumers could be expected to find reasonable substitutes for the product produced and sold by the merging firms.

Once the relevant product and geographic markets have been defined, the next step (1b) is to identify participants producing and selling in this market and to determine their respective market shares. The HMG indicate that participants may also be firms that, although not currently selling in the market, could, given appropriate incentives, quickly begin production and participation with little additional commitment of resources. Once the participants have been identified, their market shares (based on revenues, output, or both) are determined.

Conclusions reached in the previous steps provide the results needed to calculate the premerger and postmerger levels of market concentration and thus determine whether the merger seems likely to increase or enhance market power (1c). The measure of market concentration prescribed by the guidelines is the Herfindal-Hirschman Index (HHI), a single-value score that is a function of the number of firms in the market and their respective market shares. It is calculated by summing the squared values of the market shares of all firm participants. Higher scores indicate a more highly concentrated market. The highest possible score is 10,000 (which is 100 percent squared) for a market with a single participant (that is, a monopoly).

As Figure 8.2 shows, obviously nonproblematic mergers are those with postmerger HHIs of

- Less than 1,000 (an unconcentrated market)
- Between 1,000 and 1,800 (a moderately concentrated market) but with an increase of less than 100
- Greater than 1,800 (a highly concentrated market) but with an increase of less than 50

These are classified as falling into "safe harbors"—that is, in general they will not be challenged as mergers likely to increase market power. On the other hand, mergers that result in postmerger HHI scores of between 1,000 and 1,800 (with an increase of at least 100) and of over 1,800 (with an increase of over 50) raise concerns about adverse competitive consequences. These are targeted for further analysis, using criteria set out under Stage 2 of the HMG.

Figure 8.2 also lists the other factors to be considered under Stage 2 in determining whether mergers producing highly concentrated markets, as judged by the HHI, should be challenged. There are a number of other important industry-specific characteristics that should be taken into account. The HMG specifies four major factors to be considered when further analyzing potentially problematic mergers.

The first additional factor (2a) is the potential for anticompetitive effects resulting from collective action by a number of participants or unilateral action by the merged firm, or both. Collective action refers to the ability of firms to coordinate their behavior to jointly maintain excess profits, such as by colluding to fix prices. Even without cooperative behavior that reduces competition, the merged firm may display unilateral actions that have anticompetitive effects.

The second factor to consider when assessing whether increased market concentration contributes to enhanced market power (2b) relates to the ease with which new competitors can enter the market in the event that the merged firm experiences excess profits as the result of anticompetitive practices. According to the HMG, if market entry is "timely, likely, and sufficient in its magnitude, character and scope," the presence of high profits can encourage other firms to enter the market, thus deterring anticompetitive behavior. The guidelines specify that entry must occur within two years, sales of the relevant product must be profitable at premerger prices, and the assets required for entry must be available to entrants as well as incumbents. If ease of entry is assured, firms in even highly concentrated markets should not be able to exercise market power without the threat of attracting competitors.

Two other factors can be considered in defense of a merger that raises market concentration and possibly enhances market power. One (2c) is the ability of the merger to improve efficiency of operations, particularly by taking advantage of economies of scale in firm specific or joint operation of the merged firms. However, the guidelines recognize that improved efficiencies related to a merger are frequently very hard to demonstrate. Although the guidelines note that greater efficiencies are likely to be passed on to consumers in the form of lower prices, it nowhere specifies that this need be the case. The demonstration of increased efficiency at the firm level is considered a sufficient merger defense. Finally, under 2d it is expected that a merger will not substantially create or enhance market power if it can be shown that one of the merging firms is in danger of imminent failure.

HMO Mergers and Recent Merger Policy

Before turning to the case of the merger between United Health-Care and MetraHealth, it may be helpful to provide some background on HMO mergers and HMO merger policy. Table 8.1 shows the number of HMO mergers per year, the average size of HMO acquired by year, and the total number of HMOs at the start of each year for the period 1985 to 1992. There have been two major waves of HMO mergers. The first occurred in the late 1980s. This wave can be attributed to "industry shakeout" and was related to the large number of small HMOs that entered the rapidly expanding market in the early and mid 1980s. Since many of the HMOs that were acquired in that era were probably in financial trouble and were quite small, this merger wave did not have serious antitrust implications.

Although comparable recent data are not readily available, we are clearly in the midst of a second wave of HMO mergers that began in 1991. The underlying motivations appear to be very different from those of the first wave (Anders and Winslow, 1995). Rather than the mainly reactive and opportunistic acquisition of failing HMOs that characterized the first merger wave, the current wave appears to result from a self-conscious effort both to expand geographic market areas and to engage in regional consolidation, thus increasing local market shares. For example, four large California HMOs—Foundation, FHP, Pacificare, and Health Systems International—have been entering other state markets, primarily through acquisition. In a move involving market extension, market

Table 8.1. HMO Mergers.

Year	Number of Mergers[1]	Average Size of HMO Acquired	Total Number of HMOs[2]
1985	3	7,128	491
1986	10	15,815	663
1987	9	18,178	695
1988	27	30,367	680
1989	13	17,469	606
1990	3	26,210	572
1991	5	23,802	565
1992	11	53,757	555

Source: Feldman, Wholey, and Christianson, 1995.
1. Mergers are defined here as the number of HMO acquisitions.
2. This refers to the total number of HMOs at the beginning of each year.

expansion, and local consolidation, MetLife and Travelers merged to become MetraHealth. The national merger of United Health-Care and MetraHealth, as well as the proposed merger of Aetna and U.S. Healthcare, reflects a similar strategic pattern (Eaton, 1996).

Until very recently there have been few direct antitrust challenges to HMO mergers. However, in the past year both private and public parties have raised concerns about their anticompetitive implications. Corporate benefit managers are worried that consolidation in certain areas will leave consumers with fewer choices (Stutz, 1995). State governments have also expressed concern (Findlay, 1995). In 1994 the state of Minnesota, following a period of rapid consolidation in all sectors of the health care industry, enacted a moratorium on HMO mergers. In New Hampshire the proposed acquisition of the Matthew Thornton Health Plan by Harvard–Pilgrim Health Plan was delayed eighteen months by various state agencies so that regulators could ascertain whether the planned exclusive contracting arrangement with primary care providers would create future barriers to entry.

The Proposed St. Louis–Area Merger

In June 1995 United HealthCare announced that it planned to spend $1.65 billion to acquire MetraHealth, a health insurance–managed care company created in January of the same year from the health insurance components of the Metropolitan and Travelers Insurance companies ("Merger Would Create Health Care Colossus," 1995). This merger would create the country's largest managed care company, with almost 6 million full-service managed care enrollees and another 35 million in specialty managed care and traditional indemnity plans.

This acquisition would also enable United HealthCare to expand its HMO operations into new geographic areas, gaining entry to markets in Arizona, California, Colorado, Texas, Washington State, and on the East Coast. From a national perspective this appeared to be primarily a conglomerate (that is, market extension) merger. But from the perspective of some local markets, where both firms already existed and sold similar managed care products, this was clearly a horizontal merger. This case study describes the experience of one local market, the St. Louis, Missouri, metropolitan statistical area (MSA), where the merger raised antitrust concerns. Here the proposed merger would have combined the United HealthCare subsidiaries GenCare and Physicians Health Plan (PHP) with a MetraHealth-owned plan, MetLife Health Care Network, Inc.

In 1995 the Missouri part of the St. Louis MSA had a total population of about 2.5 million, with about half enrolled in some form of managed care. Based on preliminary calculations by the Missouri Department of Insurance (MDI), acquisition of the MetLife plan would have given United HealthCare 60 percent of the HMO market and 35 to 40 percent of the managed care market, where managed care was defined as including both HMO and preferred provider organization (PPO) insurance products (Kertesz and Moore, 1995).

One of the responsibilities of the director of MDI is to protect competition in the market for insurance services; as a result, he or she may review and, if necessary, prohibit acquisitions of insurance companies (including HMOs). Disapproving a merger requires demonstrating that the merger would have anticompetitive effects. The director of MDI must also hold a public hearing where all involved parties (including the proposed merger partners, suppliers, consumers, and competitors) have the opportunity to present evidence on the likely effects of the merger on competition in the local market. If MDI halts a merger, the director must specify a plan to remedy the anticompetitive effects, typically one that specifies the conditions for divestiture of one of the firms (HMOs).

In this case, the process of assessing the potential anticompetitive effects of the merger included the following steps. The firms proposing to merge first informed the appropriate federal and state authorities of their intent to merge. A variety of evidence was gathered. This included both written and oral testimony by various interested parties, including representatives of the firms contemplating the merger, their competitors, their suppliers of inputs, and the consumers of HMO services. However, since interpretation of antitrust law with respect to horizontal mergers is based to a great extent on the economic principles laid out in the HMG, the most important evidence came from the economic analyses presented by economic experts employed by the opposing sides in the case.

As one would expect, the economic experts differed in their conclusions as to the merger's possible anticompetitive consequences. Those retained by United HealthCare (UHC) concluded that the merger raised no concerns (Harris, 1995; Salkever, 1995). Experts retained by MDI reached the opposite conclusion (Given, 1995; Leven, 1995). Not surprisingly, their economic analyses differed considerably on the nature and relative importance of underlying factors as outlined in the HMG.

Table 8.2 provides a summary of the positions held by each side on the most important issues in this case, grouped by stage of the evaluation process suggested by the HMG. Common ground between the opposing experts was relatively limited: both sides agreed that the Missouri portion of the St. Louis MSA should be considered the appropriate geographic market. Also, since neither side explicitly raised the following issues, there was probably agreement that the merger would not be expected to produce any operational efficiencies and that neither of the firms involved was in danger of imminent failure.

Table 8.2. Economic Issues and Positions in the St. Louis MSA Merger.

Relevant Issues/Factors from the Horizontal Merger Guidelines	United HealthCare (pro-merger)	Missouri Dept. of Insurance (anti-merger)
Stage 1:		
Definition of Product Market	All "health care financing," including HMO, PPO, and FFS indemnity coverage, both risk bearing and self-insured.	Risk-bearing HMO and PPO coverage only— explicitly excludes any FFS indemnity and self-insured coverage.
Definition of Geographic Market	Missouri counties in the St. Louis MSA.	Missouri counties in the St. Louis MSA.
Stage 2:		
Ease of New Market Entry	New market entry is expected to be *easy*— major focus is on access to production inputs (lack of evidence of exclusive provider contracting).	New market entry is expected to be *difficult*—major focus is on access to channels of distribution (the large employer groups) and the presence of demand-side economies of scale.
Efficiency Defense	No efficiencies to be gained from the merger.	No efficiencies to be gained from the merger.

It is interesting to note that the UHC expert did not advance one of the strongest arguments in favor of permitting a merger, that it would lower average costs, even if only to the firm and not to the direct consumers. The failure to address this issue seriously undercut one of the most compelling reasons for the approval of the merger. The MDI experts did not explicitly address this issue, but they did cite recent research on economies of scale for HMOs that suggests that only much smaller HMOs than those involved in this case can reap efficiency benefits from a merger (Given, forthcoming; Wholey, Feldman, and Christianson, forthcoming).

The Main Issues Raised by the Economic Analyses

There were, however, two extremely important areas of disagreement between the experts retained by each side. These involved the relevant definition of the product market, and ease of market entry.

Product Market Definition

The preliminary screening test for the potential anticompetitive effect of a merger involves reaching a threshold level of market concentration deemed problematic. Key to the determination of industry concentration (and thus change in the level of concentration) is the definition of both the product and the geographic market. Since the experts agreed on the definition of the geographic market, this section will focus on their disagreements on the definition of the product market, the identification of participants, and the assignment of market shares.

UHC's Position. UHC's argument that the merger would not result in a dangerous increase in the level of industry concentration relied on its assertions that there were many substitute products for consumers in this market and that current market shares were not very meaningful in assessing the potential anticompetitive consequences of mergers in this industry. UHC claimed that the relevant product market should be very broadly defined to include all forms of "health care financing," including HMOs (including HMO coverage with a point-of-service [POS] option), PPOs, and all fee-for-service (FFS) indemnity products. UHC felt that the relevant product market should be defined to include not only fully insured products but also those that provide access to PPO networks, as well as administrative services to large employers who then assume the insurance risk themselves.

The major assumptions underlying this product market definition were that the various types of products were reasonably good substitutes for each other and that consumers could readily switch back and forth among them in the event of anticompetitive changes in price and quality brought about by firms trying to exercise monopoly power and that in the case of specifying non-risk-bearing substitutes, consumers would be willing and able to bear the risk or provide the insurance function themselves. Using this very broad definition, UHC concluded that the proposed merger would not cause the HHI to rise above the critical threshold that would trigger the need for further analysis.

Moreover, UHC claimed that the product market so defined had no real capacity constraints, since it was composed primarily of insurance companies that contracted with providers. The HMG, in a footnote, stipulate that in certain industries where output levels change quickly on a regular basis, it is appropriate *not* to use current market shares in calculating the HHI but is instead appropriate to simply divide up the market into "equal shares." This may be a reasonable procedure for industries with a great deal of flexibility in production, since they do not require major planning or fixed capital investment, and there are few barriers to entry.

UHC claimed that the managed care market in St. Louis could be characterized in this way and thus asserted that the merger would not produce an increase in concentration that would create or enhance monopoly power and anticompetitive practices. Applying the equal shares rationale was useful because it produced a very low HHI score, even when using the more restrictive definition of the product market proposed by MDI (see below). UHC suggested that with about ten managed care firms currently in the market, using the equal shares criterion would result in a postmerger HHI score of 1,000, falling well within the safe-harbor range.

MDI's Position. MDI defined the product market much more narrowly, including only HMO products (including those with a POS option) and PPO products. It explicitly excluded FFS indemnity products and products that require the purchaser to bear the risk. Past HMO antitrust cases had typically used the broader definition of product market adopted by UHC. MDI's rationale for defining the product market more narrowly was based on a number of considerations. FFS indemnity insurance was excluded primarily because of the fact that, although consumers might see this type of coverage as a reasonable substitute for managed care plans, employers are less likely to do so since they have found it increasingly difficult to control the benefit costs under such plans (Loomis, 1994). Employers, who are the major purchasers of health insurance benefits, are increasingly restricting employee choice to managed care (Foster Higgins, 1996). The director of the St. Louis Area Business Health Coalition underscored this point when he testified at the public hearing that employers were shunning FFS indemnity coverage in favor of more intensely controlled products in order to control costs (Stutz, 1995).

Although not discussed explicitly in the experts' analyses, one of the problems with considering these two types of insurance as substitutes stems from the problematic nature of insurance itself. The price of insurance, unlike the price of many other types of goods and services, reflects costs and risks associated with the consumer. There is a certain amount of evidence that when managed care is offered to price-sensitive consumers, lower-risk, lower-cost enrollees abandon higher-priced FFS indemnity insurance, leaving FFS plans with a pool of high-risk, high-cost enrollees. This in turn drives up the average cost and price of FFS coverage. The price increases cause continued selective disenrollment of the least costly enrollees, who can expect to get lower prices outside the increasingly high-risk, high-cost FFS group. This has been referred to as the death spiral of adverse selection. In this situation, FFS insurers will increasingly abandon the market. As a result of this dynamic, it is unlikely, contrary to what the UHC experts argued, that there can be much back-and-forth switching by customers (that is, switching simply based on what they see as the perceived net benefits of FFS indemnity coverage vis-à-vis more managed care).

MDI's experts' rationale for excluding products where the purchaser bears the risk (self-insurance by employers) is that this is not a feasible option for small employers or individuals. The major benefit they acquire in the insurance market is access to the insurance or risk-sharing function; this, of course, they lose through self-insurance. Although assumption of risk, purchase of administrative services only (ASO), and "rental" of provider networks may make sense for large employers, they are not reasonable substitutes for the approximately 40 percent of the employed population who are in firms with fewer than 100 employees (Piacentini and Cerino, 1990; Krampf, 1995). Ultimately, the appropriate product definition was therefore held to be not "health care financing" but instead the more narrow definition of "insured, managed care services."

MDI experts identified market participants as firms providing these products and calculated their market shares based on current enrollees in the area. In doing so, they rejected UHC's contention that market shares were so volatile as to render the current distribution of sales meaningless. The MDI analysis indicated that the premerger HHI score was thus about 1,630, rising to 1,780 postmerger, just under the definition of a highly concentrated market. Thus, in contrast to UHC's analysis, which implied that there was no reason to proceed with the evaluation, MDI's analysis indicated that further consideration of possible anticompetitive aspects of the merger was warranted.

Ease of New Market Entry

Under the HMG, even if a merger results in a highly concentrated market, evidence that competitors can easily enter the market to counter any attempts by the merged firm to exercise monopoly power should be weighed in determining whether to allow a merger. Both UHC and MDI addressed the question of the ease or difficulty of new market entry at some length.

UHC's Position. UHC asserted that entry of new firms (that is, de novo entry) into this market was very easy. Therefore, even in the unlikely event that a firm engaged in anticompetitive practices, this would be quickly countered by competition from other firms entering the market. UHC's argument depended on characterizing these new firms as primarily traditional insurance companies, able to move rapidly into a new local market and to contract readily with customers, provided there was access to physician and hospital providers. The ability to contract with providers, thus gaining access to critical production inputs, was considered to be the key factor determining ease of entry. Recent antitrust cases of alleged HMO market monopolization have shown that lack of access to providers, resulting from preexisting exclusive contracting relationships, can create serious barriers to entry (Johnsson, 1996). In support, UHC presented evidence that the St. Louis area had a large number of providers, including hospitals and physicians ready and willing to contract with HMOs that wanted to enter this local market. UHC also presented statistics on the recent past enrollment growth (but not de novo entry) of managed care providers in the St. Louis area, with its examples heavily drawn from the experience of incumbent FFS indemnity insurers expanding into managed care.

MDI's Position. MDI's position was that new market entry was quite difficult; thus entry by new firms would not be able to serve the appropriate disciplinary function if the merged firms exercised monopoly power, either by raising price or reducing quality. In order to support this claim, it was necessary to show that there had been negligible entry of new firms, despite the industry's recent profitability. Although the evidence presented to support this assertion rested in part on data from the St. Louis market, most of it was derived from generalizations based on national data and observed trends in the industry.

MDI agreed that lack of access to required production inputs (providers) can create one type of barrier to entry, but it indicated that another type of barrier to entry had not been recognized by UHC. Another important condition for entry is access to the most efficient customer channels of distribution—that is, the large employer group purchasers of health benefits. This is not easy for small, start-up HMOs, since the most desirable customers—large employer groups—are generally not interested in an HMO until it reaches a certain minimum size (Rose, 1995). This can result in a catch-22: it is difficult for an HMO to develop a good network (that is, one with widespread access to efficient providers and the most favorable rates) unless it can promise its providers a large flow of patients; but it cannot guarantee its providers a large flow of patients until it has contracts with large employer groups, and as noted above, large employers are reluctant to contract with small, new health plans.

There are a number of reasons that large employers may prefer to contract with larger HMOs. In the past, contracting with fewer but larger HMOs has reduced transaction costs. Preference for larger HMOs may now also be related to what are known as "demand-side" economies of scale. These are different from the traditional supply-side economies of scale. In the latter case, firms have high fixed costs related to entry, and they must raise their output volume rapidly to reduce their average cost to the levels faced by incumbent firms. Demand-side economies of scale occur in certain industries in which larger firms may not have lower costs but are perceived to produce goods or services of higher quality than smaller firms (Keeler, 1989).

Why would larger HMOs be perceived as having higher quality? On the one hand, they have greater geographic scope (Rose, 1995). This is an attractive feature for large employers with employees distributed across a wide area (Miller, 1996). But size may also be an indicator of higher-quality care, or at least of the ability to invest in the high-fixed-cost systems needed to measure and monitor quality (Cerne, 1995; Moore, Reynolds, and Rey, 1995). As large employers and purchasing coalitions have been able to radically reduce HMO premiums, concerns have arisen that HMOs may be cutting costs in ways detrimental to quality (Kertesz, 1995; Freudenheim, 1995). Therefore, even with lower prices, it may be hard for smaller, start-up HMOs to get access to large employers because of concerns about their ability to ensure high quality, especially if market prices are low to begin with. In the future the high fixed costs related to demonstrating quality will be associated primarily with the need to invest in yet-to-be-developed integrated cost and clinical information systems (Morrissey, 1995).

The evidence regarding difficulty of new market entry presented by MDI relied on the fact that very little entry into mature HMO markets has been observed. The form of expansion that is currently observed is entry through the purchase of incumbent HMOs at very high prices per enrollee. Recent market-extension mergers of California HMOs involved prices per enrollee of $800 to $1,500; the recently announced merger of Aetna and U.S. Healthcare appears to involve a price of approximately $3,000 per enrollee (Freudenheim, 1993; Gomez and Olmos, 1994; Eaton,

1996)! These prices seem high in light of the fact that there is usually little in the way of tangible assets involved, only "contracts" with purchasers and providers. But the willingness of HMOs to pay these prices to enter markets implies that the alternative, de novo entry, is considered to be more costly or even impossible. This type of evidence for the existence of barriers to entry in the health care industry has been suggested previously. Expansion by acquisition rather than de novo entry was considered an indication of barriers to entry in the hospital industry in the early 1980s. At that time, barriers to entry for hospitals were mainly related to state regulation—specifically, certificate of need (CON) rules that severely limited new construction (Alpert and McCarthy, 1984).

Summary of the Economic Analyses

The differences in the economic arguments presented stemmed primarily from the following two issues: identification of the relevant substitutes for the products sold by the firms involved (that is, definition of the product market) and the ease with which other firms could enter the market to counter any threat of anticompetitive behavior. UHC asserted that the product market should be defined very broadly, to include non-risk-bearing, nonmanaged, indemnity health insurance products as well as insured managed care products. MDI argued that it was no longer reasonable to consider indemnity coverage (risk-bearing or not) as a substitute for managed care insurance (HMOs, HMOs with a POS option, and PPO products).

On the issue of potential barriers to entry, UHC indicated they were minimal and emphasized the evidence on ease of access to providers in the area. It argued that new competitors in the St. Louis area would not have trouble setting up provider networks, because there was currently no evidence of exclusive contracting. Even with an anticompetitive increase in prices, ease of new firm entry would preclude the development of an anticompetitive environment. MDI strongly disagreed, contending that the evidence instead supported the existence of substantial barriers to new market entry in the industry in general as well as in this particular local market. Therefore, entry could not be guaranteed to occur in the event of anticompetitive actions.

Outcome of the Case

After considering the evidence, the director of the Missouri State Department of Insurance determined that the merger raised serious anticompetitive concerns and therefore should not be allowed to proceed. He issued an order for United HealthCare to divest its MetraHealth subsidiary in the St. Louis area. In responding to this order, UHC had two options—appealing the decision to the local district court or acquiescing. Although UHC disagreed with the conclusion that the merger raised anticompetitive concerns, it did not appeal the ruling. It agreed to divest.

How can we interpret this response? On the one hand, the fact that UHC decided not to appeal suggests that it believed the case against the merger was too strong to challenge. However, the relative unimportance of this local merger compared to the goal of a national merger between the two firms may have been a factor. As noted above, the major benefit of UHC's acquisition of Metra-Health was the opportunity to expand into new metropolitan markets throughout the United States. Increasing local concentration in the St. Louis area would have been an attractive side effect of the national merger, but it would have been incidental to UHC's larger goals. Hence, sacrificing the St. Louis–area merger in order to not delay or jeopardize the national merger may have seemed the most prudent strategy. If this conjecture regarding UHC's motive for settlement is correct, UHC's action provides additional support for MDI's claims of barriers to entry in the managed care market. The major benefit of the national merger would be the opportunity to enter many new markets quickly—acquisition of the MetraHealth plans provided immediate access to the most efficient channels of distribution because of its preexisting contracts with many large employer groups.

The role of the government is not merely to forbid problematic mergers but also to further actions that promote future competition (Sunshine, 1996). Therefore, the director of MDI was required to specify the conditions for the sale of the original acquisition target, the MetraHealth subsidiary. His decision had to specify the roles to be played by the various parties, the government's authority over the choice of purchaser, the deadlines for completing the different steps in the divestiture process, and sanctions for not meeting the various conditions.

This dual responsibility of the regulator provides the opportunity not only to block "bad" mergers but also to promote "good" mergers. As described above, some mergers do indeed have positive effects, giving merged firms the ability to exploit economies of scale (symbolized in Figure 8.1 by the area in rectangle B). Some have negative consequences—that is, the greater market power of the merged firm will enable it to price its goods or services above the cost of production (symbolized in Figure 8.1 by the area in triangle A). Ideally, the government regulator wants to disapprove mergers where A is greater than B and approve mergers where B is greater than A. In a situation where there are barriers to market entry, an increase in market concentration as indicated by the HHI provides an indication (albeit imperfect) of increasing market power. The regulator must decide whether the increasing market power of merged firms is outweighed by the efficiency-enhancing potential of the merger. This raises the question of how one can measure a merger's efficiency-enhancing effect.

This can be done by examining evidence presented by the merging firms about specific examples of economization in inputs or by considering empirical studies on economies of scale in the industry in question. Economies of scale reflect the ability of a firm to reduce its average or per-unit cost of production as it increases its volume of output. Firms that display sizable economies of scale are usually those with very high fixed or start-up costs. High start-up costs make the average cost of producing the first few units of output high, since these costs must be allocated over a small number of units. As production increases, however, the average cost of production drops, until a point known as the minimum efficient scale (MES) is reached.

Figure 8.3 shows a typical relationship between firm size (that is, quantity of output) and average cost of output. In this example average cost is very high for the first few units of output, but it rapidly decreases with increasing scale. MES is shown by the point on the graph where the average cost curve ceases to decline and becomes flat. Note that in this example all firm sizes above MES are equally efficient. However, we are most interested here in the

Figure 8.3. The Relationship Between Long-Run Average Cost and Firm Size.

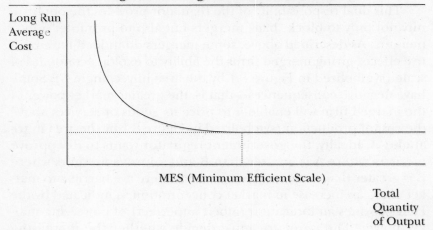

minimum size that a firm must attain to benefit from economies of scale.

Good information on the increase in efficiency that comes with an increase in firm size is not always readily available when evaluating mergers. Fortunately for the St. Louis case, recent research results were available on the presence and magnitude of economies of scale in the HMO industry (Given, forthcoming; Wholey, Feldman, and Christianson, forthcoming). Figure 8.4 relates these findings of HMO economies of scale to changes in average cost per member and the value of MES for the industry, in the same format as Figure 8.3. These studies found that HMOs do experience economies of scale but that these efficiencies are exhausted at a fairly small size; in the case of a multimarket HMO, this probably occurs at an enrollment level of thirty thousand for each of the local markets in which it operates.

This information is very useful in evaluating the proposed merger discussed in this case study. First of all, it is clear that the proposed St. Louis–area merger between United HealthCare (270,000 enrollees) and MetraHealth (30,000 enrollees) would not result in any gains in efficiency. Since both firms were already on the flat, or constant, average-cost portion of the average-cost curve

Figure 8.4. The Relationship Between
Long-Run Average Cost and HMO Size.

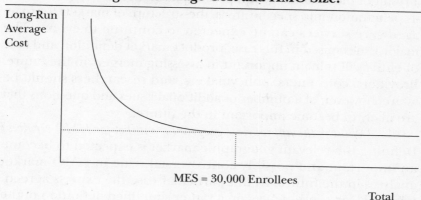

MES = 30,000 Enrollees

Total
Enrollees

shown in Figure 8.4, combining their operations would not have further lowered their average costs. A "good" merger, however, could occur if the MetraHealth subsidiary were to be purchased by a substantially smaller HMO, one operating in the region below 30,000 enrollees.

In fact, the merger partner chosen by United HealthCare and approved by the director of the Missouri Department of Insurance was Principal, an incumbent HMO with very low enrollment (approximately 2,000) in the St. Louis market (Loomis, 1994). Acquisition of MetraHealth would be expected to reduce substantially its average operating costs. Thus, by disapproving the United HealthCare–MetraHealth merger and approving the Principal–MetraHealth merger, government intervention had turned a "bad" merger into a "good" merger. The net effect was an increase in market efficiency rather than an increase in market concentration expected to enhance the merged firms' market power and thus reduce market efficiency.

Issues for Future Research

Because of expected cost savings for purchasers (employers) and profits for managed care companies, enrollment in managed care is expected to expand considerably over the next decade. Partly as a result of the national geographic expansion of managed care and its penetration into specific areas, the structure of markets for managed care services can be expected to continue to evolve. The major issues raised in this case, product market definition and ease of entry, will remain important in assessing mergers in the future. Providers, consumers, policymakers, and researchers should be aware, however, of a number of additional issues and questions that are likely to become important in the future.

1.   *What is the appropriate geographic market for HMO services?* Defining the relevant geographic market is expected to become an important and possibly controversial issue in HMO market analyses in the future. In this particular case the experts agreed, primarily for convenience, on a rather simplified definition of the geographic market for HMO services. However, this decision ignored the influence of access to providers (in terms of geography) on consumers' perceptions of quality and what are considered to be reasonable substitutes. As a result, the geographic market definition employed was undoubtedly too broad. A more appropriate definition could use the standards developed by HMO regulators in the state of California, where HMOs wanting to expand into new geographic areas must provide all prospective enrollees access to both outpatient and inpatient services within fifteen miles or a thirty-minute journey from their homes.

2.   *Should HMOs be considered natural monopolies in some markets, and if so, what should the role of government be in ensuring efficiency in these areas?* If MES for a multiple-market HMO is about thirty thousand enrollees per geographic market, it is clear that there will be large parts of the United States that will be unable to support a competitive number of HMOs. Many areas will barely be able to support more than one HMO operating at MES. If HMO services in these areas are considered a natural monopoly, how will efficiency be ensured (Enthoven and Singer, 1996)? Economic regulation with administrative pricing pegged to competitive pricing in other parts of the country is one possibility. On the other hand, if HMOs continue their practice of avoiding less densely populated areas, these regions may come to represent the last bastion of fee-for-service medicine.

3.   *Are large HMOs a necessary evil?* This question stems from two underlying concerns. We need to remember that HMO consolidation is not occurring in a vacuum but in the midst of a wave of mergers that has been sweeping through all industrial sectors producing health care goods and services. Although HMO mergers may have anticompetitive effects, it may not make sense to restrict HMO consolidation while allowing those who supply inputs to HMOs, such as physicians and hospitals, to merge. Recent rulings on proposed hospital mergers, as well as discussions in Congress about allowing physicians antitrust exemptions, suggest that much consolidation will occur in these sectors in the next few years. Given these possibilities, HMO mergers resulting in higher concentration than was previously acceptable in local markets may be justified in terms of the need for countervailing market power (Findlay, 1995).

A second reason for regarding large HMOs as a necessary evil is related to the serious problem of measuring and monitoring quality. The substantial uncertainty of medical knowledge makes the task of assessing the quality of all health care very difficult. To do so effectively requires access to huge databases. Smaller HMOs may not be able to achieve the statistical power needed to provide meaningful information on quality. Moreover, smaller HMOs may not be able to invest in the fixed information-systems costs required to collect, process, and report information on quality of care.

4.   *Will further changes in the technology of HMO production (especially a continued move to vertical integration) affect the nature of HMO costs, economies of scale, and thus MES for the HMO industry?* MES values for the HMO industry are based on an analysis of a time period when most HMOs were not very vertically integrated and could take advantage of the substantial overcapacity in the hospital industry. The HMOs that were studied had very little in the way of fixed costs for plant and equipment. However, there are indications that HMOs in the future may be required to invest in massively expensive clinical information systems. To ensure that the returns on these systems accrue only to themselves and not also to their competitors, HMOs may be required to establish and use more exclusive provider networks. If HMO production evolves in this way and large, vertically integrated systems again become the norm, our

current estimates of MES for the industry will no longer apply. In general, as fixed costs increase, MES will also increase. As a result, if maximum operational and technical efficiency is our societal goal, we may find it necessary to accept large HMOs as a necessary evil. However, this will mean that fewer local markets will be able to support a competitive number of HMOs and that there will be more regions of the country where HMO services should be considered a natural monopoly.

Conclusion

The case discussed in this chapter provides an example of government intervention to prevent the problem of a particular type of market failure, that resulting from reduced competition and increased concentration. This case is one of the first in which antitrust regulators challenged an HMO merger. It highlights two of the most fundamental economic issues relevant to determining the anticompetitive consequences of a merger in this evolving industry: the appropriate definition of the product market and the presence and magnitude of barriers to new market entry (Lerner, 1996). Considerable change has occurred over the past decade in the way health care is financed and delivered. There is growing evidence that the past conventional wisdom about product market definition and entry barriers for the managed care industry is no longer valid (Brush, 1996; Findlay and Meyeroff, 1996). Because the industry continues to consolidate at a rapid pace, it will be particularly important for antitrust regulators to understand the implications of this evidence for HMO market efficiency and to use this information in assessing the possible positive and negative consequences of future HMO mergers.

References

Alpert, G., and McCarthy, T. R. "Beyond Goldfarb: Applying Traditional Antitrust Analysis to Changing Health Markets." *Antitrust Bulletin*, Summer 1984, pp. 165–203.

Anders, G., and Winslow, R. "The HMO Trend: Big, Bigger, Biggest." *Wall Street Journal*, March 30, 1995, p. B1.

Brush, M. "For Oxford Health, Vital Signs Are Fine." *New York Times*, Mar. 31, 1996, p. F3.

Cerne, F. "Capital Decisions: Where Is the Smart Money Being Invested?" *Hospitals and Health Networks,* June 5, 1995, pp. 33–42.

Eaton, L. "Aetna to Buy U.S. Healthcare in Big Move to Managed Care." *New York Times,* April 2, 1996, p. A1, C1.

Enthoven, A. C., and Singer, S. J. "What to Regulate and by Whom." In H. J. Aaron (ed.), *The Problem That Won't Go Away: Reforming U.S. Health Care Financing.* Washington, D.C.: Brookings Institution, 1996.

Feldman, R., Wholey, D., and Christianson, J. "A Descriptive Economic Analysis of HMO Mergers and Failures, 1985–1992." *Medical Care Review and Research,* 1995, *52*(2), 279–304.

Findlay, S. "Will Big HMOs Stamp Out the Competition?" *Business and Health,* Oct. 1995, pp. 52–61.

Findlay, S., and Meyeroff, W. J. "Health Costs: Why Employers Won Another Round." *Business and Health,* Mar. 1996, pp. 49–51.

Fisher, F. M. "Horizontal Mergers: Triage and Treatment." *Journal of Economic Perspectives,* 1987, *1*(2), 23–40.

Flynn, J. J. "Antitrust Policy and Health Care Reform." *Antitrust Bulletin,* Spring 1994, pp. 59–133.

Foster Higgins. *National Survey of Employer-Sponsored Health Plans.* (10th ed.) New York: Foster Higgins, 1996.

Freudenheim, M. "$275 Million Merger for 2 HMOs: California's Health Net Deal with Qual-Med." *New York Times,* Aug. 31, 1993, p. D4.

Freudenheim, M. "A Bitter Pill for the HMOs." *New York Times,* Apr. 28, 1995, p. C1.

Given, R. S. Prefiled testimony in Missouri Department of Insurance administrative proceeding, docket no. 95–07–13–0006, 1995.

Given, R. S. "Economies of Scale and Scope as an Explanation of Merger and Output Diversification Activities in the HMO Industry." *Journal of Health Economics,* forthcoming.

Gomez, J. M., and Olmos, D. R. "FHP Will Acquire Rival TakeCare in HMO Industry's Largest Merger." *Los Angeles Times,* Mar. 5, 1994, p. D1.

Harris, B. Prefiled testimony in Missouri Department of Insurance administrative proceeding, docket no. 95–07–13–0006, 1995.

Johnsson, J. "States Ask High Court to Hear Marshfield Antitrust Case." *American Medical News,* Mar. 4, 1996, pp. 1–6.

Kassirer, J. P. "Mergers and Acquisitions—Who Benefits? Who Loses?" *New England Journal of Medicine,* 1996, *334*(11), 722–723.

Keeler, T. E. "Deregulation and Scale Economies in the U.S. Trucking Industry: An Econometric Extension of the Survivor Principle." *Journal of Law and Economics,* 1989, *32*, 229–253.

Kertesz, L. "Solving the Cost-Quality Equation." *Modern Healthcare,* May 31, 1995, p. 22.

Kertesz, L., and Moore, J. D. "United, MetraHealth Merger Creates Huge Managed Care Player." *Modern Healthcare,* Oct. 9, 1995, p. 17.

Klein, D. "Limits of Competition." *Inquiry,* 1995, *32,* 369–370.

Krampf, L. "Do You Have What It Takes to Self-Insure?" *Business and Health,* December 1995, pp. 17–26.

Lerner, A. N. "Federal Trade Commission Antitrust Activities in the Health Care Services Field." *Antitrust Bulletin,* Summer 1984, pp. 205–224.

Lerner, A. N. "Mergers of HMOs and Payors." Presentation at the National Health Lawyers Association Conference on Antitrust in the Healthcare Field, Washington, D.C., Feb. 1996.

Leven, C. Prefiled testimony in Missouri Department of Insurance administrative proceeding, docket no. 95–07–13–0006, 1995.

Loomis, C. "The Real Action in Health Care." *Fortune,* July 11, 1994, pp. 149–157.

"Merger Would Create Health Care Colossus." *Los Angeles Times,* June 27, 1995, p. D2.

Miller, R. H. "Competition in the Health System: Good News and Bad News." *Health Affairs,* 1996, *15*(2), 107–120.

Moore, G. B., Reynolds, B. E., and Rey, D. A. "Information Architects: Data by Design." *HMO Magazine,* May/June 1995, pp. 29–35.

Morrissey, J. "Building Networks to Stay Competitive." *Modern Healthcare,* Aug. 21, 1995, pp. 150–154.

Piacentini, J., and Cerino, T. *EBRI Handbook on Employee Benefits.* Washington, D.C.: Employee Benefit Research Institute-Education and Research Fund, 1990.

Rose, J. R. "Do Employers Really Care About Quality?" *Medical Economics,* December 26, 1995, p. 15.

Salkever, D. Prefiled testimony in Missouri Department of Insurance administrative proceeding, docket no. 95–07–13–0006, 1995.

Scherer, F. M., and Ross, D. *Industrial Market Structure and Economic Performance.* (3rd ed.) Boston: Houghton Mifflin, 1990.

Stiglitz, J. "Doctors Aren't Immune to Antitrust Laws." *Wall Street Journal,* October 31, 1995, p. A22.

Stutz, J. Public testimony in Missouri Department of Insurance administrative proceeding, docket no. 95–07–13–0006, Sept. 15, 1995.

Sunshine, S. C. "How Does Antitrust Enforcement Fit In?" In H. J. Aaron (ed.), *The Problem That Won't Go Away: Reforming U.S. Health Care Financing.* Washington, D.C.: Brookings Institution, 1996.

U.S. Department of Justice and Federal Trade Commission. *Horizontal Merger Guidelines.* Washington, D.C.: U.S. Government Printing Office, 1992.

Wholey, D., Feldman, R., and Christianson, J. B. "Scale and Scope Economies Among Health Maintenance Organizations." *Journal of Health Economics,* forthcoming.

Williamson, O. E. "Economies as an Antitrust Defense: The Welfare Tradeoffs." *American Economic Review,* March 1968, pp. 18–36.

Chapter Nine

State-Sponsored Health Insurance Purchasing Cooperatives

California's "HIPC"

Thomas C. Buchmueller

With the demise of health care reform at the national level, reform efforts at the state level have taken on increased importance. While recent state-level policy initiatives have been substantially more modest than President Clinton's proposed Health Security Act and various plans offered as alternatives to the Clinton plan, many contain components of those more ambitious proposals. In particular, several states have enacted legislation to establish publicly sponsored health insurance purchasing cooperatives that in many ways resemble the "health alliances" the Clinton plan would have established. California was the first state to do so, with legislation passed in 1992 and enacted in July 1993.

California's purchasing cooperative is known as the Health Insurance Plan of California (HIPC). By most accounts, in its first two-plus years the HIPC has been a successful venture. There is little evidence of the unwieldy bureaucracy envisioned by critics of

I am grateful to the Henry J. Kaiser Family Foundation for financial support and to Sandra Shewry for providing data on the HIPC and answering numerous questions.

the Clinton plan's health alliances, nor of the severe problems of adverse selection that others argued would be inevitable in a voluntary purchasing cooperative. While the HIPC represents a very small fraction of the small-group insurance market, enrollment continues to grow at a fairly steady rate, and disenrollment has been low. Satisfaction appears to be high among enrollees, participating insurers, and insurance brokers and agents.

This chapter reviews the HIPC's early experience, emphasizing the policy decisions and outcomes that are most relevant to public and private sector policymakers involved with or contemplating similar programs elsewhere. The chapter is organized as follows. The next section briefly summarizes the context in which the HIPC developed and describes the program's design. Next, I evaluate the HIPC in terms of several outcomes: enrollment, premiums, competition among plans, and risk selection. Concluding comments appear in the final section.

The Economics of Small-Group Health Insurance

Health insurance in the United States is largely employment-based: nearly nine out of ten Americans with private insurance are covered through their employer or the employer of a family member. The likelihood of having employer-sponsored insurance increases with income and with the size of one's employer; accordingly, employees of small firms and their dependents make up a large fraction of the uninsured. In 1993, forty-nine percent of uninsured workers were in firms with fewer than one hundred employees; an additional 16 percent were self-employed (Employee Benefit Research Institute, 1994).

The problems with the small-group market are well known (see, for example, Helms, Gauthier, and Campion, 1992; Zellers, McLaughlin, and Frick, 1992; Thorpe, 1992; Morrissey and Jensen, 1996). Because they lack economies of scale in purchasing insurance, small employers face higher per-employee marketing and administrative costs than larger firms. When one or more employees of a small firm has a serious health condition or when a firm is deemed a high risk by virtue of its industry or employee demographics, premiums are even higher, and coverage may be difficult to obtain at all.

In addition to these supply-side considerations, demand-related factors are important in explaining the low rate of insurance provision by small employers. Economic theory predicts that whether or not the employer writes the premium check, it is the worker who pays for employer-sponsored health insurance. A disproportionate number of workers in small firms have low incomes and are unable to afford private insurance at current rates. Also, while most uninsured workers are in firms that do not provide health benefits, not all workers in such firms are uninsured. Many receive coverage through a spouse or parent and do not wish to receive insurance (and thus lower wages) from their employer (Monheit and Vistness, 1994; Chernew, Frick, and McLaughlin, 1995). On top of the unwillingness (or inability) of small-firm employees to trade wages for health benefits, many small employers are simply opposed to playing a role in financing health insurance for their employees. Some have philosophical objections to such a role (McLaughlin and Zellers, 1994). Others may be reluctant to commit to a benefit that has the potential to grow significantly in cost and that carries burdensome administrative costs.

Small-group health insurance reform initiatives have focused primarily on supply-side factors. State policies proposed or enacted in the early 1990s have consisted mainly of underwriting and marketing reforms, the establishment of small-group purchasing cooperatives, or, as in the case of California, both. Some states have also enacted legislation allowing the sale of bare-bones insurance policies—that is, plans not subject to state-mandated benefits. A small number of states have established premium subsidies, though such programs have been quite limited in scope (Morrissey and Jensen, 1996). The main argument for small-group cooperatives is that they give small employers the advantages enjoyed by large employers—economies of scale in administration and marketing, more comprehensive benefits, and a choice of plans. (See Pauly, 1993, for a dissenting view on the potential for lowering administrative costs by pooling small groups.) Premiums may also be reduced if cooperatives can use their size to negotiate lower rates from insurers or if greater consumer choice leads to increased price competition among plans. Pooling employees from many small groups has also been seen as a way to overcome the problems of risk selection endemic to the small-group market.

Small-Group Purchasing Cooperatives

Purchasing cooperatives can be publicly or privately sponsored, and current examples differ in the relative roles played by the public and private sectors (General Accounting Office, 1994). (For more on private cooperatives, see Sullivan, 1993, Chapter Three; McLaughlin and Zellers, 1994.) The main rationales for government sponsorship are fairness, public accountability, and regulatory oversight (Lipson and De Sa, 1995). Privately sponsored cooperatives need not extend coverage to all groups, and they in fact have an incentive to exclude high-risk groups. While there are examples of very successful private cooperatives, many other cooperative purchasing arrangements, particularly those organized as multiple-employer welfare arrangements, have failed due to problems of instability, insolvency, and fraud (Leibowitz, Damberg, and Eyre, 1992).

To the extent that purchasing cooperatives can reduce administrative costs and increase price competition among health plans, they may make insurance more affordable for many small employers. However, the cost savings are likely to be small relative to the amounts required to substantially expand insurance coverage. While previous studies suggest that employers' decisions to offer health insurance are sensitive to price, the degree of sensitivity is fairly low (Leibowitz and Chernew, 1992). Research on the effect of health insurance subsidies suggests that even large subsidies would have a limited effect on the provision of insurance by small employers (Hogan and Woodbury, 1992; Thorpe and others, 1992; McLaughlin and Zellers, 1994; Chernew, Frick, and McLaughlin, 1995). Thus it is unlikely that the establishment of purchasing cooperatives alone will greatly expand the provision of employer-sponsored insurance.

Nonetheless, small-group purchasing cooperatives have the potential to provide important benefits to consumers in the small-group health insurance market. First, while the cost savings generated by cooperatives may not entice many noninsuring firms to begin offering insurance, they represent an important benefit to participating firms. Perhaps as important as the financial savings is the potential reduction in the time small employers must spend shopping for insurance and dealing with agents and insurers.

Another important benefit of purchasing cooperatives is their effect on consumer choice. The majority of small firms that do offer health benefits do not offer their employees a choice of plans. Morrissey, Jensen, and Morlock (1994) estimate that in 1993 only 2 percent of insurance-providing firms with fewer than fifty employees offered a choice of plans. In the ten states studied by Cantor, Long, and Marquis (1995), only 14 percent of firms of this size offered a choice of plans. In a health insurance market dominated by traditional indemnity insurers, this lack of plan choice is not a major issue, because traditional indemnity insurance allows patients an unfettered choice among providers. In a market like California that is dominated by managed care plans, however, individuals whose employers offer only one plan may be dissatisfied with the constraints placed on their choice of physician and hospitals. Health insurance purchasing cooperatives like California's "HIPC" provide a much wider range of choices than otherwise would be available to employees of small firms.

A publicly sponsored small-group purchasing cooperative may produce spillover benefits as well. Since rates charged within the cooperative are public information, competitive pricing by plans within the cooperative may also stimulate price competition in the general small-group market as well. A June 1994 *New York Times* article quoted a representative of California Blue Cross (a carrier that chose not to participate in the HIPC) who said that competition from the HIPC caused Blue Cross to lower its small-group premium twice between 1993 and 1994 (Quinn, 1994).

California's "HIPC"

California's "HIPC" was one component of small-group health insurance reform legislation passed in 1992. That legislation, California Assembly Bill 1672 (AB1672), evolved from several years of debate and represented a compromise among various interest groups, including those advocating more comprehensive health care reform and those preferring a more laissez-faire approach (Dowell and Oliver, 1994b).

The provisions of AB1672 correspond closely to model legislation proposed by the National Association of Insurance Commissioners and reform legislation passed recently in other states

(General Accounting Office, 1995). AB1672 entitles firms with three to fifty employees guaranteed issue and renewability of insurance (the lower limit began at five and was lowered to four in 1994 and three in 1995). To discourage cream skimming, insurance agents are required to show prospective customers summary plan brochures for all insurance products they sell or service. Underwriting on the basis of occupation or health status is prohibited, though premiums are allowed to vary by age, family size, and geographic region. For each cell defined by these factors, health plans must define a standard premium. (The standard rate need not be an average rate. For example, insurers are free to charge the majority of customers a "20 percent under" rate while charging a minority of high-risk firms a "20 percent over" rate. In such a situation, the rate charged to high-risk groups would exceed the median rate by 50 percent.) Actual premiums cannot be more than 20 percent above or below the standard rate. In July 1996, the rate bands go to 10 percent above and below the standard rate. Coverage for preexisting conditions can be denied for a maximum of six months. Individuals with prior insurance coverage can apply the time with prior coverage toward any exclusionary period, with the result that insurance is essentially portable for anyone with at least six months of continuous coverage.

AB1672 also provided for the establishment of the HIPC. The overarching goal in establishing the HIPC was to provide employees of small firms with health benefits that were similar in cost and quality to those enjoyed by employees of larger firms. In terms of its design and operation, the HIPC resembles the purchasing cooperatives proposed by Alain Enthoven (1993) and others and the health alliances of the Clinton health plan. (The two obvious differences between the HIPC and the Clinton plan's health alliances are that in the HIPC enrollment is voluntary and limited to small firms.)

The HIPC is managed by the California Managed Risk Medical Insurance Board (MRMIB), an independent public agency created in 1989 to manage the state's high-risk insurance pool. The MRMIB's staff, in conjunction with the HIPC's five-member board, is responsible for major policy development, negotiating with health plans, and generally overseeing the operations of the HIPC. The basic administration of the HIPC—for example, enrollment and premium collection—is subcontracted to a private firm on a competitive-bid basis. This arrangement allows the MRMIB staff to remain small and to focus on policy issues rather than on day-to-day administrative matters.

HIPC eligibility is limited to firms with three to fifty employees, the same size as is covered by the general insurance market reforms. Within firms, eligibility is limited to full-time employees (thirty or more hours per week), and a 70 percent minimum participation rate is required. Employers must contribute a minimum of 50 percent of the lowest single coverage premium; there is no minimum contribution for dependent coverage. When the employer pays 100 percent of the premium, 100 percent of eligible workers are required to participate.

One hotly debated aspect of the Clinton administration's Health Security Act concerned the types of health plans that would be available through the health alliances. The managed competition models on which the Clinton plan was loosely based envisioned consumers' choosing from a set of integrated managed care plans. However, in response to political pressure from physicians and indemnity insurers, the Clinton plan would have required the alliances to include at least one fee-for-service plan "in which patients have the option of consulting any health care providers subject to reasonable requirements" (White House Domestic Policy Council, 1993, p. 67). That the HIPC includes only health maintenance organizations (HMOs) and preferred provider organizations (PPOs) and that the vast majority of HIPC enrollees are in the former (as will be discussed below) reflects the degree to which managed care currently dominates the California health care market.

For each type of plan there are two levels of benefits: standard and preferred. The main difference between the standard and preferred plans for HMOs is that the standard plans require a higher copayment per office visit ($15 rather than $5). The standard plan also requires a $100 payment for inpatient mental health treatment, whereas there is no payment required under the preferred HMO benefit plan. Both types of PPOs have coinsurance rates of 20 and 40 percent for in-panel and out-of-panel providers, respectively. Standard PPOs have a higher annual deductible than preferred PPOs ($500 per person versus $250). Within a plan category, benefits are completely standardized. Premiums vary across enrollees according only to age, family size, and geographic region, and carriers are prohibited from selling the same coverage at a lower rate outside the HIPC. Two carriers with a large presence in the small-group market—Blue Cross and Blue Shield—noted this restriction as one reason they chose not to participate in the HIPC when it was first established. Their fear was that the premiums they would have to charge in the HIPC would exceed those charged to many existing customers, and they were reluctant to raise rates for those customers ("Insurers Divided on Joining HIPC," 1993).

While a large number of insurers offer plans through the HIPC, access to the program is not automatic. Rather, it is the outcome of negotiations between the plans and the MRMIB. This active approach to "managing competition" among health plans resembles that of the California Public Employee Retirement System (CalPERS), the large purchasing cooperative that is a model for the HIPC and other recently established cooperatives. In contrast, in other states, the public agencies responsible for managing purchasing cooperatives are given less power and autonomy. The most notable example is Florida, where the managing agency has limited authority, and all insurers wishing to sell in the small-group pool are guaranteed access (Herrman, 1994).

Another important policy issue for government-sponsored purchasing cooperatives concerns the role of brokers and agents. To some, such intermediaries represent unnecessary administrative costs. The obvious counterargument is that brokers and agents perform valuable educational and informational functions. In particular, while the number of choices available through the HIPC is one of the program's main selling points, so much choice may be overwhelming to some employers and employees, particularly since it is quite uncommon for small firms to offer a choice of health plans. The job of educating employees about the choices available to them is one for which brokers and agents are well suited. On a more practical level, insurance brokers and agents are important players in the small-group market and can have an important influence on how small employers view a cooperative.

Different states have placed different weight on these various considerations. When the state of Washington established its Basic Health Plan, a low-cost health insurance program for individuals, it decided to market it directly to consumers rather than through brokers or agents (Hoare, Mayers, and Madden, 1992). In contrast, in Florida small groups *must* go through brokers or agents to enroll in the government-sponsored purchasing cooperative established there in 1993 (Ross, 1995).

California's approach represents a compromise between these two extremes. Employers can enroll in the HIPC directly or through an agent. That roughly 70 percent of firms enrolling in the HIPC have chosen the latter and that over 90 percent of those who used an agent to initially enroll continued to use the agent's services when reenrolling (Haggerty, 1994) indicate the important role that insurance agents and brokers play in the small-group market.

Agents' fees in the HIPC consist of a fixed monthly amount per group plus $4 per enrollee per month. The per-group fees vary with the size of the group. Market research conducted by the MRMIB has suggested that the fees paid for smaller groups were competitive with those in the general market, though the fees for larger groups were slightly less than what agents could make out-side the HIPC. While an argument can be made that enrolling firms in the HIPC is easier than helping them purchase insurance in the general market—for example, no time is spent negotiating over premiums—there has been some concern that the relatively low fees for larger eligible groups has discouraged agents from enrolling such firms. Because of this, starting in July 1996 the HIPC will increase the monthly per-group charge for firms with more than twenty enrollees. Also, firms not enrolling through an agent will pay a fee to offset the cost to the HIPC of servicing the group.

Another important policy decision concerns the geographic size and scope of the purchasing pool. Although economies of scale should be greatest in one statewide cooperative, the fact that market conditions can vary substantially within a state, particularly one as large and diverse as California, suggests an argument for organizing purchasing pools at a more local level. Again, the approach taken with the HIPC represents a compromise solution. While the program is managed at the state level and a uniform set of rules applies statewide, the state is divided into six regions for the purpose of setting premiums. Carriers need not offer coverage in all six regions, but they must offer coverage in their entire licensed service area.

Evaluation of Early Results

My evaluation of the early experience of the HIPC focuses on enrollment, characteristics of the firms enrolled in the plan, premiums, competition among plans, and risk selection.

Enrollment

As of January 1996 there were 5,529 small groups enrolled in the HIPC, representing over one hundred thousand employees and dependents. Figure 9.1 presents the number of new groups enrolled for each of the HIPC's first thirty months. The monthly figures suggest a seasonal pattern in new enrollment activity. There are pronounced spikes in new enrollment in June, just after new rates are announced and just prior to when they become effective, and December, when many firms presumably are arranging for insurance coverage for the new year. Activity is lowest in the months of March, April, and May. Adjusting for these seasonal oscillations, the data indicate that new enrollment activity is declining slightly over time.[1] As a result, the HIPC continues to grow, but at a slightly decreasing rate.

It has been estimated that firms enrolled in the HIPC represent less than 2 percent of those eligible (Lipson and De Sa, 1995). Given that HIPC premiums are very competitive relative to the outside market (see below) and that the initial indications are that HIPC enrollees are satisfied with their coverage, it is natural to ask why the HIPC has not gained greater market share.

One explanation is that a large fraction of small employers in California are unfamiliar with the HIPC. In the summer of 1995 I conducted a survey of small employers in California. The survey, which was focused on small firms' health insurance decisions, asked respondents if they knew about the HIPC. Only 24 percent said they did. (To the extent that the interviewers were not always able to identify and interview the most knowledgeable person in each firm, the results from this survey may understate small employers' awareness of the HIPC.) While it is a significant issue, this low level of awareness is not unique to the HIPC. McLaughlin and Zellers (1994) studied privately sponsored cooperatives in Cleveland, Tampa, and Denver. They found that only 10 percent

Figure 9.1. Number of New Groups Enrolled in the HIPC, July 1993 to December 1995.

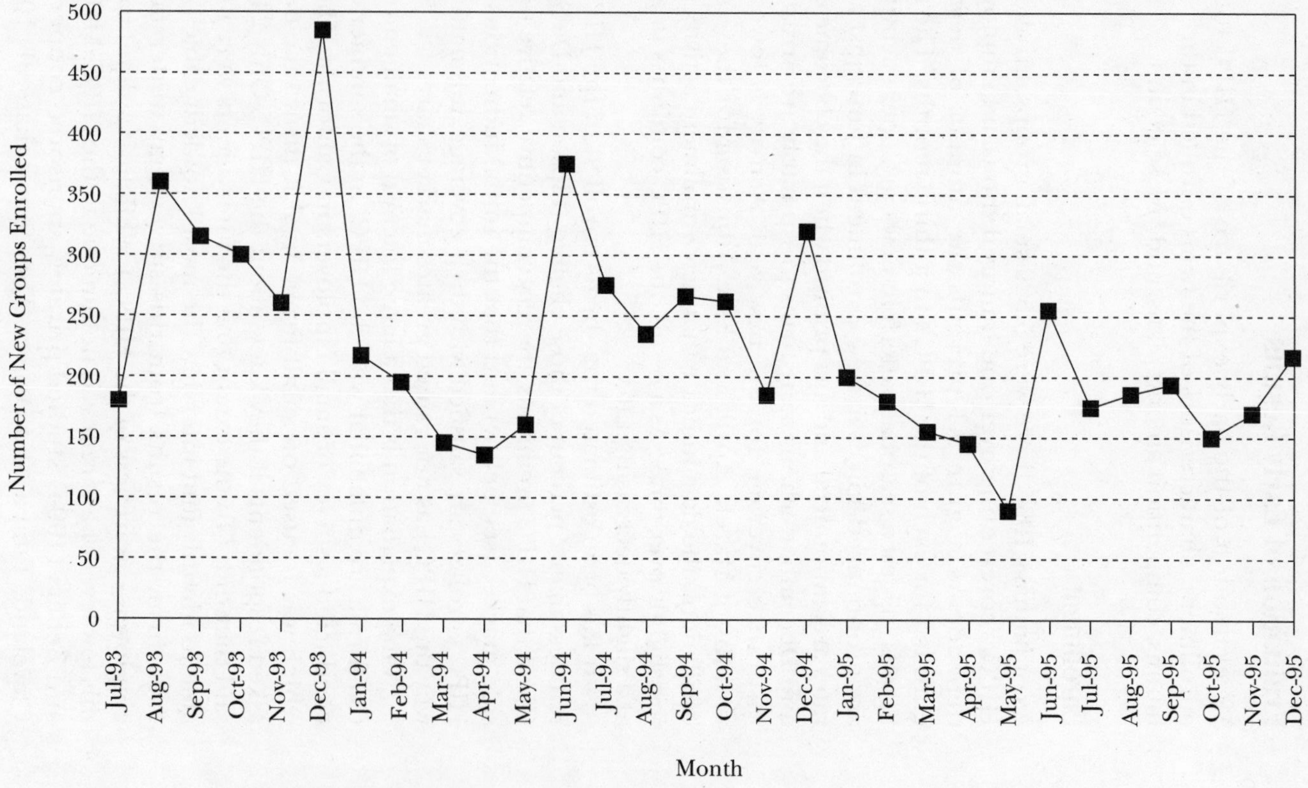

of Cleveland employers, 44 percent of Tampa employers, and 32 percent of Denver employers were aware of the cooperative in their city. Morrissey and Jensen (1996) surveyed employers nationally about their knowledge of health insurance reform legislation in their states. They found that only 9 percent of employers in states with reforms were aware of those reforms.

Awareness of the HIPC varies across firms in predictable ways. Firms that offer health insurance to their employees were more likely than those not offering insurance to be familiar with the HIPC (26 versus 17 percent). As a gauge of their overall level of knowledge about health benefit issues, survey respondents were asked how many hours they spent in the typical week on employee benefits. Only 13 percent of respondents reporting zero hours were familiar with the HIPC, compared to 19 percent who reported one hour per week and 35 percent who reported spending two or more hours per week on benefit-related issues. There were no clear patterns with respect to firm size.

The survey went on to ask employers offering non-HIPC insurance why they had chosen not to enroll in the HIPC. Respondents were read seven possible reasons and were asked to rate the importance of each reason on a scale of 1 (not at all important) to 5 (extremely important). Table 9.1 gives the percentage of respondents who said each reason was the most important relative to the others (because of ties, these figures do not add up to 100 percent) and the percentage giving a rating of 4 or 5.

Not surprisingly, the most important reason given for not enrolling was that the firm was satisfied with its existing coverage. For employers who are satisfied with their current insurance, the cost of switching—including the inconvenience to both employer and employees—will likely outweigh whatever benefits the HIPC has to offer. This will be particularly true when premiums are flat or falling, as has been common in California in the years since the HIPC was established. Switching costs are particularly high for firms whose current insurance carrier is not available in the HIPC. As will be shown below, this is likely to be the case for many firms purchasing PPO coverage. Also, for firms that already offer their employees a choice of plans, the benefit of switching to the HIPC is relatively low.

A relatively small proportion of employers said that their main reason for not enrolling in the HIPC was that HIPC premiums

Table 9.1. Employers' Reasons for Not Enrolling in the HIPC.

Reason	Percentage for whom this is most important reason	Percentage for whom this is very important
Satisfied with current coverage	62.2	61.4
Firm already offers employees a choice of plans	47.2	37.0
HIPC is less convenient for managers	33.9	28.4
Current insurer not available within HIPC	33.1	23.6
Premiums are lower outside HIPC	29.9	20.5
Agent or broker advised against joining HIPC	28.3	22.8
Not enough information	25.2	17.3

Survey respondents were read seven potential reasons for their not enrolling in the HIPC and were asked to rate the importance of each on a scale of 1 (not at all important) to 5 (very important). The first column gives the percentage of respondents for whom each reason was at least as important as any of the others. Since respondents may have given the same rating for more than one reason, these figures do not sum to 100 percent. The second column gives the percentage who rated each reason as a 4 or 5.

Source: 1995 California Small Employer Survey, Graduate School of Management, University of California, Irvine.

were too high compared to the outside market. The survey responses provided little evidence that insurance agents were strongly advising their clients against enrolling in the HIPC.

Characteristics of Enrolled Firms

The descriptive data in Table 9.2 on firms enrolled in the HIPC give a fuller picture of how the HIPC fits into California's small-group insurance market and provide some indication of the challenges facing the HIPC in terms of increasing enrollment over time. The first thing to note is that most firms enrolled in the HIPC are quite small. Seventy-one percent have ten or fewer employees, and 94 percent have fewer than twenty-five. There are very few firms near the upper limit on group size. (This is not to

Table 9.2. Characteristics of Firms Enrolled in the HIPC as of November 1995.

	Percentage of Total Groups	Percentage Previously Uninsured	Percentage Using a Broker/Agent
By Group Size			
3 to 10 employees	71	46	60
11 to 25 employees	23	16	74
26 to 50 employees	6	5	81
All Groups	100	20	67

Source: Author's calculations based on unpublished data provided by the HIPC.

say that the size distribution of firms enrolled in the HIPC is unrepresentative of all eligible firms. The firm size distribution is highly skewed—there are many more firms with three to ten full-time employees than, say, twenty-five to fifty.)

The firms eligible for the HIPC make up a very diverse group in terms of their health insurance offerings. While discussions of the small-group market often give the impression that very few small firms offer insurance at all, the reality is that a majority of firms with twenty-five to fifty employees offer insurance to their employees (Health Insurance Association of America, 1991; Morrissey, Jensen, and Morlock, 1994). Ninety-five percent of the firms in this size category that joined the HIPC had previously offered insurance. The California small-group market has been sufficiently competitive in recent years that the premiums paid by these firms compare favorably to the health care costs of much larger firms. To the extent that the other AB1672 reforms will drive disreputable insurers and agents from the market, they will make the general small-group market even more hospitable to small firms. In other words, while the HIPC may offer attractive coverage to firms with twenty-five to fifty employees, the outside options are also fairly attractive. It remains to be seen whether the increases in the fees paid to agents for larger eligible groups will increase their enrollment.

Roughly half of the firms with three to nine employees who have enrolled in the HIPC began offering insurance for the first time when they did so. Since firms offering insurance for the first time do not face the type of switching costs that already-insured firms do, the HIPC is likely to look relatively more favorable compared to outside options. However, growth in the enrollment of firms with ten or fewer employees is likely to be limited by the demand-side factors mentioned above. While the HIPC, the other AB1672 reforms, and the general increase in price competition in the California small-group market may have lowered premiums and other barriers to insurance coverage, it is unlikely that the changes have been great enough to induce a large fraction of the smallest firms to begin offering insurance for the first time.

Premiums and Competition Among Plans

Table 9.3 lists the number and type of plans available to enrollees in the HIPC's first three years. In the first year, twenty plans were offered (seventeen HMOs and three PPOs). While not all HMOs were available statewide, in each of the six rating regions at least seven HMOs were available. The HMOs include a mix of large, well-established plans—including the Northern and Southern California Kaiser-Permanente plans, the two largest HMOs in the United States—and some very small plans with limited geographic coverage.

In the second year (beginning July 1994) three new HMOs entered, and several existing plans expanded their geographic coverage. One of the new entrants was PacifiCare, the fourth largest HMO in California (fifth largest in the United States). Prior to 1993 PacifiCare had a fairly limited presence in the small-group market. After the passage of AB1672, PacifiCare publicly announced its interest in expanding its small-group business, though initially it chose to stay out of the HIPC. The reason given for staying out was that doing so would allow the company more flexibility, particularly in setting premiums. PacifiCare's decision to enter the HIPC one year later may reflect an assessment that being required to charge the same rates within and outside the HIPC was not as much of a handicap as the company initially feared. In other

Table 9.3. The Number and Type of Health Plans Available Through the HIPC, 1993–94 to 1995–96.

	1993–94	1994–95	1995–96
HMO Plans			
Total number available	17	20	26
Most available in one region	11	14	17
Fewest available in one region	7	12	11
PPO Plans			
Total number available	3	3	2
Most available in one region	3	3	2
Fewest available in one region	3	3	1

Source: Author's calculations based on unpublished data provided by the HIPC.

words, PacifiCare may have concluded that business gained within the HIPC would not come at the cost of reduced business in the outside market.

There were greater changes in plan offerings in July 1995, the start of the HIPC's third year. Two carriers stopped offering PPO coverage, while Blue Shield of California began offering PPO coverage for the first time, though not in all regions. Since Blue Shield's premiums are substantially higher than the other PPO (which in turn charges more than most of the HMOs), it has captured virtually no market share in its first six months. Two HMOs dropped out of the HIPC, though four new ones entered. Some of the new entrants are smaller plans with niche marketing strategies. For example, one of the new plans is the Chinese Community Health Plan, which operates in San Francisco and Los Angeles and is dedicated to meeting the health care needs of the Asian community.

The entry of new carriers and the geographic expansion of existing ones reflects positively on how insurers view the HIPC. Although it is too early to tell which plans will be most successful, the size diversity of HMOs currently participating indicates that plans of all sizes see market opportunities in the HIPC. At the same time, however, the evidence also suggests that not all types of carriers view the HIPC as an attractive vehicle for selling insurance in the small-group market. The pattern of entry and exit, combined with the premium trends and enrollment figures discussed below, has resulted in an internal market dominated by HMOs.

In 1993 program administrators estimated that the initial HIPC premiums were, on average, between 10 and 15 percent below standard rates for comparable coverage outside the HIPC (Dowell and Oliver, 1994a; Lipson and De Sa, 1995). While precise comparisons are difficult, informal evidence suggests that since then HIPC premiums have remained competitive and may even have fallen relative to the general market.

Between 1993 and 1994, health insurance costs for groups of all sizes were generally flat or falling. An annual survey by the consulting firm Foster Higgins showed that per-employee health expenditures fell by 1.1 percent nationwide, largely due to a shift in enrollment toward less expensive plans (Service, 1995). In July 1994 CalPERS announced that its average premiums for the coming contract year were 1.1 percent below those of the prior year. Other large employers, such as Stanford University, the University of California, members of the Pacific Business Group on Health (PBGH), and the federal government saw their premiums fall by even greater percentages (Enthoven and Singer, 1996). Taking a straight average across all plans, HIPC premiums fell by 6.3 percent; weighting by plan enrollments, premiums declined by 3.2 percent.

Between 1994 and 1995, employer health care costs nationwide remained essentially flat. According to the Foster Higgins Survey, the cost of indemnity and point-of-service plans increased in nominal dollars by between 3 and 4 percent, while the mean cost of HMO coverage fell by a comparable amount (Findlay and Meyeroff, 1996). Weighted average premiums for CalPERS, Stanford, PBGH, and HMOs in the Federal Employee Health Benefit Program fell for the second year in a row, while there was a slight increase for the University of California (Enthoven and Singer, 1996). Average HIPC premiums fell by just under 3 percent over this period.

While these figures on the changes in average premiums are useful for establishing that the HIPC has remained competitive relative to the general market, a more disaggregated examination is required to better understand the market dynamics unfolding *within* the HIPC. Since premiums for a particular plan vary by age, region, and coverage type, there are actually dozens of premiums for each carrier. In order to make meaningful comparisons across plan categories and over time, I constructed for each plan a composite (weighted average) premium based on the "employee-only" rates for each of the seven age categories. The age-specific premiums are weighted by the percentage of all HIPC enrollees in each age category. Separate composite premiums are calculated for each plan in each region. In other words, for a carrier offering standard and preferred HMO coverage in each of the six regions, twelve composite premiums are calculated. Table 9.4 presents descriptive statistics on these composite premiums, tabulated by year and coverage type. The means are not weighted by enrollment.

The figures in Table 9.4 show that the mean HMO premium fell by an average of 11 percent between 1993–94 and 1994–95 and by an additional 5 percent in the following period. The median and minimum HMO premiums also fell over these three years. The ratio of preferred HMO to standard HMO premiums remained fairly constant over this period.

Premiums for the PPOs show a different pattern. As with the HMOs, average PPO premiums fell between 1993–94 and 1994–95, though by a smaller percentage (roughly 4 percent). Because of this difference in the rate of decline, the mean composite premium for standard PPO coverage went from being $4 higher than the mean for the standard HMOs to being $13 higher. In some age categories the mean PPO premium was actually lower than the mean HMO premium in the first year, but for all age groups the mean PPO premium was higher in the second year.

As noted, two PPOs exited the HIPC before the start of the 1995–96 rating period. The PPO that remained raised its rates, and the one that entered came in with rates far exceeding all other plans. As a result of these developments, the mean composite premium for standard PPO coverage went from $130 in 1994–95 to $152 in 1995–96, an increase of 16 percent. This further widened the gap between HMO and PPO rates. Whereas in 1993–94 premiums for the standard PPOs were comparable to the standard HMOs, by 1995–96 the mean composite PPO premiums

Table 9.4. Trends in "Employee-Only" Premiums by Plan Type, 1993–94 to 1995–96.

	1993–94	1994–95	1995–96
Standard HMO			
mean	131.90	117.33	110.83
median	133.73	115.39	111.83
standard deviation	12.77	10.72	9.76
range	102–162	95–144	92–153
number of plans	64	78	88
Preferred HMO			
mean	145.48	130.17	123.67
median	145.54	129.24	124.00
standard deviation	13.65	12.35	9.88
range	118–176	110–163	107–166
number of plans	64	79	88
Standard PPO			
mean	136.31	130.37	151.75
median	137.12	124.41	167.38
standard deviation	23.55	21.31	24.24
range	97–195	102–195	112–184
number of plans	18	18	10
Preferred PPO			
mean	150.01	143.31	169.36
median	154.72	141.18	175.48
standard deviation	26.31	22.71	29.09
range	106–208	111–204	123–202
number of plans	18	18	10

The figures represent composite premiums calculated as a weighted average of seven age-group premiums, where the weights are the percentage of total HIPC enrollment in each age group. Separate composite premiums are calculated by carrier, coverage type (standard or preferred), and region.

Source: Author's calculations based on unpublished data provided by the HIPC.

were *37 percent higher.* A similar trend is evident for preferred PPO coverage.

A ranking of plans by their monthly premiums provides further evidence on the change in market structure within the HIPC. In 1993–94, the lowest-cost PPO was among the three lowest-cost plans in four of the six regions. In the other two regions, the lowest-cost PPO ranked twelfth and thirteenth. In 1995–96, in four of the six regions there were between twenty-five and thirty-five HMO options (counting standard and preferred coverage from a single carrier as separate plans) with lower premiums than the lowest-cost PPO.

Price Competition Among Plans: A Case History

Several aspects of the HIPC's design should cause the internal market to be quite price-competitive. The standardization of benefits across plans should reduce nonprice competition while emphasizing differences in premiums across plans. The fact that employers' premium obligations are defined in terms of the premium for the lowest-cost plan means that most individual enrollees bear the incremental cost of choosing a more expensive plan. In addition, the fact that the program is new should reduce the effects of the persistence some researchers claim is characteristic of people's health plan choices (Neipp and Zeckhauser, 1985).

A brief case history of trends in plan rates and market share provides a sense of the highly competitive nature of the HIPC's internal markets. For the sake of clarity, I will focus primarily on one HIPC region, that encompassing the San Francisco Bay Area. Below I present a snapshot of market shares and other indicators of competitiveness for all six regions.

In the HIPC's first year, carriers had to set premiums with virtually no information on the characteristics of enrollees or the rates of their competitors. That year, Aetna's HMO premiums were the lowest in each of the five regions where it offered coverage. In the San Francisco Bay Area, Aetna's composite single premium for preferred HMO coverage was $6 lower than the nearest competitor, Qual Med ($124 versus $130) and $22 lower than Kaiser North, the plan that historically has had the greatest market share in that area. The difference between Aetna's rates and those of its nearest competitors was even greater in other regions. As a result, by the end of the first contract year roughly 30 percent of HIPC enrollees statewide were in Aetna HMOs. In terms of market share, the next-closest HMO was Kaiser North, with roughly 11 percent. (This figure is misleading, however, because Kaiser North does not compete in southern California. In 1993 the combined enrollment of Kaiser North and Kaiser South—which are separate plans—was between 15 and 18 percent of total HIPC enrollment.)

Between the first and second contract years, while Aetna kept its HMO rates for the Bay Area constant, Kaiser North and other plans reduced their rates dramatically. The Kaiser North composite premium for that region fell by $27. As a result, during the 1994–95 contract year, Kaiser North's composite premium was $5 lower than Aetna's. Two other HMOs competing in the Bay Area, PacifiCare and MetLife, also had composite premiums that were as low or lower than Aetna's. As a result of this price competition and similar changes in other regions, Aetna began losing market share to its rivals. In December 1994, Aetna's share of total HIPC enrollment had declined to 22 percent, while Kaiser North's share had increased to 14 percent.

In the third contract year, Aetna's composite premium for preferred HMO coverage in the Bay Area increased by $4 (from $124 to $128), while Kaiser North's composite premium continued to fall (from $119 to $116). Five other preferred HMOs in that market had lower composite premiums than Aetna. By the end of 1995 Aetna's overall market share was roughly half what it had been two years prior. Despite competing in fewer regions, Kaiser North's market share was now higher than Aetna's (18 percent compared to 16 percent).

Differences in Competition and Enrollment Patterns Across Regions

The HIPC's six rating regions are fairly diverse, and so have been their experiences in terms of plan competition. In particular, because of California's size and diversity, different market dynamics across regions provide useful evidence concerning the argument that competition among managed health care plans may succeed in controlling costs in urban areas but not in sparsely populated rural areas (Kronick and others, 1993).

While the majority of California's population lives in urban or suburban areas, the state has vast areas that are quite sparsely populated. The HIPC's Region 1 spans roughly half the length of the state and incorporates thirty rural counties. Health care and labor market conditions are quite different in those counties than in the two most urban regions, Region 3, which consists of the San Francisco Bay Area, and Region 5, which consists of Los Angeles County. Region 2 is mixed in the sense that it includes two fairly large cities—Fresno and Sacramento—as well as several fairly rural counties in central California. Region 4 includes counties directly north and south of Los Angeles—Santa Barbara, Ventura, and Orange. Region 6 includes San Diego, San Bernardino, and Riverside.

Table 9.5 presents information on enrollment patterns within each of the six regions as of March 1996. The top panel gives the enrollment distribution by type of plan. Differences across the regions in the percentage choosing HMOs versus PPOs are relatively small. Given the differences in PPO and HMO premiums noted above, it is not surprising that most HIPC enrollees are in HMOs. The combined HMO market share ranges from a low of 87 percent (Region 1) to a high of 97 percent (Region 2). Overall, 91 percent of HIPC enrollees are in HMOs. It is interesting to note that individuals choosing HMO coverage show a slight preference for preferred coverage over standard coverage. As shown in Table 9.4, preferred coverage costs roughly $13 more per month than standard coverage. The main difference between the two benefit designs is a $10 difference in the copayment required for an office visit and for prescriptions. Standard plans also require a $100 charge per inpatient admission, whereas preferred plans do not.

The figures in the middle and bottom panels of Table 9.5 are presented to give a sense of the importance of price as a determinant of market share in each of the six regions. The middle panel gives the market share for the plan with the lowest composite premium and the combined market share of all plans with composite premiums that are within $10 and $20 of the lowest one. The bottom panel compares the composite premium for the plan with the greatest market share in each region with the lowest composite premium in the market. Since the market leader in each region is a

Table 9.5. Plan Market Shares and Premium Differences by HIPC Region, March 1996.

	Region					
	1	2	3	4	5	6
By Type of Plan						
HMOs	87 percent	97 percent	91 percent	91 percent	92 percent	95 percent
Standard HMOs	34 percent	39 percent	39 percent	45 percent	42 percent	44 percent
Preferred HMOs	53 percent	58 percent	59 percent	46 percent	50 percent	51 percent
PPOs	13 percent	3 percent	3 percent	9 percent	8 percent	5 percent
Standard PPOs	5 percent	1 percent	1 percent	2 percent	2 percent	1 percent
Preferred PPOs	8 percent	2 percent	2 percent	7 percent	6 percent	4 percent
By Relative Premium						
lowest-cost plan	5 percent	10 percent	12 percent	6 percent	12 percent	9 percent
plans within $10 of lowest	7 percent	18 percent	27 percent	34 percent	28 percent	9 percent
plans within $20 of lowest	20 percent	51 percent	72 percent	65 percent	60 percent	52 percent
Difference Between Composite Premium of Plan with Greatest Market Share and:						
lowest-cost plan (all plans)	$55	$13	$13	$10	$17	$26
lowest-cost plan (same type)	$42	$0	$4	$10	$3	$10

Region 1 consists of thirty rural counties in northern and central California. Region 2 consists of fourteen counties in northern and central California. The counties are mostly rural, though the cities of Sacramento, Santa Cruz, and San Luis Obispo are also in this region. Region 3 consists of the San Francisco Bay Area (Alameda, Contra Costa, Marin, San Francisco, San Mateo, and Santa Clara Counties). Region 4 consists of Orange, Santa Barbara, and Ventura Counties. Region 5 consists of Los Angeles County. Region 6 consists of Riverside, San Bernardino, and San Diego Counties.

Source: Author's calculations based on unpublished data provided by the HIPC.

preferred HMO, the price difference with the lowest-cost preferred HMO is also presented.

The market share figures in the middle panel of Table 9.5 suggest that price competition is much less vigorous in Region 1 than in the more densely populated areas. In Regions 2 through 6, a majority of enrollees are in plans with monthly premiums falling within $20 of the lowest-cost plan. In the San Francisco Bay Area and Los Angeles, the figures are 72 percent and 60 percent, respectively. In contrast, only 20 percent of enrollees in Region 1 are in plans with such low premiums (as compared to the lowest-cost plan). The figures in the bottom panel create a similar impression. In Region 1, the plan with the greatest market share costs $55 per month more than the lowest-cost plan.

One explanation for this pattern is that because plans offering coverage within a region need not be available in all the areas within the region, the total number of plans offered in a region (as reported in Table 9.3) may overstate the number of plans actively competing in a particular county or area of a county. This is the case for Region 1. While in 1995–96 a total of thirteen plans were available in the region overall, in several counties only one or two HIPC plans are available. In some counties no HIPC plan is available at all. Thus, plans that do operate in Region 1 enjoy more market power than plans in more compact urban areas.

A breakdown of premium changes by region also suggests a greater degree of price competition in the more urban markets. While average premiums fell in all regions between 1993–94 and 1994–95, the decline was greatest in Regions 3 and 5 (San Francisco and Los Angeles) and lowest in Region 1. Between 1994–95 and 1995–96, composite premiums averaged across all available plans fell everywhere but in Region 1. (There, constant HMO premiums combined with rising PPO rates meant that the mean composite premium rose by 1.5 percent.)

Risk Selection

In a program like the HIPC, purchase decisions are made at two levels, and biased risk selection is a potential problem at both. The first decision is the employer's decision to participate in the cooperative. If underwriting rules are significantly more restrictive inside the cooperative than outside, it may attract firms that are more costly to insure. The basic idea is that insurers operating outside the pool will offer lower-than-pool rates to low-risk groups and higher-than-pool rates to high-risk groups. The former will purchase insurance directly from the outside carriers, while the latter will find they get the best deal inside the cooperative. Over time, sorting of this nature will cause premiums inside and outside the cooperative to diverge. It is possible that the cooperative will become in effect a high-risk pool. If the remaining enrollees cannot afford the premiums that reflect their higher-risk status, either the state will be left to subsidize the program, or it will be driven completely out of business.

The HIPC was well designed to avoid this worst-case scenario. The HIPC's most important protection against adverse risk selection is that it was established within the context of greater market reforms. The limits on preexisting-condition exclusions and rules on guaranteed issue and renewability are the same within the HIPC and the general small-group market. While premiums are allowed to vary more outside the HIPC than within it, the variation is constrained by the rate bands introduced as part of AB1672. Thus, the rates available to low-risk groups are not so low that these groups have an obvious incentive to shun the HIPC. Indeed, because of the HIPC's low administrative costs and success in bargaining with plans, its community-rated premiums are likely to compare favorably to the general market for even low-risk groups. Since the rate bands are scheduled to become even tighter over time, the ability of non-HIPC carriers to cream-skim will be reduced further. The prohibition on HIPC carriers' underpricing their HIPC plans in the outside market reduces the potential for biased selection.

In the HIPC's first three years there has been no evidence that its enrollees are, on average, more costly to insure than employees of small firms purchasing group insurance in the general market. The average age of HIPC enrollees is actually lower than the program's actuaries had expected (Lipson and De Sa, 1995). The entry of new carriers in the second and third year of operation and the decline in premiums both suggest that carriers do not view the HIPC on balance as being plagued by adverse selection.

The second purchase decision, and the second point at which risk selection becomes a potential issue, is the individual's choice of plan. As Luft (1995) points out, even if biased risk selection is not a problem at the group level, it may be a problem when individuals within a group are allowed to select among plans. Several strategies have been suggested for minimizing the potential for biased risk selection within a setting like the HIPC. These include guaranteed issue and renewability, third-party management of enrollment, a standardized benefit package, a modified community rating system, oversight of health plan marketing materials and strategies, and the publication of information on consumer satisfaction and plan quality (Kronick, Zhou, and Dreyfus, 1995). In other words, experts argue that to minimize biased risk selection, large multiple-option insurance programs should look like the HIPC. (This is not to say that advocates of managed competition believe these design elements will completely eliminate the problem of biased risk selection. These are necessary, but not sufficient, conditions.)

Despite these checks, however, there is some evidence of biased selection across plans within the HIPC. In particular, it appears that HIPC enrollees with higher expected medical expenditures have disproportionately chosen PPO coverage. The data on premiums and plan exit provide indirect evidence of such sorting. The large increase in the ratio of PPO to HMO premiums over the first three years resembles a classic adverse selection premium spiral. The exit of two of the three PPOs, along with the fact that the PPO that entered the market in 1995 came in with extremely high rates, suggests that PPOs are being adversely selected against. It is particularly interesting to note that Aetna, one of the carriers withdrawing its PPO, continues to offer an HMO in the HIPC. This suggests that Aetna views the HMO component of the HIPC favorably as compared to the general market but finds the PPO component to be unprofitable, presumably because of risk-selection issues.

The potential for risk-selection problems was anticipated by the HIPC's developers. Not only was the program designed to minimize the problem, the original legislation contained a provision that would allow the use of a prospective risk-adjustment process to compensate plans that receive a disproportionate share of high-cost individuals. In 1994 the MRMIB received a grant from the Robert Wood Johnson Foundation to study the issue of risk selection and to develop an appropriate risk-adjustment mechanism.[2] Working with Coopers and Lybrand, they conducted a risk assessment of all carriers participating in the HIPC. For each carrier they calculated a "risk assessment value" (RAV) based on three cost factors that are not incorporated into the HIPC rating scheme: the gender mix of the carrier's enrollees, the family size mix, and the diagnosis mix. The diagnoses were ones that are relatively costly, reasonably predictable, and subject to a limited degree of discretion.

Claims data from each HIPC health plan were used to weight the values for gender, family size, and diagnosis to construct overall RAVs. The RAV for the entire pool is defined to equal 1, so plans that receive a higher-than-average proportion of "high-risk" enrollees have an RAV greater than 1. The results of this exercise provide no evidence of biased selection on the basis of gender or family size. In contrast, the diagnosis mix results confirm that the PPOs covered a disproportionate number of people with the identified high-cost diagnoses. Just over 1 percent of the individuals choosing PPO coverage had one of the marker diagnoses, compared to 0.2 percent to 0.3 percent of HIPC HMO enrollees. (To be counted as having a marker diagnosis, an enrollee must have been hospitalized for the diagnosis some time during a twelve-month reporting period. Thus these figures understate the proportion of enrollees with one of the marker conditions.)

Beginning in the 1996–97 contract year, the results from this risk assessment will be used to redistribute funds among carriers to compensate for an uneven risk distribution. The procedure is as follows. Carriers are ranked according to their risk mix. If any plan is either 5 percent above or below the mean risk level, funds will be transferred among plans. In this case, a calculation is made to determine the funds needed to move high-end outliers to the 1.05 threshold and low-end outliers to the .95 threshold. The sum of these two amounts is considered the risk transfer pool. If the amount from the low-end outliers is not enough to fully compensate the high-end outliers, funds are taken from the carriers with the next-lowest risk values. The results of this risk-adjustment process were made available to carriers during the period when

HIPC rates were negotiated for the upcoming (1996–97) rating year so that carriers could factor risk-adjustment transfer payments into their premium-setting decisions.

The risk assessment based on 1995 data found one PPO with a risk value above the 1.05 threshold and two HMOs below the .95 threshold. Because the transfer amount required to compensate the high-end outliers was more than the amount required to bring the low-end outliers up, five other HMOs were required to pay into the transfer pool. Seventeen plans (one PPO and sixteen HMOs) were unaffected by the risk-adjustment process. The amount ultimately transferred represented slightly more than 1 percent of total premiums for the entire program.

Conclusion

In recent years there has been a flurry of health care reform activity at the state level. In addition to other initiatives, several states have enacted legislation either establishing or allowing for publicly sponsored small-group health insurance purchasing cooperatives. Since California was among the first states to do so, the early experience of its program has important implications for similar voluntary cooperatives being formed or considered elsewhere.

In its first two and a half years, the HIPC has proven to be a viable component of a competitive small-group insurance market. The initial evidence suggests that employers, individual employees, and participating insurance carriers are satisfied with their experience in the HIPC. Since the program was established in July 1993, HIPC premiums have fallen, the number of available plans has expanded, and enrollment has grown at a fairly steady rate.

Despite this growth, however, the HIPC remains a very small part of the small-group health insurance market. Most firms enrolled in the HIPC had already offered insurance prior to joining the HIPC. Further increases in the enrollment of such firms are limited by the fact that the current small-group insurance market in California is currently very price-competitive, and small employers have many attractive alternatives to the HIPC. Another, and perhaps more important, constraining factor is that the HIPC has evolved into a program that is heavily dominated by HMOs.

Thus, for employers who prefer other types of plans, the outside market offers a better range of options.

Beginning in 1996–97, the HIPC will offer several point-of-service plans, which will provide enrollees with greater provider choice than the HMO plans. The rates for these plans will be higher than the rates for most HMO plans but lower than the PPO rates. It remains to be seen whether these new products will attract employers that stayed out of the HIPC because of an aversion to HMOs.

Increased enrollment of firms that do not currently offer insurance is likely to be limited as well. An important motivation for both the establishment of the HIPC and the broader small-group reforms enacted as part of AB1672 was a desire to reduce the number of uninsured persons by making health insurance more affordable and accessible to small employers. Most small firms that do not offer insurance cannot afford coverage at going rates. Other employers do not offer insurance because either their employees have insurance coverage from other sources, they are afraid to commit to a benefit that could increase greatly in cost, or they simply do not feel it is necessary to offer health benefits. While the reforms and the increase in market competition have lowered premiums and reduced other nonprice barriers, the changes have been small. California's experience, and that of other states instituting similar legislation, indicates that as long as the purchase of insurance is voluntary and nothing is done to subsidize individuals who cannot afford it, small-group insurance reform will do little to reduce the problem of the uninsured.

The HIPC's design resembles the models that advocates of managed care competition have suggested for years. The early results from the HIPC are consistent with many of the predictions made by these advocates and with the experience of large employers that have instituted similar purchasing arrangements. The evidence suggests that when choices are structured appropriately, individuals will make cost-conscious decisions, and insurers will have an incentive to compete on the basis of price. The HIPC's results, however, suggest two important caveats. First, differences across the HIPC's six rating regions are consistent with the argument that competition among managed care plans works best in densely populated areas and less well in sparsely populated regions. In Los Angeles and the San Francisco Bay Area, where HIPC enrollees have many plans to choose from, price appears to be an important determinant of plan market share, and premiums have declined substantially in the HIPC's first three years as carriers have fought for market share. In contrast, while the HIPC is also available in California's most rural counties, the choices there are substantially more limited, and price appears to matter less as a determinant of plan market share.

The second caveat is that with freedom of choice comes the possibility of biased risk selection. An important reason that benefits are standardized across plans is to reduce the possibility that some plans will be more attractive to high-risk individuals. While this approach makes all plans in a broad category (for example, HMOs or PPOs) look alike, important differences across categories remain. The early evidence from the HIPC suggests that individuals with higher expected medical expenses prefer the freedom of provider choice offered by PPOs. The result has been that two PPOs have exited the program, and those remaining have raised premiums substantially. This suggests that without some type of risk adjustment, plans offering broader provider choice will have difficulty competing in a managed competition environment.

HIPC administrators have responded to this problem by designing a risk-adjustment mechanism that will compensate plans receiving a disproportionate share of high-cost individuals. This mechanism will go into effect during the 1996–97 contract year. Risk adjustment in a multiple-option insurance program is a topic on which much has been written but little has been done. Thus, of all aspects of the HIPC, the outcome of this process may have the most important and far-reaching policy implications.

Notes

1. I estimated a simple regression of new enrollment on a time trend (that is, the number of months the HIPC has been in existence) plus dummy variables for January-February, March-April-May, June, and December. The estimated coefficient on the time trend was -5.10 (absolute t-statistic = 5.44). This implies that new enrollments are declining by sixty-one groups per year.

2. This discussion of risk-assessment and adjustment methodologies is drawn largely from two reports compiled by HIPC staff (Health Insurance Plan of California, 1995a, 1995b). The HIPC's approach

to risk assessment and adjustment is also described in a recent article by Shewry, Hunt, Ramey, and Bertko (1996).

References

Cantor, J., Long, S. H., and Marquis, M. S. "Private Employment-Based Health Insurance in Ten States." *Health Affairs,* 1995, *14*(2), 199–211.

Chernew, M., Frick, K., and McLaughlin, C. G. *The Effectiveness of Health Insurance Subsidies.* Ann Arbor: University of Michigan, School of Public Health, 1995.

Dowell, E., and Oliver, T. "Small Employer Health Alliance in California." *Health Affairs,* 1994a, *13*(1), 350–351.

Dowell, E., and Oliver, T. "Interest Groups and the Political Struggle over Expanding Health Insurance in California." *Health Affairs,* 1994b, *13*(2), 123–141.

Employee Benefit Research Institute. *Sources of Health Insurance and Characteristics of the Uninsured: Analysis of the March 1993 Current Population Survey.* EBRI Issue Brief no. 145. Washington, D.C.: Employee Benefit Research Institute, 1994.

Enthoven, A. C. "The History and Principles of Managed Competition." *Health Affairs,* 1993, *12*(Suppl.), 24–48.

Enthoven, A. C., and Singer, S. J. "Managed Competition and California's Health Care Economy." *Health Affairs,* 1996, *15*(1), 39–57.

Findlay, S., and Meyeroff, W. J. "Health Costs: Why Employers Won Another Round." *Business and Health,* March 1996, pp. 49–51.

General Accounting Office. *Access to Health Insurance: Public and Private Employers' Experience with Purchasing Cooperatives.* GAO/HEHS-94–142. Washington, D.C.: General Accounting Office, 1994.

General Accounting Office. *Health Insurance Regulation: Variation in Recent State Small Employer Health Insurance Reforms.* Washington, D.C.: General Accounting Office, 1995.

Haggerty, A. G. "California's HIPC Marketing Support Pleases Agents." *National Underwriter,* Oct. 24, 1994, pp. 11, 22.

Health Insurance Association of America. *Critical Distinctions: How Firms That Offer Health Benefits Differ from Those That Do Not.* Washington, D.C.: Health Insurance Association of America, 1991.

Health Insurance Plan of California. *Methods for Calculating and Applying Risk Assessment and Risk Adjustment Measures, Results of Simulation #2.* Sacramento: Health Insurance Plan of California, 1995a.

Health Insurance Plan of California. *Risk Assessment and Risk Adjustment Calculations, Results for 1996/97 Contract Year.* Sacramento: Health Insurance Plan of California, 1995b.

Helms, W. D., Gauthier, A., and Campion, D. "Mending the Flaws in the Small Group Market." *Health Affairs*, 1992, *11*(2), 7–27.

Herrman, J. "Health Insurance Purchasing Alliances in Florida and California." *Health Systems Review*, 1994, *27*(5), 22–25.

Hoare, G., Mayers, M., and Madden, C. "Lessons from Implementation of Washington's Basic Health Plan." *Health Affairs*, 1992, *11*(2), 212–218.

Hogan, A. J., and Woodbury, S. A. "Small Employer Health Insurance Pools." In J. H. Goddeeris and A. J. Hogan (eds.), *Improving Access to Health Care: What Can the States Do?* Kalamazoo, Mich.: W. E. Upjohn Institute for Employment Research, 1992.

"Insurers Divided on Joining HIPC." *Orange County Business Journal*, May 24, 1993, p. 3.

Kronick, R., Zhou, Z., and Dreyfus, T. "Making Risk Adjustment Work for Everyone." *Inquiry*, 1995, *32*(1), 41–55.

Kronick, R., and others. "The Marketplace in Health Care Reform—The Demographic Limitations of Managed Competition." *New England Journal of Medicine*, 1993, *328*(2), 148–152.

Leibowitz, A., and Chernew, M. "The Firm's Demand for Health Insurance." In U.S. Department of Labor, *Health Benefits and the Workplace*. Washington, D.C.: U.S. Department of Labor, Pension and Welfare Benefits Administration, 1992.

Leibowitz, A., Damberg, C., and Eyre, K. "Multiple Employer Welfare Arrangements." In U.S. Department of Labor, *Health Benefits and the Workplace*. Washington, D.C.: U.S. Department of Labor, Pension and Welfare Benefits Administration, 1992.

Lipson, A., and De Sa, J. *The Health Insurance Plan of California: First Year Results of a Purchasing Cooperative*. Washington, D.C.: Alpha Center, 1995.

Luft, H. "Potential Methods to Reduce Risk Selection and Its Effects." *Inquiry*, 1995, *32*(1), 23–32.

McLaughlin, C. G., and Zellers, W. *Small Business and Health Care Reform: Understanding the Barriers to Employee Coverage and Implications for Workable Solutions*. Ann Arbor: University of Michigan, School of Public Health, 1994.

Monheit, A. C., and Vistness, J. P. "Implicit Pooling of Workers from Large and Small Firms." *Health Affairs*, 1994, *13*(1), 301–313.

Morrissey, M., and Jensen, G. "State Small Group Insurance Reform." Unpublished manuscript, January 1996.

Morrissey, M., Jensen, G., and Morlock, R. "Small Employers and the Health Insurance Market." *Health Affairs*, 1994, *13*(5), 149–161.

Neipp, J., and Zeckhauser, R. "Persistence in Health Plan Choice." In R. M. Scheffler and L. F. Rossiter (eds.), *Advances in Health Economics and Health Services Research.* Vol. 6: *Biased Selection in Health Care Markets.* Greenwich, Conn.: JAI Press, 1985.

Pauly, M. V. "Killing with Kindness: Why Some Forms of Managed Competition Might Needlessly Stifle Competitive Managed Care." In R. B. Helms (ed.), *Health Policy Reform: Competition and Controls.* Washington, D.C.: AEI Press, 1993.

Quinn, M. "California's Health Pool: Limits, but Lower Rates." *New York Times,* June 11, 1994, p. 1.

Ross, N. L. "Health Insurance Purchasing Cooperatives: How Does Your Cooperative Grow?" *Journal of the American Association of CLU & ChFC,* Sept. 1995, pp. 72–81.

Service, M. "Why Health Costs Got Smaller in 1994." *Business and Health,* Mar. 1995, pp. 20–28.

Shewry, S., Hunt, S., Ramey, J., and Bertko, J. "Risk Adjustment: The Missing Piece of Market Competition." *Health Affairs,* 1996, *15*(1), 171–181.

Sullivan, S. "Collective Purchasing and Competition in Health Care." In R. B. Helms (ed.), *Health Policy Reform: Competition and Controls.* Washington, D.C.: AEI Press, 1993.

Thorpe, K. E. "Expanding Employment-Based Health Insurance: Is Small Group Reform the Answer?" *Inquiry,* 1992, *29,* 128–136.

Thorpe, K. E., and others. "Reducing the Number of Uninsured by Subsidizing Employment-Based Health Insurance—Results from a Pilot Study." *Journal of the American Medical Association,* 1992, *267*(7), 945–948.

White House Domestic Policy Council. *The President's Health Security Plan.* New York: Times Books, 1993.

Zellers, W., McLaughlin, C. G., and Frick, K. D. "Small-Business Health Insurance: Only the Healthy Need Apply." *Health Affairs,* 1992, *11*(1), 174–180.

Chapter Ten

Managing the Managed Care Revolution

States and the New Medicaid

Michael S. Sparer

States are key players in nearly every aspect of health care policy. Sometimes state discretion is nearly unfettered. For example, each state operates its own medical education and licensure system, medical malpractice system, and workers' compensation system. States also own and operate health care institutions (usually for the mentally ill or developmentally disabled). In other policy arenas, states share authority with different levels of government. The obvious example is Medicaid, the nation's health insurance program for the poor. Under Medicaid, states determine, within federal guidelines, who in their state receives Medicaid coverage, what services Medicaid will cover, and how much Medicaid providers will be paid.

Despite the state-based nature of the American health care system, there is a bipartisan consensus that states should be delegated even more policymaking authority. The debate over Medicaid again illustrates the point. The Republican majority in Congress has passed legislation that would convert Medicaid from an entitlement program (under which persons meeting basic federal criteria are entitled to coverage) into a block grant (under which states would have total control over who receives coverage, what coverage they receive, and how much providers are paid). The Democrats (including President Clinton) oppose the block grant proposal, but they also offer legislation to increase state control over the program. For example, states must now receive federal permission before requiring Medicaid beneficiaries to enroll in managed care. The president's proposal would permit mandatory managed care without such a waiver. Similarly, the president's proposal would increase state authority over Medicaid eligibility policy (by eliminating mandatory coverage for certain groups), and it would enable states to ratchet down provider reimbursement.

Republican support for increased state authority has been prompted by three factors. First, Republicans generally oppose a large centralized government, and they hope to dismantle (or at least reduce) the federal role in public policy. Second, federal spending under a block grant is capped (and controlled). Third, conservatives (and governors) argue that state officials are better able to develop practical solutions to difficult problems than are their counterparts in Washington.

Democratic support for increased state authority grew following the defeat of the various national health insurance proposals in 1993 and 1994. The goal is to support state programs for the uninsured. The hope is that innovative state programs will become models emulated elsewhere. The strategy is encouraged by the handful of states now implementing major reform initiatives. Tennessee, for example, is implementing a program called TennCare, which offers a choice of publicly subsidized managed care plans to nearly 1.5 million low-income persons, a third of whom were previously uninsured. Minnesota provides state-subsidized insurance to families with incomes below 275 percent of poverty and to individuals with incomes below 100 percent of poverty. Hawaii requires most employers to provide health insurance to their workers.

Given this bipartisan alliance, Congress is likely to increase state authority over health care. Even if Medicaid is not converted to a block grant, for example, state flexibility under the program will undoubtedly increase. Congress also may amend the Employee Retirement Income and Security Act (ERISA), which today prohibits states from regulating or taxing those companies that self-insure (and nearly 70 percent of all employees now work for companies that do). States might even become responsible for certain aspects of the Medicare program (the nation's health insurance program for the elderly and disabled, which today is nationally administered and financed).

The likelihood is, however, that few states will respond to the new era with either comprehensive insurance expansions or innovative cost-containment measures. The obstacles to insurance expansion include the cost of reform (at a time when federal funding is dwindling and antitax ideology remains strong), interest group opposition (including the threat of a business exodus), and the (antigovernment) Republican revolution in many statehouses. Meanwhile, no state has demonstrated the political will to impose a draconian cost-containment regime. Even Minnesota, perhaps the most innovative of all states, is retreating from its plan to impose a statewide global budget. Moreover, it is the federal government, not the states, that is imposing the Medicaid cutbacks that are about to ensue.

States will instead implement a host of incremental initiatives, many of which are already under way. The focus will be on three groups. First, states will enact programs to make insurance more attractive and affordable for small employers. Second, some states will establish insurance subsidy programs for uninsured women and children. Third, states will encourage or require Medicaid clients to enroll in managed care delivery systems.

The most popular of the three strategies is the movement toward managed care in Medicaid. The assumption is that managed care will improve access to care and quality of care while simultaneously reducing costs. The argument is straightforward. Most Medicaid clients do not have access to a primary care physician. These clients instead receive health care in the emergency rooms of large safety net hospitals. Treating sore throats in emergency rooms is inefficient, inappropriate, and unnecessarily expensive. Once in managed care, however, each client will have a primary care provider. Care will be managed. Emergency room visits will decline. Costs will be reduced. Access and quality will be improved.

Despite its promise, the transition to managed care for Medicaid beneficiaries is difficult. They must be educated about how to pick a health plan, and a primary care provider within that plan, and about the terms and conditions of managed care enrollment. Health maintenance organizations (and private physicians) that have traditionally treated a commercially insured middle-class population need to learn to care for a low-income and vulnerable population. Safety net providers (including hospitals and community health centers) need to compete successfully for healthy Medicaid clients, if only to subsidize the uninsured and high-cost Medicaid clients. State officials have to regulate and supervise the emerging system, complying all the while with governing federal law.

In this chapter I consider a dozen questions that Medicaid managed care initiatives must answer. I then consider the relationship between these substantive issues and the more general issues of federalism, especially the question of how much discretion states should have. First, however, I consider more carefully why nearly every state is moving so rapidly toward managed care in Medicaid.

Setting the Stage: Medicaid and Managed Care

The history of Medicaid can be divided into three eras. The first era, which lasted from the program's enactment in 1965 until around 1983, was characterized by significant state discretion and wide interstate variation. The second era, which lasted from around 1984 until the early 1990s, was characterized by increased federal mandates, rising costs, and intergovernmental disputes. The third era, which is now in place, is a time of increased state authority and an emphasis on managed care.

During the first Medicaid era, states had enormous discretion to set eligibility policy, benefit coverage policy, and reimbursement policy. For example, while states were required to provide Medicaid coverage to all beneficiaries of the Aid to Families with Dependent Children (AFDC) cash assistance program, it was the states themselves that determined which persons received AFDC. Similarly, while states had to cover a small handful of medical services, states also had the option of covering another two dozen or so benefits. Finally, while states were generally required to reimburse hospitals for their reasonable costs, states had significant discretion in setting rates for physicians, nursing homes, and other providers.

For all of these reasons, state Medicaid programs evolved quite differently from one another. The interstate variation remains today, even between states that seem similarly situated. In Vermont, a family of three with a monthly income below $900 can receive coverage, while a similar family in Maine can have a monthly income of no more than $458 (Congressional Research Service, 1993). In New Jersey, a hospital receives from Medicaid about 105 percent of the cost of care; a similarly situated hospital in Pennsylvania receives about 79 percent of the cost of care (Prospective Payment Assessment Commission, 1995). In California, Medicaid spends approximately $2,801 per beneficiary; New York spends almost three times as much—$7,286 (General Accounting Office, 1995a). Throughout the nation, similar states have dissimilar programs.

During the 1980s, however, the federal government significantly increased its control over state Medicaid policy. For example, Congress required states to provide coverage to millions of new enrollees, mainly pregnant women and young children. These mandates increased total program enrollment from around 22 million in 1988 to well over 33 million in 1993 (Kaiser Commission on the Future of Medicaid, 1995a). Congress also expanded mandatory benefit coverage, again with a focus on young children: states now must provide youngsters with all needed services, even if such services are not available to adults. Finally, Congress limited state control over reimbursement policy, requiring, for example, that states pay community health centers for all of their reasonable costs.

By the early 1990s, Medicaid costs were rising rapidly, growing from $54.1 billion in 1988 to $131 billion in 1993. State officials blamed the increases on the new federal mandates. This accusation was partly true. The eligibility mandates increased costs, though most of the new enrollees were pregnant women and children, who were low-cost clients. One study suggests that between 1988 and 1992 these populations accounted for nearly 50 percent of new Medicaid enrollees but only 9.3 percent of Medicaid spending growth (Holahan, Rowland, Feder, and Heslam, 1993). Federal reimbursement mandates also increased costs. The best example is the so-called Boren Amendment, a federal law that regulates the rates states pay to hospitals and nursing homes. The benefit mandates also raised costs.

The federal mandates were not, however, the only explanation for the rapid increase in costs. One factor was general health care inflation. Another was a sicker Medicaid population (many have diseases like AIDS or tuberculosis that are costly to treat). Still another factor was the recession of the late 1980s.

The rising costs were due also to illusory financing schemes developed by states to generate billions in additional federal dollars. The following hypothetical example illustrates the point. Assume New York pays hospitals $100 for a particular procedure. The state and federal governments would split the cost of the bill evenly. Assume further that New York decides to pay $110 for the procedure. The state and federal governments will now pay $55 each. But assume finally that the hospitals either pay a special state tax of $5 or simply donate $5 to the state treasury. The hospitals would end up with a $5 rate increase (the $110 payment minus the $5 donation), funded entirely by the federal government.

By 1992 the states were using this technique to collect an estimated $7 billion in provider taxes or provider donations and to generate almost $11 billion in additional federal dollars (Holahan, Rowland, Feder, and Heslam, 1993). Not surprisingly, these initiatives generated significant federal opposition. Congress eventually enacted legislation to curb the practice.

This made it even harder for states to cope with rising Medicaid costs, however. The traditional options—cutting eligibility, benefits, or reimbursements—were unavailable, and the nontraditional option of transferring rising costs to the federal treasury had been limited as well. The only plausible alternative was to promote more cost-effective health care, and the preferred strategy was managed care.

By the mid 1990s, nearly every state was encouraging (or requiring) Medicaid clients to enroll in managed care. Medicaid managed care enrollment grew from 750,000 in 1983 (or 3 percent of all enrollees) to 11.6 million in 1995 (36 percent of all enrollees). At the same time, the Medicaid program has entered a third phase: there are few (if any) new federal mandates, it is much easier for states to get waivers from restrictive federal rules, and national policymakers (from President Clinton to Newt Gingrich) agree that states need more flexibility in implementing Medicaid programs. Indeed, while the president and the Republicans have (as of this writing) yet to agree on a Medicaid reform law, both sides would eliminate the rule that states need federal permission before mandating managed care for Medicaid beneficiaries.

Managing Managed Care: A Dozen Questions

Increased state flexibility in administering Medicaid will lead inevitably to increased interstate variation in managed care initiatives. This is one clear lesson of Medicaid history. The question then is whether managed care variation is good or bad (or somewhere in between). In considering this question, I examine a dozen Medicaid managed care issues on which there already is significant interstate variation. I then consider the implications of this variation on the current debate about managed care and Medicaid.

1. *Which beneficiaries should participate in managed care?* Medicaid is a health insurance program for three distinct low-income populations: families with children, the blind and disabled, and the aged. Medicaid officials generally treat these groups differently when developing Medicaid managed care initiatives. For example, while nearly every state encourages (or requires) families with children to enroll in managed care, very few include the aged or disabled.

The emphasis on families with children is prompted by three factors. First is the (debatable) assumption that managed care benefits this population the most. The argument is that managed care supplies what these beneficiaries do not have: a primary care provider. No longer will mothers need to bring their feverish children to hospital emergency rooms. Instead, the child's primary care provider will treat the fever, prescribe an antibiotic, and manage the care. Costs will be reduced and care improved. In contrast, the benefits of managed care for the aged and disabled are less obvious. The aged, for example, are likely to have an established relationship with a primary care provider (if only because Medicare generally pays better than Medicaid). Similarly, the disabled rely less on primary care providers and more on specialists (who may not belong to a Medicaid managed care plan).

To be sure, it is not always the case that families with children are better suited to managed care. For example, beginning in the late 1980s, most states increased significantly the reimbursement paid to OB-GYNs and primary care providers. Client access to care increased. At the same time, many aged and disabled beneficiaries either have trouble finding the right specialist (and thus go without needed care) or see too many specialists (and thus receive unco-ordinated and unmanaged care). Under either scenario, a managed care gatekeeper could well improve access and quality while reducing cost.

Nonetheless, care outcomes are not the only factor driving Medicaid managed care eligibility decisions. A second variable is administrative simplicity. It is easier to set capitation rates that cover general health care services for pregnant women or children than it is to set rates for the chronically ill. It may also be easier to monitor quality of care and to regulate marketing and enrollment, though these are more controversial propositions.

The emphasis on families with children is due also to politics. There are few groups with less political influence than welfare moms and their children. The aged and disabled, in contrast, are often organized, influential, and unhappy about efforts to mandate managed care. The point is illustrated by the interest group politics in California that persuaded state officials to scuttle a plan to require San Diego County's elderly beneficiaries to enroll in managed care. The point is illustrated also by the contentious politics of Medicare managed care.

To be sure, some states are experimenting with managed care for the aged, disabled, and other clients with special needs (such as the mentally ill, substance abusers, and the chronically ill). Minnesota, for example, requires the aged (but not the disabled) to participate in its managed care initiative. Even in California, San Mateo and Santa Barbara Counties succeeded where San Diego County did not, and the aged and disabled in those counties are now required to enroll in managed care. In addition, the On Lok program in San Francisco provides medical care and social services to the frail elderly in exchange for a capitated payment from both Medicaid and Medicare. Organizations in a dozen communities around the country are trying to replicate the On Lok model.

Moreover, fiscal pressure is sure to encourage other states to experiment with managed care for the aged and disabled. After all, these are by far the most costly Medicaid populations: 27 percent of enrollees are aged or disabled, but 59 percent of expenditures are on behalf of these populations (Kaiser Commission on the Future of Medicaid, 1995b). Despite these numbers, the emphasis on families with children is likely to continue: states will move first to enroll families with children and only later turn to the aged and disabled.

2. *Should managed care be mandatory?* Under federal law, Medicaid beneficiaries generally have the right to seek care from any willing provider. States therefore cannot require beneficiaries to enroll in a managed care plan unless they receive from the federal government a waiver from the freedom of choice mandate. Without such a waiver, managed care enrollment can be encouraged but not required.

The most common managed care waivers are those authorized by Section 1915(b) of the Social Security Act. As of early 1995, forty-two states operated 1915(b) waiver programs, most of which require groups of beneficiaries to have a physician gatekeeper, generally paid on a fee-for-service basis (General Accounting Office, 1995b).

Over the last few years, however, states have increasingly bypassed the 1915(b) route, seeking instead a waiver under section 1115 of the Social Security Act. These waivers are preferable for two reasons. First, and most importantly, states have far more flexibility under the provisions of 1115 than under 1915(b). For example, under 1115 states can require beneficiaries to stay in one health maintenance organization (HMO) for twelve months, they can limit beneficiaries to a restrictive benefit package, and they can contract with HMOs that serve only Medicaid clients. None of these options are available under the 1915(b) program. Similarly, under 1115 states can provide eligibility to groups previously ineligible for Medicaid (on the theory that the managed care savings will offset the cost of the expansion). This option also is unavailable under 1915(b). A second reason for the popularity of the 1115 option is that these waivers are good for five years, versus the two-year renewal process for 1915(b) waivers.

To be sure, the first 1115 waivers were granted nearly fifteen years ago, to Arizona (to implement a statewide managed care initiative) and to half a dozen other states (California, Florida, Minnesota, Missouri, New Jersey, and New York, to require managed care in one or more counties). Until recently, however, there were few other 1115 applications, and none that replicated Arizona's statewide initiative. Instead, most states experimented with fee-for-service gatekeeper programs, limited in scope and authorized under 1915(b).

Since 1992, however, twenty-two states have applied under 1115 to implement statewide mandatory managed care programs. As of late 1995, federal regulators had approved eleven applications and were reviewing the rest (General Accounting Office, 1995b).

Even when managed care is mandatory, most states have a process by which persons can seek an exemption from enrollment. The mandatory program in southwest Brooklyn, New York, illustrates this point. Under this 1915(b)-approved program, AFDC-related beneficiaries in the community need to enroll in managed care. Nonetheless, the following group of clients are exempt: those who have received ongoing care from a primary care provider for more than one year; those with chronic medical conditions; those receiving mental health, alcohol, or substance abuse services on more than an incidental basis; those receiving care from a provider who speaks a language not currently available through a health plan; and those receiving prenatal care from a nonparticipating provider (New York City Human Resources Administration, 1993).

3.   *Should clients receive a period of guaranteed eligibility?* Medicaid eligibility for most beneficiaries hinges on AFDC or Supplemental Security Income (SSI) eligibility. For these clients, Medicaid recertification occurs at the same time as welfare recertification, which happens every six months or so. For a variety of reasons, however, many clients fail to appear at their welfare recertification (or they appear without needed documents). These clients then lose their program eligibility. More often than not, the loss of eligibility (and the missing cash assistance check) prompts the client to come to the welfare office. If the client comes quickly, retroactive eligibility is often possible. Eventually the paperwork will be filed, and the client will get her check.

The high incidence of client churning is quite problematic for managed care enrollees. Not only are these clients terminated from Medicaid, they are also terminated from their managed care plan. Restoring managed care eligibility is administratively burdensome for the state and the managed care plan, and churning is potentially dangerous for the client, who may miss out on needed care during the suspension period.

States have two options to deal with this problem. One option is to provide six months of guaranteed eligibility to all beneficiaries who enroll in federally qualified HMOs. (States are not permitted to offer six months of guaranteed eligibility to other Medicaid clients.) This helps some clients (those that lose eligibility in the first six months). A better option is to offer clients one month of additional Medicaid eligibility whenever termination is due to a failure to recertify. This approach would help all clients who temporarily lose eligibility, and it would ease the administrative burden on states and managed care plans.

Most states are reluctant to adopt either option; their concern is that benefits will be provided to ineligible persons. Other states are willing to provide such coverage, concluding that on balance the benefits (for beneficiaries, managed care plans, and state administrators) outweigh the costs. Minnesota's 1115 waiver program, for example, includes a one-month extended-coverage provision. Similarly, New York's 1915(b) program provides six months of guaranteed eligibility to enrollees in federally qualified HMOs.

4.   *What should be the content of the managed care benefit package?* Federal Medicaid law stipulates certain health care services that state programs must cover, others that states can cover with federal matching funds, and still others that states can cover only at their own expense. Different states thus cover different services. For example, thirty-nine states pay for dentures, thirty-four cover occupational therapy, and twenty-seven include chiropractor services. Moreover, many states impose limits on the amount, scope, or duration of covered benefits. Louisiana, for example, covers no more than fifteen days of inpatient hospital care per calendar year. Other states have similar restrictions. In short, the options for states are plentiful, and the result is that no two states offer an identical benefit package.

Despite the interstate variation in Medicaid benefit packages, states generally are required to offer the same package to beneficiaries within the state, although they can seek a federal waiver to offer somewhat different benefits to different groups or beneficiaries in different areas of the state. Clients in San Francisco are entitled to the same benefits as their counterparts in Los Angeles. States also are required to ensure that beneficiaries in managed care receive the same benefit package as those remaining in the fee-for-service program. Clients shouldn't be penalized (or rewarded) for enrolling in managed care.

In theory, the conversion to managed care should thus contain few benefit issues. States should simply require managed care plans to provide whatever services are already required in their fee-for-service program. In practice, however, the conversion is far more problematic. Indeed, no state requires managed care plans to provide every Medicaid-covered service. Instead, some services are delivered through the plans and others remain part of the traditional fee-for-service system. There are three reasons for this mixed-model approach. First, federal law entitles beneficiaries to receive certain services (such as family planning services) from any available provider. Second, most managed care plans are unable to provide certain services (such as nursing home care), and states are unwilling to force the plans to add them. Third, and most importantly, state policymakers sometimes decide that certain services (such as mental health or dental services) should be carved out of the managed care initiative and delivered through an alternative delivery system (either the fee-for-service system or a separate and specialized managed care system—see Chapter Eleven).

Given this background, state policymakers need to decide how comprehensive their managed care benefit package should be. At one extreme is the so-called comprehensive benefit approach, under which a managed care plan receives a capitated fee to provide nearly all of the services covered in the state's benefit package. This is the model most states are moving toward. A second strategy is the partial benefit model, under which the managed care plan provides a quite limited set of services, sometimes in exchange for a capitated fee and sometimes for a fee-for-service reimbursement. The most common partial benefit programs, called primary care case management programs, provide primary care and gatekeeper (or case management) services.

The debate over the content of the managed care benefit package is often quite fierce. Consider mental health services in New York State. Should New York beneficiaries receive mental health services through their managed care plan or through the traditional fee-for-service mental health system? The issue first arose in 1991, following the enactment of state legislation that encouraged beneficiaries to enroll in managed care. The players were state officials (committed to managed care), managed care plans (anxious to provide and be paid for mental health services), county mental health organizations and other mental health providers (desperate to retain their patient base), and advocates for the mentally ill (concerned that the transition to managed care would be disruptive for clients). After months of negotiations, there was a compromise: managed care capitation rates would cover routine mental health services provided on an intermittent basis. The capitation rates would not cover care for services received on more than an incidental basis: clients could seek those services from any available provider, and the provider would be paid on a fee-for-service basis. More recently, the state submitted an 1115 waiver application, under which the mentally ill would receive mental health services from newly created "special needs" health plans. The state's application is pending.

5.   *What are the Medicaid managed care plans, and what difference does their organizational structure make?* The Medicaid managed care market, like the general managed care market, is extraordinarily difficult to characterize. It is easy to fall back on the traditional typologies. One approach is to classify by ownership (for-profit, nonprofit, or public). Another strategy is to divide by organizational structure (there are, for example, several types of HMOs, PPOs, and a host of plans especially established for the Medicaid program). A third strategy is to focus on how plans are paid (by full capitation, partial capitation, or fee-for-service reimbursement) or how plans pay their own providers (by capitation or fee-for-service reimbursement).

Perhaps the most useful typology, however, begins by dividing participating plans into two generic groups: those that have traditionally cared for a commercially insured middle-class population but are now entering the Medicaid market and those that are composed of medical providers that traditionally served the Medicaid population (but worry that they'll lose patients and revenue to the more-established health plans). The question for state officials then becomes whether to favor one type of plan over the other or simply to let the market determine the winners and losers.

Consider the mainstream managed care organizations that until recently ignored the Medicaid market but now participate aggressively. Why the strategic change? First, many states passed (or threatened to pass) legislation that penalized health plans with too few Medicaid enrollees. New York, for example, imposed a 9 percent surcharge on the hospital bills of HMOs not active in the Medicaid market. Second, the 1994 national health reform debate also encouraged health plans to expand into the Medicaid market (if only to be well positioned when national health insurance was enacted). Third, once in the market, HMOs discovered that enrolling Medicaid beneficiaries generates profits (especially in states, like New York, that are generous payers). Fourth, managed care plans that have large numbers of enrollees can persuade hospitals (and other providers) to offer deep discounts on price.

For all of these reasons, many well-established managed care plans now compete in the Medicaid market. This trend threatens the fiscal viability of the traditional Medicaid providers (such as hospitals located in low-income communities, community health centers, and even individual providers with large numbers of Medicaid patients). The fear is that the mainstream health plans will attract the low-cost Medicaid client, and the safety net providers will be left with the high-cost Medicaid beneficiary and the uninsured (a recipe for financial disaster).

One option for safety net providers is to persuade HMOs to refer patients to their facilities. This strategy works especially well for primary care providers with a large Medicaid clientele, and mainstream HMOs often aggressively court these providers. The strategy works less well, however, for safety net hospitals and community health centers. Many HMOs, for example, prefer to contract with low-cost private hospitals than with generally high-cost public hospitals or academic medical centers.

A second option is for safety net providers to themselves establish a managed care entity. The newly created plan could be composed of a public hospital system, a group of community health centers, or simply a cadre of individual providers. It could compete primarily (or exclusively) in the Medicaid market, or it could seek Medicare and commercial business as well.

6. *Should states establish safety net protection plans?* Safety net providers are often threatened by the movement toward Medicaid managed care. This is particularly true for hospitals that rely heavily on Medicaid revenue generated through their emergency rooms. These hospitals must cope with lower revenue (as Medicaid, Medicare, and the private sector all cut back), fewer staff (as Congress threatens to scale back funding for graduate medical education), and a costlier and sicker patient population (as mainstream HMOs attract the low-cost Medicaid client but leave the hospital with the high-cost client and the uninsured).

The outlook is equally bleak for community-based specialty clinics (such as those that provide women's health services, mental health services, or substance abuse services) and for some federally qualified community health centers. HMOs often prefer not to contract with specialty clinics (or to refer only the most difficult patients). Meanwhile, while HMOs often contract with the more primary care–oriented community health centers, they are generally unwilling to pay the cost-based reimbursement that the centers now receive. (In 1989, Congress enacted legislation requiring Medicaid programs to reimburse community health centers for 100 percent of their reasonable costs. Several states have now filed 1115 applications that would waive this requirement. Congress is also considering legislation that would eliminate the mandate.) In this environment, state officials must decide whether to develop a safety net protection program or to instead let the market alone determine winners and losers.

One option is to require managed care organizations to contract with "essential community providers." Minnesota's 1115 waiver program, for example, would require all health plans to contract with essential community providers for five years (the first three years with cost-based reimbursement). A less onerous approach is to encourage but not require contracts with safety net providers. This works especially well where managed care contracts are awarded through a competitive bid process (health plans that have contracts with essential community providers would presumably have an advantage in the bidding process).

States also can encourage and support those safety net providers that choose to form their own managed care plans. One option is to change the laws governing managed care to accommodate such newly forming plans. New York, for example, created a new type of HMO that could enroll Medicaid and other publicly funded beneficiaries but could not compete in the commercial market. These new HMOs could receive start-up and transition funding from the state. Similarly, California hopes to temporarily exempt safety net health plans from the state's stringent cash reserve and capitalization requirements.

The California rule on cash reserve requirements is part of the nation's most aggressive safety net protection plan. Under the so-called Two-Plan model (recently approved by the federal government. Medicaid beneficiaries in twelve California counties will have to choose between two managed care plans, a mainstream (or private sector) plan and a government-run plan that will feature the county-run public hospital system. Clients who do not choose would be assigned to the government-run plan, at least until that plan achieves its minimum enrollment targets. This will not only ensure the survival of the public plan, it would also enable county hospitals to maintain most or all of their federal disproportionate-share income. Federal legislation requires states to take into account the situation of those hospitals that serve a disproportionate number of low-income persons. In 1992, for example, this requirement provided safety net hospitals with an additional $17.4 billion (General Accounting Office, 1995a). Most hospitals use this funding to pay for care rendered to the uninsured.

7.   *How should marketing and enrollment be conducted?* With rare exceptions, managed care initiatives offer beneficiaries a choice of managed care plans. The marketing and enrollment process is thus critical. There is, however, wide interstate variation in the ways that states handle both processes. (There are some managed care initiatives that require all beneficiaries to enroll in the same managed care plan. In San Mateo, California, for example, all beneficiaries are required to enroll in the County Organized Health System, a publicly administered managed care network.)

In some mandatory managed care programs (like the one in Minneapolis), county Medicaid workers inform beneficiaries of their managed care options during a face-to-face presentation. The county worker reviews the basic principles of managed care, describes the competing managed care plans, and answers questions. Health plan marketers are not permitted to participate in the process or to engage in any direct marketing, though county workers do hand out brochures and provider lists produced by the plans. Nearly all beneficiaries select a managed care plan (and a primary care provider affiliated with the plan) during that initial presentation.

By all accounts, the Minneapolis model works well. Despite its success, the model is rarely replicated. States (and managed care plans) are often concerned that county workers will be biased in favor of the county-administered plan. State officials also worry about the high cost of a county-administered face-to-face system.

Smaller health plans particularly dislike the model, arguing that the prohibition on direct marketing puts them at a competitive disadvantage (after all, most beneficiaries have heard of Blue Cross or U.S. HealthCare, but few recognize the names of smaller and newer organizations).

For all of these reasons, several states permit health plans to engage in direct marketing and enrollment of beneficiaries. In these unregulated states, health plan marketers sometimes knock on doors in low-income communities. They often attend health fairs and other community gatherings, and they market to beneficiaries in local welfare offices. Oftentimes, however, unregulated marketing and enrollment lead to allegations of fraud and abuse. Back in the early 1970s, for example, some door-to-door marketers in California told beneficiaries that enrollment was mandatory (it wasn't). Others promised benefits and perks well beyond the Medicaid package (Chavking and Treseder, 1977). While the California legislature enacted legislation designed to reduce such marketing problems, door-to-door marketing is still permitted in much of the state. Allegations of abuse continue (Sparer, Gold, and Simon, 1996). Similar allegations have surfaced in New York City as well (Sparer and Chu, 1996).

In response to claims of fraud and abuse, both California and New York now plan to have third-party contractors handle the marketing and enrollment functions. The contractor strategy avoids the bias of a county-administered program and the dangers of an unregulated system. Nonetheless, the strategy has its own pitfalls, particularly if the contractor is expected to convert clients to managed care through the mail (instead of in face-to-face meetings).

Consider the fiasco that occurred in Sacramento, California, when state officials hired a private contractor to convert 150,000 beneficiaries to managed care in early 1994. The first problem was that clients were not adequately informed about their options under the new program: the written materials did not include directories listing the providers associated with each health plan. This omission made it very difficult for beneficiaries to learn which doctors were in which plan. Beneficiaries also had trouble accessing the contractor's toll-free telephone number; they instead asked their doctors for guidance. Doctors (and clinics) often responded by giving their patients enrollment forms designating themselves as primary care provider (in whatever plan they belonged to). As a result, approximately 16 percent of all clients signed up two or more times and chose two or more health plans. The contractor eventually received over 400,000 enrollment forms from approximately 150,000 clients. The result was confusion for clients, providers, and plans (Sparer, Gold, and Simon, 1996). The lesson is that marketing and enrollment by mail are problematic, particularly if implemented quickly and with inadequate resources.

8. *How much should Medicaid pay health plans?* There are three key reimbursement decisions for Medicaid managed care regulators. First, should plans be paid a capitated fee (whether full or partial capitation) or a case management fee for service? Second, should Medicaid develop a single statewide rate, regional rates, or plan-specific rates? Third, how much should Medicaid pay, and is there a way of adjusting the payment to take into account the risk status of plan enrollees?

The trend today is toward capitation payment systems, under which plans are capitated for all but a few medical benefits (such as long-term care and care for the chronically mentally ill). The goal is to shift away from the inflationary incentives of the fee-for-service model and toward a more cost-conscious capitation approach. To be sure, several states still operate primary care case management programs, under which providers receive a separate fee for providing case management services. These programs are especially common in rural communities, where there often are too few medical providers to support a competitive managed care market. Where there is an option, however, Medicaid officials are clearly moving toward full capitation.

The question of whether to have a statewide rate, regional rates, or plan-specific rates is more controversial. Tennessee uses a single statewide rate for all plans, with some demographic adjustments (Gold, Frazier, and Schoen, 1995). In contrast, Minnesota officials divide the state into three regions and develop a separate rate for each (Sparer, Ellwood, and Schoen, 1996). (Medicaid officials actually issue several rates for each region, with different rates for children, adults, and so on. Moreover, the state has recently begun giving those Hennepin County plans with high medical education costs and high disproportionate-share hospital payment costs a slightly higher capitation rate.) Finally, New York's program develops plan-specific rates. New York officials first determine for each of eight geographic regions the average amount spent on different groups of Medicaid clients under the fee-for-service system (the groups are divided by age and sex). Health plans cannot under any circumstances receive more than 95 percent of the average fee-for-service rate. Each plan then uses the fee-for-service data to develop a proposed premium for each of the different client categories. At that point, state and plan officials negotiate final rates.

Whatever the payment methodology, there is often controversy over the amount actually paid. A hypothetical example illustrates the point. In 1995, state X spent $100 per Medicaid beneficiary per month. In 1996, the state pays a health plan $95 to provide enrollees with a comprehensive set of medical benefits. Is this a reasonable amount to pay? Maybe yes and maybe no. If the health plan enrolls a low-cost client, who would have cost the state only $80 in the old fee-for-service world, then Medicaid has paid too much; it has lost $15. Conversely, if the plan enrolls a high-cost client, who would have cost the state $120, then Medicaid has saved $35.

Given this variation, Medicaid officials are working hard to develop accurate risk-adjustment systems under which the amount paid depends in part on the risk status of the beneficiary. So far, however, the technology of risk adjustment is in its infancy. States can (and do) pay separate rates for separate categories of clients (more for the disabled, less for young children), but no state effectively differentiates within these categories (more for the high-risk youngster, less for the low-risk).

The optimum payment rate is affected by a variety of other factors as well. First, state fee-for-service expenditure patterns vary dramatically. New York spends approximately $7,286 per beneficiary, while California spends only $2,801. So long as managed care rates are established by referring to local fee-for-service expenditure patterns, managed care rates will also vary dramatically. As a result, New York managed care plans often produce significant profits even when paid only 80 to 85 percent of the average fee-for-service rates. Profits are less likely in states such as California. Second, well-run health plans spend time and money trying to alter beneficiaries' patterns of health care use. They hire new staff (from social workers to interpreters), provide additional services (from transportation services to special immunization programs), and then seek additional reimbursement from Medicaid for these start-up costs. Finally, states often require health plans to provide some of these additional services (requiring, for example, that materials be translated into several languages). Plan officials complain that the compensation for these cultural and linguistic requirements is usually inadequate.

9.   *Do beneficiaries get access to mainstream providers?* Medicaid has generally disappointed those who had hoped that the program would provide poor people with health care equal to that of the nonpoor. Nearly half of the nation's poor are not even eligible for coverage. Moreover, most Medicaid clients have neither their own physician nor ready access to a private physician's practice. For these clients, medical care is received most often in the emergency rooms of large hospitals.

One goal of Medicaid managed care is to improve client access to mainstream health care. For this reason, states generally encourage the participation of those managed care plans that have traditionally served a privately insured middle-class population. The assumption is that these plans will provide clients with access to providers that previously saw few, if any, Medicaid clients. In Minneapolis, for example, Medicaid clients who enroll in Medica (a large HMO with both commercial and Medicaid clients) can select any primary care provider affiliated with the plan.

In some cases, however, health plans develop two lists of providers: one for commercial enrollees and another for Medicaid clients. The New York City public advocate's office recently released a report alleging that this practice is common in New York (Public Advocate of the City of New York, 1996). Obviously this practice reduces the likelihood that clients will see anyone but traditional Medicaid providers.

To be sure, even if a commercial health plan has only one provider list, clients are unlikely to choose a provider located in a distant neighborhood. Similarly, non-English-speaking clients are unlikely to select a provider who neither speaks their language nor is familiar with their culture. In these cases, clients are often better off choosing a traditional Medicaid provider who speaks their language, knows their culture, and lives nearby. These providers are often better able to provide useful primary care and to manage access to other forms of care. Unfortunately, however, there

are too few primary care providers who live in low-income neighborhoods, speak a language other than English, and accept Medicaid clients. Moreover, even when such providers are available, some
clients want the freedom to choose others (even if it requires them
to leave their home neighborhood), which again raises the need
to encourage more doctors to accept Medicaid clients.

Medicaid officials deal with the provider capacity problem
with two general strategies. The first and most common strategy
is to shift the burden to the health plans. For example, states
require participating plans to demonstrate that they have enough
providers (conveniently located) to serve their Medicaid members. The expectation is that health plans will do a better job of
encouraging provider participation than did the traditional
Medicaid program. The second strategy is for the state itself to
encourage additional provider participation. Tennessee, for example, requires any provider that treats state employees to also treat
Medicaid clients. Under either scenario, states are increasingly
requiring both health plans and providers to demonstrate sensitivity to the special needs of the Medicaid population. Some states
require plans to hire interpreters if more than a certain minimum
number of enrollees speak a particular language. Most states
require plans to develop a health promotion and education program. All states require plans to establish a patient grievance
process. Put simply, the goal is to both encourage more participation by mainstream providers and to ensure that the newly participating providers deliver good health care.

10.   *Do beneficiaries receive high-quality care?* Capitated payment
systems contain an economic incentive to underserve. The health
plan (or provider) receives the same fee regardless of the amount
(or quality) of the care delivered. If the plan (or provider) delivers health care costing more than the predetermined fee, there is
an economic loss. The plan (or provider) profits, however, if
health care costing less than the capitated fee is delivered. The
incentive (at least in the short term) is thus to deliver as little care
as possible.

To be sure, there also are (long-term) incentives to provide
good and timely care, particularly primary and preventive care.
The short-term costs of promptly providing primary care are sometimes less than the long-term costs of delaying the onset of care.

The commonly cited example is prenatal care for pregnant women. The cost of a single low-birthweight baby far exceeds the cost of providing good prenatal care to hundreds of women. Managed care supporters typically rely on this long-term focus. The assumption is that managed care companies will manage the care of clients, discouraging unnecessary care, encouraging appropriate care, reducing overall health costs, and improving the quality of care. This assumption seems especially valid in the Medicaid context. After all, many Medicaid clients receive care, if at all, in expensive hospital emergency rooms. By providing these clients with a primary care physician, the expectation is that managed care will provide both better and less-expensive care.

There are, however, three problems with this rosy assumption. First, some health plans lack the money to focus too much on the long term. Many health plans composed of safety net providers are in this tenuous financial position. Moreover, states, anxious to ensure safety net plan participation, are often willing to permit these plans to participate even if they cannot meet the financial requirements generally applied to the managed care industry. Second, many health plans, especially those for-profit plans created solely to tap the Medicaid market, are simply more interested in short-term profits than in long-term viability. Third, many Medicaid clients churn on and off the Medicaid rolls or in and out of Medicaid managed care plans. This pattern of client churning makes it less likely that health plans will focus on the long term. This does not mean that health plans discourage the delivery of prenatal care; the time period between the onset of pregnancy and birth is short enough to avoid this problem. Nonetheless, health plans are less likely to pursue long-term prevention strategies (treatment regimens that are not likely to save money for years).

Given the mixed incentives, states need to carefully monitor the quality of care provided by managed care plans. Can clients get timely access to their primary care provider? Is the provider network-adequate? Does the plan have a good patient education system? Are there programs to encourage clients to receive primary and preventive care? Are clients able to have their grievances resolved quickly and fairly? Are plans adequately capitalized? Does the plan have an adequate system for supervising its providers? Do providers themselves have a fiscal incentive to underserve?

There are at least three strategies states use to answer these and similar questions. First, states require health plans to submit their internal quality-of-care protocols for state approval. By reviewing a plan's internal procedures, the state can sometimes influence its external outcomes. Second, states themselves conduct quality-of-care audits. Third, states are required by federal law to hire an independent evaluator to conduct annual quality-of-care reviews.

Not surprisingly, however, there is significant variation in how states pursue these three strategies. Two issues are particularly important. First, which state agency should be in charge of assessing quality of care? Some states (like Minnesota) assign the task to the agency generally in charge of the managed care industry (usually the health department or the insurance department). Other states (like California) assign a bigger role to the agency directly in charge of the Medicaid program. Second, states differ in their choice of measurement tool for monitoring plan performance. Some states use criteria established by the National Commission on Quality Assurance in their Health Plan Employer Data and Information Set (HEDIS). Other states participate in the Quality Assurance Reform Initiative, a project funded by the Henry J. Kaiser Family Foundation, which is developing quality assurance standards for Medicaid managed care systems. Still other states use their own systems. In all states, however, while the task of encouraging high-quality care is high on the policy agenda, the oversight systems now in place are still in their infancy. The key unknown about Medicaid managed care remains its impact on quality of care.

11.   *Is the transition to managed care occurring too quickly?* The recent growth in Medicaid managed care is extraordinary. In 1983 there were 750,000 enrollees (3 percent of the total Medicaid population). By 1994 the number of enrollees was up to 7.8 million (23 percent), and by mid 1995 the number was up to 11.6 million (36 percent). By the turn of the century, nearly all Medicaid clients may well be enrolled in managed care.

Even in states with a preexisting managed care infrastructure, the rapid conversion to managed care is often problematic. California illustrates the point. California has long had a thriving managed care industry, and state officials argue both that managed care in California is mainstream care and that the state has the managed care infrastructure to accommodate the influx of Medicaid beneficiaries. Despite these advantages, however, the state's effort to convert 150,000 Sacramento beneficiaries in just a few months was problem-filled. Clients were confused by the marketing and enrollment procedures, the enrollment contractor was unable to respond adequately to client questions, and neither health plans nor providers engaged in significant client education (Sparer, Gold, and Simon, 1996).

Rapid implementation is even more problematic in states, like Tennessee, with little managed care experience or infrastructure. Before the state's Medicaid managed care initiative began, one Tennessee health plan served thirty-five thousand Medicaid clients (all other clients were in fee-for-service Medicaid). A year later, twelve health plans were serving over one million clients. By most accounts, many of the new health plans had limited provider networks, inadequate provider payment systems, and too few client education programs (Gold, Frazier, and Schoen, 1995).

The better approach is to develop an incremental managed care initiative. Minnesota provides a good example. Minnesota has taken ten years to enroll 140,000 of its 400,000 Medicaid clients into managed care, and it is now slowly enrolling the rest. The slow growth is helpful to all participants. Commercial health plans need time to develop programs to meet the special needs of the Medicaid population. Safety net providers need time to successfully transition to a managed care environment. Beneficiaries need time to learn about managed care and about the changes in the health care delivery system. State officials need time to develop effective and unbiased enrollment and marketing procedures.

12.   *What are the spillover effects of managed care initiatives?* Medicaid managed care initiatives have an impact well beyond the Medicaid program. The impact is most obvious in states that use the savings from Medicaid managed care to subsidize health insurance for previously uninsured residents. Tennessee and Oregon each subsidize health care for the uninsured with savings (presumably) garnered from Medicaid managed care.

More generally, however, managed care initiatives have a significant impact on states' entire health care delivery systems. Safety net and traditional Medicaid providers are required either to contract with health plans, form their own health plan, or suffer serious fiscal consequences. Managed care companies are encouraged to expand and serve new clients in new communities with new providers. Health care providers are encouraged (and sometimes required) to accept Medicaid clients. Nonprofessional health care workers will likely be shifted from (often unionized) jobs in hospitals to (nonunionized) positions in other health care settings.

Conclusion

The ongoing debate over the federal budget revolves, in large part, around the future of Medicaid: Republicans propose converting the program into a block grant (under which states would have nearly unfettered discretion) while Democrats seek to keep in place certain minimum federal standards (governing, for example, program eligibility). While the Washington debate proceeds, however, the states have already engineered a Medicaid managed care revolution, persuading or (requiring) millions of Medicaid clients to enroll in managed care delivery systems. Moreover, despite the partisan bickering in Congress, the movement toward Medicaid managed care is certain to continue: both the Republicans and the Democrats support proposals to make it even easier for the states to convert beneficiaries into managed care.

The movement toward managed care impacts every actor in the Medicaid policy arena. Commercial HMOs, which have traditionally served a commercially insured middle-class population, are now competing to serve low-income populations. Primary care physicians, who previously accepted few Medicaid clients, are now pressured to expand their client base. Safety net providers, which have traditionally cared for low-income populations, are now learning to become insurers. Medicaid beneficiaries, who are accustomed to relying for care on the local hospital emergency room, are now sifting through and evaluating the terms and conditions of various managed care plans. And state (and sometimes local) officials must organize and supervise the entire initiative, determining which beneficiaries are to be enrolled, developing marketing and enrollment procedures, establishing benefit packages, setting capitation rates, supervising quality of care, ensuring that the medical safety net is not eliminated in the transition, and performing a host of other implementation activities.

As the managed care revolution proceeds, a few observations seem pertinent. First, there is extraordinary variation in every aspect of Medicaid managed care policy. Some states cover only women and children, others are now including the aged and disabled. Some states mandate managed care, others still rely on voluntary enrollment. There is also variation in the managed care benefit package, the methodology used to develop reimbursement rates, and required quality-of-care protocols. In short, Medicaid managed care initiatives vary as much as (or more than) traditional Medicaid programs.

Second, since Congress is likely to increase state discretion over Medicaid managed care initiatives, the interstate variation in such initiatives is also likely to increase.

Third, the value of interstate variation itself varies. For example, different states have different managed care infrastructures. States with minimal managed care infrastructures should move more slowly than states where managed care is well established. Similarly, variation in the content of a managed care benefit package is also appropriate. For example, whether mental health coverage is included in a managed care package should depend, in part, on the state's preexisting mental health delivery system.

On other issues, however, the value of variation is less apparent. Some states (such as New York) have only a minimal safety net protection plan, while others (such as California) have a more aggressive approach. This interstate variation is problematic: every state should be required to develop an aggressive safety net protection plan. Why? First, the profitability of the Medicaid client may diminish, encouraging commercial HMOs to withdraw their participation. Safety net plans (and providers) are less likely to abandon the program. Second, commercial HMOs, even when willing participants, rarely market to the uninsured or the high-cost Medicaid client. Until and unless universal insurance is enacted, the safety net will be needed to care for these populations.

Fourth, and finally, the federal government should not abandon the Medicaid managed care arena. Federal oversight is useful, if only to minimize inappropriate interstate variation and maximize useful interstate variation. The block grant approach is thus unwise. States already have significant policymaking authority and have exercised their discretion to enact extraordinarily diverse managed care initiatives. States do not need additional policy-making authority. Although states' rights remains a rallying cry for most politicians, rational federal supervision of state Medicaid programs remains the best policy choice.

References

Chavking, D., and Treseder, A. "California's Prepaid Health Plan Program: Can the Patient Be Saved?" *The Hastings Law Journal,* 1977, 28, p. 685.

Congressional Research Service. *Medicaid Source Book: Background Data and Analysis (A 1993 Update).* Washington, D.C.: U.S. Government Printing Office, 1993.

General Accounting Office. *Medicaid: Spending Pressures Drive States Toward Program Reinvention.* GAO/HEHS-95-122. Washington, D.C.: U.S. Government Printing Office, 1995a.

General Accounting Office. *Medicaid Section 1115 Waivers: Flexible Approach to Approving Demonstrations Could Increase Federal Costs.* GAO/HEHS-96-44. Washington, D.C.: U.S. Government Printing Office, 1995b.

Gold, M., Frazier, H., and Schoen, C. *Managed Care and Low-Income Populations: A Case Study of Managed Care in Tennessee.* Washington, D.C.: Kaiser Family Foundation and the Commonwealth Fund, 1995.

Holahan, J., Rowland, D., Feder, J., and Heslam, D. "Explaining the Recent Growth in Medicaid Spending." *Health Affairs,* 1993, *12*(3), 177–193.

Kaiser Commission on the Future of Medicaid. *Medicaid and Managed Care: Lessons from the Literature.* Washington, D.C.: Kaiser Commission on the Future of Medicaid, 1995a.

Kaiser Commission on the Future of Medicaid. *Medicaid Policy Brief.* Washington, D.C.: Kaiser Commission on the Future of Medicaid, 1995b.

New York City Human Resources Administration. "Exemptions from Medicaid Managed Health Care Program." New York: New York City Human Resources Administration, 1993.

Prospective Payment Assessment Commission. *Medicare and the American Health Care System: Report to Congress.* Washington, D.C.: Prospective Payment Assessment Commission, June 1995.

Public Advocate of the City of New York. "Two Lists: Commercial and Medicaid Managed Care Providers." New York: Public Advocate of the City of New York, 1996.

Sparer, M., and Chu, K. *Managed Care and Low-Income Populations: A Case Study of Managed Care in New York.* Washington, D.C.: Kaiser Family Foundation and the Commonwealth Fund, 1996.

Sparer, M., Ellwood, M., and Schoen, C. *Managed Care and Low-Income Populations: A Case Study of Managed Care in Minnesota.* Washington, D.C.: Kaiser Family Foundation and the Commonwealth Fund, 1996.

Sparer, M., Gold, M., and Simon, L. *Managed Care and Low-Income Populations: A Case Study of Managed Care in California.* Washington, D.C.: Kaiser Family Foundation and the Commonwealth Fund, 1996.

Chapter Eleven

The Challenges of Implementing Market-Based Reform for Public Clients

Kelly J. Devers

As discussed in Chapter Ten, states are rapidly moving ahead with Medicaid managed care programs. Like employers in the private sector, state governments are searching for effective cost-containment strategies. Medicaid expenditures as a percentage of total state general expenditures increased from an average of 3 percent in 1966, when the Medicaid program began, to 17 percent in 1995 (Kaiser Commission on the Future of Medicaid, 1995). Between 1990 and 1992 the average annual rate of growth for Medicaid was 28.1 percent, compared to 7.2 percent for private insurance and 10.7 percent for Medicare (Coughlin, Ku, and Holahan, 1994). Besides controlling costs, state governments are attempting to resolve the endemic problems of reduced access and inappropriate utilization. To achieve these goals, state governments are borrowing strategies and techniques from the

I acknowledge the assistance of several individuals in the preparation of this chapter. John Wilkerson and Susan Giaimo both read earlier drafts and offered helpful suggestions for revision. Joan Bloom, Nancy Wilson, and Teh-wei Hu also read drafts and provided very useful comments. Finally, and most important, I thank those individuals involved in the state of Colorado's capitation program, in particular Bill Bush, capitation program manager; Tom Barrett, director of mental health services; and Gary Toerber, director of hospital services, Office of Direct Services. I am grateful for their input. Any factual errors remain my own.

private sector. Specifically, they are changing from passive purchasers to active buyers of services, and they are increasingly using
managed care techniques.

At the heart of these efforts is the idea that state governments
can either adapt private managed care practices to the public sector or use the private market to insure and care for Medicaid beneficiaries. Is it possible for state governments to become active
buyers of managed care services? On the surface the answer seems
to be an unequivocal yes. Upon closer reflection, however, several
assumptions underlying this idea are more complex than is initially
apparent. These assumptions can be framed as sets of questions.

First, are there any special features of state governments that
constrain them from acting like private purchasers? If so, what are
they? Second, do state governments have a unique power to shape
the emerging managed care market? If so, what factors do state
governments consider when they attempt to shape the market?
Finally, what must state governments do to implement Medicaid
managed care initiatives? What processes do state governments use
to implement Medicaid managed care programs? What organizational and technical capabilities are required at each phase of the
process, and how does the process ultimately affect the programs'
operations?

This chapter explores these questions and their implications
for state governments, traditional public providers, beneficiaries,
and the promise of managed care (to reduce costs while improving access and quality). I begin by examining state governments'
traditional role in the Medicaid program and the power they possess to reshape it. In answer to the first set of questions, I argue that
the political nature of state governments and their social welfare
function constrain them from acting like the aggressive purchasers
at work in the private market. Next, in answer to the second set of
questions, I argue that state governments have a unique authority
to determine how the emerging managed care market will be organized. I examine two general strategies states can employ to reform
Medicaid through managed care, and their similarities and differences from an implementation and a policy perspective. With
respect to existing problems with the Medicaid program and views
about how best to address them, I argue that market and political
factors play a key role in determining which strategy states pursue.

Finally, in answer to the third set of questions, I explore the challenges of implementing Medicaid managed care programs. In particular, I examine the process by which state governments implement managed care programs and the organizational and technical challenges inherent in that process.

Throughout the chapter I use the development of Colorado's Medicaid managed care program for mental health services to illustrate the kinds of decisions state governments face in formulating and implementing managed care programs for special Medicaid populations. Medicaid is the primary source of insurance for many of the severely mentally ill because of its link to the Supplemental Security Income (SSI) program (Manderscheid and Sonnenschein, 1994; Steinwachs, Kasper, and Skinner, 1992). SSI is an income support program for individuals who are blind, aged, or disabled and who earn below a defined level of income ($500 per month in 1992). In general, individuals who are eligible for SSI are also eligible for Medicaid. In 1991, there were 596,800 Medicaid beneficiaries nationwide receiving SSI who were disabled by mental disorders (Kennedy and Manderscheid, 1994).

Colorado's managed care program for mental health services warrants special attention because it includes not only the severely mentally ill but also any Medicaid beneficiary who requires mental health services. (Dually eligible Medicare and Medicaid recipients must participate in the program if Medicaid is the primary payer.) In addition, the program places contracted organizations at full risk for the cost of both inpatient and outpatient services. (See Bloom and others, 1994a; Dangerfield and Betit, 1993; Hadley, Schinnar, and Rothbard, 1992; and Mechanic and Aiken, 1988, for summaries of other managed care initiatives.) In the quest to control costs and improve programs, state governments may follow Colorado's example and consider managed care programs for mental health services and other special Medicaid populations.

The Unique Role of State Governments

On the most general level, Medicaid, like Medicare, is a social insurance program (Folland, Goodman, and Stano, 1993). That is, the government insures individuals in the Medicaid program because the private market fails to do so. Enacted in 1965, Medicaid is a federal-state program that provides health insurance for low-income individuals (Shonick, 1995). The federal government establishes minimum benefit standards for specific categories of individuals and provides matching grants to the states. The federal government pays for 50 to 80 percent of state governments' Medicaid expenditures. The federal matching percentage is determined by a formula based on the per capita income of each state; poorer states get more matching funds. State governments determine their degreee of participation (that is, the categories of individuals included beyond those mandated) in the program and administer it. Individuals below a given income level are entitled to participate in the program.

Although Medicaid and Medicare are both social insurance programs, political scientists and welfare state theorists emphasize that Medicaid is also a social welfare program. Health insurance premiums for the very poor (including the severely mentally ill) are completely subsidized through federal and state taxes. Unlike Medicare, where premiums for the elderly are only partially subsidized through income transfers, most people who pay for the Medicaid program will never directly benefit (that is, receive support) from it. As a result, there is relatively weak public support for the Medicaid program (Cook and Barrett, 1992; Skocpol, 1992; Esping-Andersen, 1994).

The lack of public support for Medicaid has affected the program's operation. Most significantly, the rates state governments are willing to pay providers are relatively low. Although Medicaid adopted a fee-for-service reimbursement system to ensure that a separate-and-unequal system did not develop, Medicaid rates have proved insufficient to induce the majority of private providers to participate. Consequently, the primary burden of caring for Medicaid patients typically falls on the small number of providers who are willing to accept the rates. The combination of low rates and a limited number of providers has resulted in a host of problems. Freund (1984) termed this constellation of problems Medicaid Syndrome: restricted access leading to inappropriate utilization, inadequate quality of care, or both. The level of Medicaid funding varies quite markedly by state (see Chapter Ten). However, the problems with Medicaid are widespread and persistent. This is particularly true for Medicaid mental health services.

In short, governments' role in the Medicaid program has been to guarantee poor Americans health coverage. However, state governments also became heavily involved in service provision, because they could not attract sufficient numbers of private providers to participate in the program. State governments either provide services directly or through long-term contracts with a variety of public and private nonprofit providers. These are referred to as "safety net" providers because they are the place of last resort for those individuals unable to obtain health care elsewhere.

Formally, safety net providers are those providers legally required to provide health care for free or at reduced rates to those who cannot afford to pay. Informally, the safety net includes a broader array of health care providers and programs (Rovner, 1996). The array of providers and programs that make up the safety net include public hospitals, community health centers, clinics (migrant health, family planning, and rural health), the Ryan White AIDS program, health care programs for the homeless, and public health departments. Community mental health centers (CMHCs) could be included in this list as well. While they have been criticized for not adequately serving the needs of the severely and chronically mentally ill, they provide outpatient mental health services to many low-income individuals (Grob, 1994).

In Colorado, the majority of outpatient mental health services for Medicaid beneficiaries are provided by seventeen CMHCs and three specialty clinics with performance contracts from Colorado's Division of Mental Health.[1] All but one of the CMHCs are private nonprofit organizations that provide a broad range of outpatient mental health services to Medicaid and largely low-income clients in specified geographical regions (see Figure 11.1). A relatively small portion of outpatient services are provided by other private providers (such as therapists practicing in the community). Long- and short-term psychiatric inpatient services are provided through two state hospitals operated by the state (in K, Denver and R, Pueblo). Additional mental health services are provided in private facilities throughout the state, typically hospitals with inpatient psychiatric units or free-standing psychiatric facilities. Thirty states have similar delivery systems for mental health services (Frank and Gaynor, 1993; Lutterman, 1994).

If state governments wish to develop managed care programs for Medicaid, what authority do they have to do so? As noted

Figure 11.1. The Colorado Community

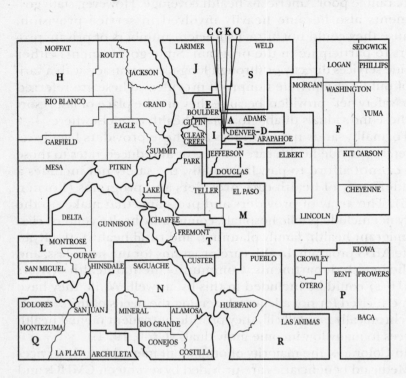

LEGEND

A. Adams County (except Aurora)

B. Arapahoe and Douglas Counties

C. Statewide (Specialty Clinic)

D. Adams/Arapahoe Counties

E. Boulder County

F. Logan, Sedgwick, Phillips, Yuma, Washington, Morgan, Elbert, Lincoln, Kit Carson, Cheyenne Counties

G. Statewide (Children's Hospital)

H. Moffat, Rio Bianco, Garfield, Mesa, Pitkin, Eagle, Grand, Jackson, Routt, Summit Counties

I. Jefferson, Clear Creek, Gilpin Counties

J. Larimer County

K. City and County of Denver

L. Gunnison, Delta, Montrose, San Miguel, Ouray, Hinsdale Counties

M. El Paso, Teller, Park Counties

N. Saguache, Mineral, Rio Grande, Alamosa, Conejos, Costilla Counties

O. Statewide (Specialty Clinic)

P. Crowley, Kiowa, Otero, Bent, Prowers, Baca Counties

Q. Dolores, San Juan, Montezuma, La Plata, Archuleta Counties

R. Pueblo, Huerfano, Las Animas Counties

S. Weld County

T. Fremont, Custer, Chaffee, Lake Counties

above, Medicaid is a joint program between the federal and state governments. As a result, certain program changes require approval from the federal government. States seek approval from the federal government to alter aspects of the Medicaid program by requesting a waiver.

In the Omnibus Reconciliation Act of 1981, the federal government granted states more flexibility in determining the scope of their Medicaid programs and setting spending levels. States were permitted to obtain waivers that required Medicaid beneficiaries to enroll in managed care plans and to develop alternative forms of managed care (section 1915b waivers). In addition, the Department of Health and Human Services permitted states, through section 1115 waivers, to develop statewide managed care systems that do not meet federal statutory requirements (Kaiser Commission on the Future of Medicaid, 1995; Physician Payment Review Commission, 1995). (See Chapter Ten for a discussion of the similarities and differences between sections 1915b and 1115 waivers and their prevalence in the states.) To date, most of these waivers have been for medical services for beneficiaries of the Aid to Families with Dependent Children (AFDC) program and low-income pregnant women and have not included mental health services.

The federal government is proposing further changes to the Medicaid program that would give states increased control over it. Medicaid reform proposals currently before the House and Senate would convert Medicaid from a federal entitlement to a block grant to states and would provide broader flexibility to states to determine coverage and benefits. In addition, the legislation would cap federal contributions to Medicaid and reduce projected federal expenditures by $182 billion from 1996 to 2002, a 19 percent reduction from baseline spending projections (Kaiser Commission on the Future of Medicaid, 1995).

While most states favor block grants, this type of reform increases the pressure on state governments to develop programs that control costs. The ability of state governments to successfully develop and implement managed care programs will in part be affected by the actions of state legislators and various state agencies. Actions by state governments are critical because they have a unique power to affect transactions among organizations.[2]

There are two unique ways in which state governments affect transactions among organizations. The first is by specifying what types of negotiations and exchanges can legally occur. State governments (in addition to the federal government) are the only agents with the institutional authority to determine the rules that govern transactions among organizations. In essence, they determine the "rules of the game" through policy and regulation. A shorthand way to acknowledge the special character of state government is simply to say that it exercises authority over other organizations (Lindblom, 1977).

The second way state government affects transactions among organizations is by directly engaging in transactions with them, extracting resources from some and providing resources to others. Along with defining and regulating economic transactions, state governments also participate in them through taxation, subsidies and grants, or the purchase of products and client services (Campbell, Hollingsworth, and Lindberg, 1991).

Because state government has these unique roles, organizations attempt to ensure that their concerns and interests are represented when laws are being formulated, implemented, or revised. As legislation is developed, organizations can testify before legislative committees, lobby, mobilize other groups, and so on. As legislation is implemented, organizations can attempt to shape program design and influence the interpretation of specific rules and the process and timing of implementation. Finally, when laws are enforced, organizations attempt to court the favor of administrative officials and seek expert legal counsel to help define and defend their interests through litigation. Ultimately, the government must "arbitrate" among competing organizations through the political and legal processes.

Because of the increased flexibility granted by the federal government, state governments will play a central role in restructuring Medicaid through managed care initiatives. Through legislation, state legislatures determine the general features of Medicaid managed care programs. After legislation is passed, state agencies are charged with further delineating key features of the program and ensuring their implementation. Given the central role of state governments in restructuring Medicaid programs, what strategies have they used to reduce costs without reducing access and quality through managed care programs?

General Managed Care Strategies

Managed care programs for Medicaid beneficiaries vary on many dimensions (see Chapter Ten; Freund and Hurley, 1995; Mechanic, Schlesinger, and McAlpine, 1995; Hurley, Freund, and Paul, 1993). However, I focus on two general strategies, and the approaches within them, for the purpose of highlighting their similarities and differences from an implementation and a policy perspective. The primary criterion for distinguishing the two strategies is whether the state government retains its role as an insurer (whether it continues to bear the risk and carry out insurance functions such as paying claims) or transfers this role to another entity (see Figure 11.2). If the state transfers the insurance function to another entity, it then becomes important to explore what kind of entity assumes that function and its relationship to traditional public providers.

State Government Finance and Traditional Public Provider Supply

The first general strategy states can employ is to retain the insurance function but to give traditional providers incentives to adopt managed care techniques. State governments can accomplish this task in two ways. The first is to use moderate financial incentives in conjunction with programs that attempt to better coordinate and integrate care. The most common example of this approach is case management, which includes primary care case management programs (PCCM), programs for physical health, and high-cost case management programs for mental health (see Surles, Blanch, and Shern, 1992; Chamberlain and Rapp, 1991, for a review of case management programs for mental health services).

In their simplest form, case management programs maintain the existing fee-for-service system but pay providers an additional case management fee to maintain treatment plans and coordinate care for Medicaid beneficiaries. Each beneficiary is assigned a primary care physician or case manager, who attempts to treat

Figure 11.2. General Managed Care Strategies.

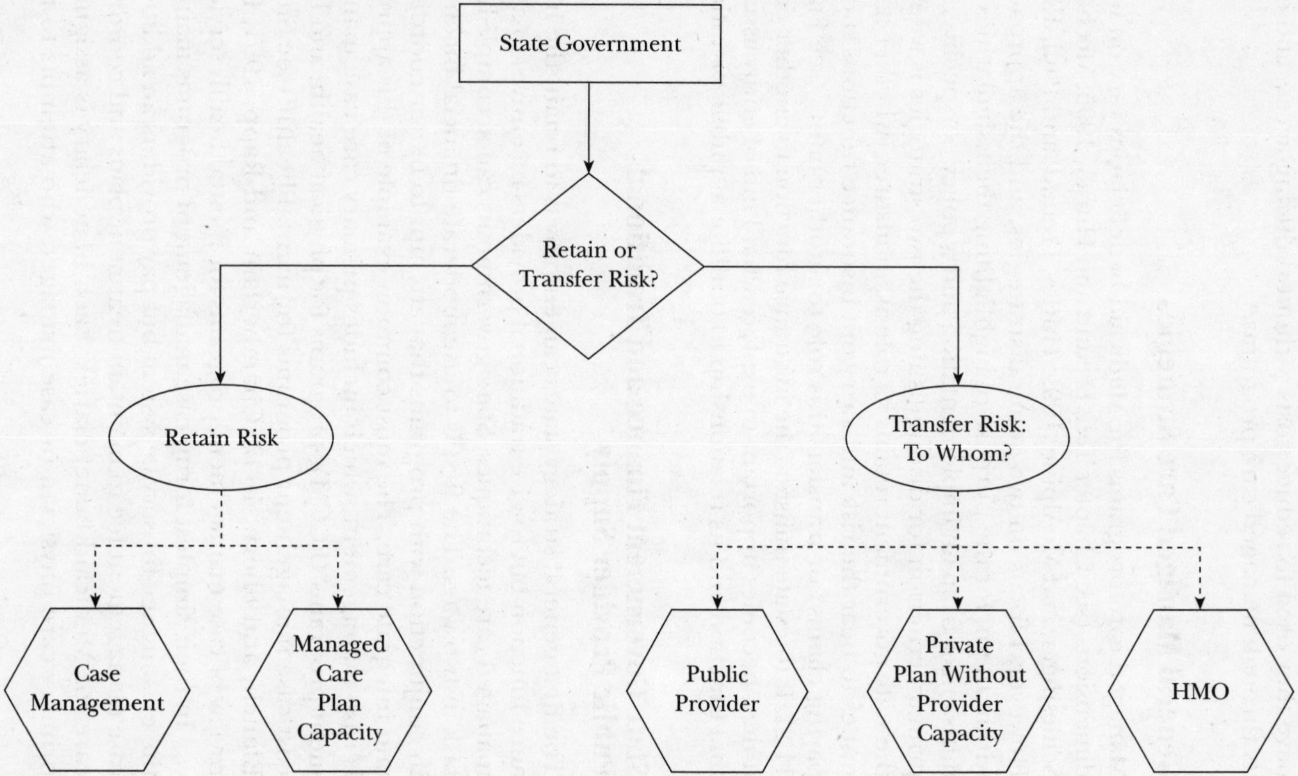

```
┌──────────────────┐
│ State Government │
└──────────────────┘
          │
          ▼
       ◇─────────◇
      │  Retain or  │
      │ Transfer Risk? │
       ◇─────────◇
       │          │
  ┌────┘          └──────────────┐
  ▼                              ▼
Retain Risk              ╭──────────────────╮
                         │ Transfer Risk:   │
                         │   To Whom?       │
                         ╰──────────────────╯
```

Retain Risk:
- Case Management
- Managed Care Plan Capacity

Transfer Risk: To Whom?
- Public Provider
- Private Plan Without Provider Capacity
- HMO

problems early and identify the most cost-effective level of care (for example, by avoiding emergency room visits for acute psychiatric episodes requiring inpatient admission). With this approach, a state government can reduce the overall costs of its Medicaid program while improving access and quality.

A case management program involves little change to the existing Medicaid system and is therefore relatively easy to implement. State governments and providers are not required to develop new financial mechanisms or organizational structures to operate the program. In addition, providers can readily take on the new case management function. PCCM programs are the most dominant type of managed care program for Medicaid beneficiaries' physical health and have also been extensively used for mental health services (Kaiser Commission on the Future of Medicaid, 1995; Mechanic, Schlesinger, and McAlpine, 1995).

The second way a state government can give traditional public providers incentives to adopt managed care techniques is for the state itself to function as a managed care plan. In this case the government retains the insurance function but works with Medicaid providers to develop and implement managed care techniques. For example, a state government could develop utilization management expertise, preauthorizing inpatient visits, certifying providers, conducting concurrent review, and so on. While never tried at the state level, several counties have developed managed care plans. Hennepin County, Minnesota, formed a county-owned health maintenance organization (HMO) ten years ago as a mechanism for insuring patients on public assistance and strengthening services at Hennepin County Medical Center (Bluford, 1994). More recently, Lancaster County, Pennsylvania, developed a community health plan for Medicaid beneficiaries, including those in need of mental health services (Montesano, 1995).

This approach involves great change for government. State governments have to develop managed care plan capability and educate providers about utilization management techniques. Despite the challenges, there are advantages to this type of program. The major advantage is that the entity ultimately accountable for insuring the poor is operating the plan. The job of writing contracts and monitoring plan performance is costly (particularly for mental health services, where outcomes are difficult to measure). A second advantage, although one vigorously debated, is that public providers serve society more equitably than do private organizations (particularly for-profit organizations) and therefore should be utilized and maintained. While proponents of the public sector lack empirical data to document this claim, ideas about the relative merits of the public and private sectors typically play a role in debates about how state government should proceed (Clark, Dorwart, and Epstein, 1994).

While the second approach is rare, it warrants mention because it is a viable option for state governments to pursue. Of interest is why this alternative has not been used more extensively, a topic I discuss below.

State Government Contracts with Managed Care Plans

The second general strategy state governments can employ is to contract with managed care plans. In essence, state government transfers the risk and the insurance function to a number of plans. State governments do this by implementing full-risk, prepaid (that is, capitated) managed care programs. Plans are paid a fixed fee per beneficiary, per month, regardless of how many individual beneficiaries become ill.

Capitation programs also require a great deal of change for state government. As noted above, state governments must learn how to purchase managed care plan services. This involves many challenges—for example, the ability to select and contract with plans, to set rates, and to monitor access and quality. The private sector continues to struggle with carrying out these tasks.

In addition, contracting for insurance raises questions about the role of the state. In particular, who is ultimately accountable for insuring Medicaid beneficiaries? Publicly funded CMHCs already operate under a crude form of managed care in that they provide care under a global budget to a defined population in a specific area. However, is there something different about passing risk on to them? If state government ultimately remains accountable for the care of the poor, what is the advantage in contracting with plans?

There are several advantages in capitated programs for state governments. First, the cost of the Medicaid program is stabilized.

The state government can use stricter global budgets to transfer financial risk to another entity. If costs during that year are higher than anticipated, the plans assume the burden, not the state government. Second, besides reducing costs by transferring risk, the state government can often negotiate rates that are less than projected fee-for-service costs. To obtain a federal waiver to implement managed care programs, state governments must demonstrate that such programs will be budget neutral (Health Care Financing Administration, 1994). States typically reduce program costs by 5 percent, anticipating that savings from increased efficiency (for example, from reduced inpatient care) will offset the reduction in total funds (Freund and Hurley, 1995). Finally, capitation gives the strongest incentive to public providers to find better ways of managing care.

The disadvantage of capitated plans is that they may create incentives to reduce access and quality. When providers are capitated, they have an incentive to make conservative judgments when they are uncertain about whether a patient requires treatment. As a result, the state must be able to measure and monitor access to and quality of care.

If states select this strategy, the issue then becomes what kind of plan to contract with and whether to attempt to structure the managed care plan's relationship with traditional public providers.

Public Provider Plans

The issue of how to structure a managed care plan's relationship to public providers is avoided if the state contracts with them. In this case, public providers develop risk-bearing (or insurer) capacity. The addition of this capacity transforms public providers into publicly sponsored insurance plans similar in structure to group- or staff-model HMOs—the plan and provider organizations are tightly linked (that is, integrated through common ownership or exclusive contract arrangements).

Becoming a prepaid health plan requires a great deal of change for public providers. (See Christianson and Gray, 1994, on challenges for community mental health centers.) Public providers have to develop both insurer and utilization management capacity. In addition, they may have to enhance provider capacity to cover the entire continuum of care. This requires capital and managed care expertise, which many public providers lack.

Despite these challenges, public providers may be willing to participate in these programs for three reasons. First, they may believe that prepayment will improve the system, integrating the financing of care with its organization and delivery. Capitation programs place dollars directly into the hands of providers, which brings new resources and increased flexibility to develop innovative programs and services. Second, prepayment may be in public providers' best interests. Not only does it increase the total amount of funds over which they have control, it also maintains their organizational autonomy. Finally, public providers may be compelled to participate in managed care programs anyway. Private managed care firms are entering the Medicaid market, and states are increasingly interested in reducing costs. In this climate, public providers must compete with organizations that have greater managed care experience.

Private Plans Without Provider Capacity

The state can also contract with private plans that do not have provider capacity. This approach (especially when the plan is already operational) has several advantages for the state besides those noted above for capitated public plans. First, states may be able to implement the program more rapidly. Effectively functioning private plans may require less start-up time. Second, since the plan already has developed a managed care infrastructure and expertise, it may be able to offer services more cheaply. In addition, bundling public beneficiaries with large numbers of private enrollees may allow private plans to negotiate for better rates from providers.

In this case (as with HMOs, which I discuss below), the state must decide whether to allow plans to subcontract with public providers as they choose or to require them to form partnerships with public providers. States' decisions in this area vary, with some states actively structuring the relationship between traditional providers and others adopting a more free-market approach. I will discuss factors states may consider when making such a decision after completing my description of strategies.

HMOs

The third approach states may employ is to purchase services from private managed care plans that have comprehensive service delivery networks—that is, HMOs. The appeal of this approach is obvious. The state contracts with a single organization that is capable of insuring and providing services to Medicaid beneficiaries. In addition, Medicaid beneficiaries would no longer be treated in a separate system but instead would be mainstreamed into private managed care plans, as the program's designers originally intended.

In theory this approach seems ideal. In reality, however, serious questions remain. First, why is managed care now viewed as the mainstream standard? Many Americans remain in fee-for-service indemnity plans. Although fee-for-service coverage is unlikely to continue, the major growth in managed care plans is in less restrictive plans that allow individuals to go outside the plans for an additional fee (see the Preface to this volume). Medicaid beneficiaries will not be able to exercise that option. Second, it is not clear that Medicaid beneficiaries will truly be mainstreamed. Just because an organization treats multiple groups does not mean that differences in care have been eliminated. Differences in care can be found inside organizations as well as between separate organizations. Third, Medicaid beneficiaries may have even more difficulty in large managed care organizations that may be unaccustomed to their problems and insensitive to their needs. Finally, as with private plans, HMOs may be likely to exit the market if rates do not remain high enough to cover their costs and produce a reasonable return on their investments (see Chapter Ten; Freund and Hurley, 1995).

Factors Affecting Strategy Selection

What determines the type of strategy, and specific approach, a state will pursue? Research on Medicaid managed care for physical health indicates that the cost savings of PCCM programs are comparable to those found in HMOs (Freund and Hurley, 1995). In addition, the impact of prepayment on the severely mentally ill population is just beginning to accumulate. Finally, it is not clear from experience to date that implementing capitated programs can occur more quickly than developing other types of managed care programs.

Given insufficient data to suggest the superiority of one of these strategies and attendant approaches over another, what factors affect a state government's strategy selection? I argue that, besides the desire to try some new means of addressing long-standing difficulties, market and political forces ultimately determine which strategy a state pursues.

Stabilization of costs has become the primary objective of state governments. As a result, capitated programs are very attractive. However, capitation strategies cannot be pursued unless there are organizations capable of assuming the insurance role. Clearly market forces are important, because they determine the range, and supply, of alternatives. Increasing competition for managed care enrollees in the private sector has resulted in new organizations' becoming interested in the Medicaid market. In 1994 there were 340 health plans that provided managed care services to Medicaid beneficiaries. Almost two thirds of these plans were HMOs or health-insuring organizations (HIOs) capable of accepting capitated payment (Kaiser Commission on the Future of Medicaid, 1995). Similarly, Medicaid is becoming attractive to the largest managed behavioral health care firms, most of which are for-profit (Oss, 1995).

If private market alternatives exist, state legislatures and agencies must determine in the policy formulation and implementation stage which strategy to pursue. Four factors may affect states' decisions in this area. The first is whether state governments believe that traditional public providers have developed any distinctive competence in working with the Medicaid population (that is, poor individuals who often have additional difficulties, such as poor housing, limited transportation, unstable families or minimal family contact, poor education, and so on). The second factor is what state governments believe are the relative merits of nonprofits and for-profits. For example, nonprofits may be viewed as less likely to shift difficult cases elsewhere, and for-profits may be viewed as more efficient. The third factor is whether, and for how long, state governments believe private plans will stay in the Medicaid market. The public infrastructure has been developed because governments cannot easily compel private firms to remain in the market. The fourth factor is who should shape the relationship between traditional public providers and newly entering plans: the private plans themselves or the government? State governments' assessments of these four factors, both in the short term and in the long term, are likely to affect the choices they make.

While it is often difficult to assess states' views of the first three factors, every state that designs and implements a managed care program makes a decision about the fourth factor. State governments have some discretion to shape the relationship between traditional public providers and entering plans, although they may be constrained by federal and state procurement laws and the federal waiver process. In particular, state and federal procurement laws may require the bidding process to be open, fair, and competitive and hence would require modification to exempt specific requests for proposals (RFPs). In addition, federal waiver rules stipulate that the bidding process must be open, fair, and competitive. However, sole-source contracts can be awarded if justified by the state.

As alluded to earlier in this chapter, there are several grounds on which state government could justify (particularly in the short term) protecting traditional public providers by awarding them sole-source contracts or by actively structuring their relationship to entering plans. Chief among them are the maintenance of a public safety net, a smooth transition from one service system to another, and a lack of information about the impact of increased competition on the public mental health and social service system. In addition, it could be argued that such a transition period may ultimately promote greater competition. When prepayment strategies are selected, the major criterion for assessing organizations becomes managed care insurance capability. Since public providers have been required to operate under a fee-for-service system, they typically have been unable to develop significant managed care experience. If they are required to compete without protections in the short run, they may not be selected and ultimately may be severely weakened. Conversely, private plans may enjoy what economists call "first mover" advantage. This raises concerns not only about the maintenance of a public safety net but also about the number of managed care organizations willing and able to compete in the long run.

Grounds for not protecting traditional public providers stem from market theory. According to the theory, markets (or, in this case, an open, fair, competitive bidding process) will result in the most efficient delivery of services. In addition to its interest in ensuring services for a vulnerable population, government has an interest in delivering services efficiently. Existing providers are not necessarily the most efficient; therefore, it is important to consider other organizations and assess them on their merits. Moreover, it could be argued that private managed care organizations should be free to structure their relationship with providers in any way they see fit as long as they comply with program requirements. In short, the relationship between traditional public providers and newly entering plans can be viewed as a business decision that each firm should be allowed to make independently. Finally, as noted above, federal and state procurement rules may require that the bidding process be open, fair, and competitive. Protecting traditional public providers through a sole-source contract or structured relationship can be viewed as unfair and anticompetitive. As a result, the government has to have strong reasons for excluding any given class of organization from the competitive bidding process.

Perhaps unlike any other institution, state agencies are faced with the difficult task of balancing potentially competing objectives (equity and access versus efficiency). With respect to mental health, several states (for example, Utah and Tennessee) have awarded sole-source contracts to existing community providers. However, there have been challenges to these contracts. For example, in Tennessee the state attorney general is conducting an investigation into a group of community mental health centers to determine whether they violated antitrust laws. Antitrust laws prohibit price fixing or efforts to eliminate competition. The investigation is in part a response to claims from a competitor that the centers sought to be the exclusive providers of case management services in ninety-three of the state's ninety-five counties (Cheeks, 1996). The strategies state governments choose in the future may be shaped by the outcome of such legal cases, in addition to the three factors noted above. At present, the general political climate in the United States is oriented toward reducing government involvement in social programs and relying more heavily on competitive market forces (Chapter Ten; Balz and Brownstein, 1996). Consequently, those approaches that involve relatively less government intervention and greater competition may be favored.

In Colorado, market changes stimulated a variety of organizations to consider alternatives to the existing fee-for-service system. As with other Medicaid programs, the cost of the Medicaid program in Colorado was rapidly rising. It grew overall by 19 percent annually from 1988 to 1993. From 1990 to 1991, mental health expenditures grew 28 percent, from $53.7 million to $69.4 million (Colorado Department of Institutions, Division of Mental Health, 1992, p. 13; Colorado Department of Social Services, 1993, p. 1).

In addition to responding to rising costs, the Division of Mental Health and the CMHCs felt that a prepaid, capitated program was the best way to address problems within Colorado's mental health system—in particular, the lack of coordination among different segments of the mental health and social services system and the prevalent use of inpatient care. In fiscal year 1991–92, most expenditures were for inpatient care (30.4 percent of expenditures for general hospitals, 20.9 percent for state hospitals, and 3 percent for under-twenty-one psychiatric facilities and inpatient care facilities designated for children). The remaining 45.7 percent was spent on outpatient care in CMHCs and offices of other private providers, accounting for 42.0 percent and 3.7 percent, respectively (Bloom and others, 1994b).

Finally, the state was considering a capitated program for physical health (Graham, 1996). Since 1983, the state had had a PCCM program for AFDC and low-income pregnant women. From the beginning of this program there was a provision stating that if a beneficiary's physician joined a Medicaid HMO, the beneficiary had to follow the physician into the plan or switch to a new physician. The rationale for this provision was to minimize risk selection. This was not much of an issue, however, because for many years there was only one Medicaid HMO in the state, and fewer than 5 percent of Medicaid beneficiaries were enrolled in it.

Mental health could have been included in this larger program. At least one other state (Minnesota) had piloted a capitated program in which beneficiaries with mental illness, including the chronically mentally ill, were rolled into HMOs. Although one of the larger participating plans (Blue Cross–Blue Shield) withdrew from the project after seven months due to adverse selection, no adverse affects on the chronically mentally ill were reported (see Lurie and others, 1992; Christianson and others, 1992). In the case of Colorado, if HMOs had been selected as the primary vehicle for the financing of mental health services, both the Division of Mental Health and the CMHCs might have lost autonomy. For the division, mental health program funds may have been placed under the control of the larger Medicaid agency. For the CMHCs, they would be farther down the Medicaid managed care "food chain," uncertain of their relationship to the plans.

In short, three key organizations—the state legislature, the Division of Mental Health, and the CMHCs—came to a consensus that a capitated program for mental health services was the best way to reduce costs while improving the mental health system. In May 1992 the state legislature passed House Bill 92–1306, requiring the state to design, implement, and evaluate a prepaid, capitated pilot program.

The Implementation Process

Other states' experience indicate that implementing Medicaid managed care programs is challenging. State governments tend to become more proficient at managed care program implementation over time, however (Freund and Hurley, 1995). Nevertheless, program implementation is still difficult. There are significant organizational and technical challenges that must be overcome.

Technical challenges include the new tasks and functions that must be carried out in order for managed care programs to operate—for example, the development of not only a managed care infrastructure (such as a management information system) but also the information and expertise needed to make informed decisions about a wide variety of program design issues. This may include designing managed care programs, setting rates, contracting for services, and measuring plan performance. Many of the technical challenges state agencies face are similar to those found in the private sector, although they may be heightened in the public sector (for example, the bidding process, rate setting, legal issues).

Organizational factors affecting policy implementation include the ability to carry out new tasks and functions. The ability of organizations to carry out new tasks depends not only on their financial and technical resources but also on their ability to change. As discussed above, some managed care strategies require more change than others.

Finally, technical decisions and organizational change occur simultaneously as part of the implementation process. In particular, there is a sequence of steps that occurs so that decisions made at one time can affect decision making later in the process. In addition, state governments are implementing programs rapidly, and this heightens the challenges of program implementation.

The remainder of this chapter illustrates the managed care implementation process and the technical and organizational challenges embedded in it, utilizing the early implementation experience of Colorado as a case study. As described above, legislation passed by the Colorado legislature defined two major features of the Medicaid managed care program for mental health services. The program would be a prepaid, capitated system, and the program would be pilot tested before being implemented statewide. The legislation did not, however, specify the strategy the state would pursue for implementation. A capitated program could be incorporated into any of the approaches described above (public plan, private plan without provider capacity, or HMO).

In other states, debate about the role of mental health in larger managed care initiatives has occurred at the policy formulation stage, resulting in a narrowing of program strategy alternatives. (See Chapter Ten for a discussion of mental health services in New York; see Speckman, 1992, and Bloom and others, 1994a, for a discussion of Utah's mental health capitation program.) However, in Colorado the legislature did not indicate who would be allowed to compete for capitation contracts or under what conditions. Consequently, the Division of Mental Health was chartered to further articulate and select the state's strategy, through a series of technical decisions concerning the delineation of key program design features and the bidding process.

Three documents produced by the Division of Mental Health in conjunction with other state agencies trace the evolution of this agency's thinking about the overall program strategy and about specific program design elements. The first document is a feasibility study submitted by the Division of Mental Health and the

Department of Social Services to the General Assembly on October 14, 1992. The second document is the waiver application the Colorado Department of Social Services submitted on July 20, 1993, to the Health Care Financing Administration (HCFA). This waiver was completed eight months after the feasibility study and was approved by HCFA three months later, on October 14, 1993. The third document is the actual RFP that the Division of Mental Health issued, on March 23, 1994. This RFP was issued seven months after the HCFA waiver application.

Who Can Compete?

The first thing a state agency must determine in developing a Medicaid managed care program is who can compete. Since the legislation did not restrict the options, the decision about whether mental health would be programmatically carved out or rolled into an HMO was left to the Division of Mental Health. The feasibility study introduced a new term, mental health assessment and service agencies (MHASAs), to broadly indicate the types of organizations that would be allowed to compete.[3] The Division let the competitive bidding process determine which organizations could serve as MHASAs.

What Are the Conditions for Competition?

Given that a variety of organizations could potentially compete for the contract, the Division had to decide the conditions under which organizations would compete. There are many conditions for participating in the program. Of most interest to the discussion in this chapter are the conditions under which new organizations entering the market would be permitted to work with traditional public providers.

There were two ways new organizations could enter the Medicaid market, which stipulated different conditions for working with traditional public providers. Bidders had to select one of two options.

Option 1 was to agree to *operate* the entire public mental health system in the geographical service area. This would include not only Medicaid services but also non-Medicaid public mental health services that CMHCs provide. New organizations entering the market under this option would in effect have to become CMHCs, accepting all the terms that current CMHCs operate under. As a result, the conditions under which newly entering plans had to work with existing CMHCs were fairly extensive. In particular, newly entering plans would be required to negotiate in good faith with existing CMHCs and describe in detail how they would assume the responsibilities of the currently operating center (Colorado Department of Institutions, Division of Mental Health, 1994b, p. 21).

Option 2 was to propose specific strategies for *coordinating* Medicaid and non-Medicaid services to achieve the state's goals. Under this option, newly entering organizations that wished to compete for Medicaid business had to articulate how they would coordinate services with CMHCs, which would continue providing non-Medicaid public mental health services. The main stipulation under Option 2 was that "The state expects that bidders choosing this option will gain the cooperation of the existing Community Mental Health Center(s) in the service area being proposed, in order to satisfactorily assure the State can deliver a coordinated mental health system" (Colorado Department of Institutions, Division of Mental Health, 1994b, p. 21).

The Division of Mental Health issued an addendum to the RFP in which it clarified what cooperation would entail. Non-CMHC bidders were not required to submit in writing (for example, through letter of intent, written agreement, subcontract agreement) that they had gained cooperation of the CMHCs. Bidders could earn the minimum required points in this area if the proposal contained strategies and procedures that the Evaluation Committee determined to be minimally acceptable and would be awarded additional points if the proposal included documentation of cooperation (Colorado Department of Institutions, Division of Mental Health, 1994a, pp. 19, 21).

All but one non-CMHC selected Option 2.

What Are Managed Care Organizations Competing For?

While state agencies are determining which organizations can compete and under what conditions, they also are considering what the organizations will be competing for: individual beneficiaries, geographical regions, or some combination of both. This decision is important for three reasons:

1. It affects the financial viability of the program—in particular, whether there are sufficient numbers of Medicaid beneficiaries for the program to be actuarially sound, overall and for any particular organization.
2. These programs have very different effects on beneficiaries. In the case where a single organization would compete for and be awarded a single geographical area, beneficiaries would only be allowed to change providers within a MHASA. If more than one agency were allowed to compete and receive a contract, beneficiaries would have a choice between organizations.
3. Finally, depending upon how state agencies attempt to deal with these problems, new challenges emerge. For example, when more than one organization is allowed to compete in a single area, state agencies have to monitor how plans are marketed to enrollees and whether one plan is getting favorable risk selection. If a single agency is awarded the contract, the state has to have mechanisms to monitor access and quality and reward performance in those areas (see Frank, McGuire, and Newhouse, 1996, on risk contracting).

Until the RFP was issued, it was not clear whether plans would compete for regions, beneficiaries, or some combination of both. It also was not clear until the RFP was issued how regions (or bidding areas) would be defined.

The feasibility study stated that MHASAs would compete for geographically defined regions and that enrollment would be mandatory in those areas included in the pilot program. However, the study did not define the geographical areas in which MHASAs would compete or if more than one MHASA would be allowed to function in a given area.

The HCFA waiver resolved the ambiguity about the definition of bidding areas, stating that the seventeen previously existing mental health service planning areas the CMHCs covered would be used. But it did not resolve the issue of the nature of competition for enrollees. The RFP clarified this issue, eliminating competition among MHASAs. MHASAs would compete for a bidding area. If one was selected through the bidding process, it would be the sole organization providing services in that area. In addition, the RFP reduced the number of bidding areas from seventeen to fifteen, combining three mental health service planning areas (areas A, B, and D in Figure 11.1). (The state combined these areas because the state database tracked beneficiaries by county. Since these three CMHCs served contiguous counties, they felt they would be unable to determine appropriate rates and accurately reimburse MHSAs.) Table 11.1 lists the bidding areas, the number of Medicaid eligibles in each, and the organizations competing for the area.

Providing What to Whom?

As discussed previously, the Colorado managed care program for mental health services covers inpatient and outpatient services for all Medicaid beneficiaries requiring mental health services. In general, three distinctive characteristics of mental illness may affect the way managed care mental health services are delivered (Mechanic, Schlesinger, and McAlpine, 1995). First, mental illness involves broad social costs borne by families, communities, and the legal system. Coordination between managed care organizations and these social institutions is critical for managed care to be effective. Second, mental illness is often a chronic condition. As a result, costs and utilization of services are likely to persist over time. This makes it difficult to measure the quality of care provided. Third, there is a stigma attached to mental illness. Not only does this increase people's fear of individuals with mental illness, it also makes it difficult for beneficiaries to advocate for their interests in a managed care system. Consumer advocacy may grow more important in the era of managed care.

Besides these general features of mental health services, when mental health services are "carved out" of broader health care services, there are new administrative and continuity-of-care challenges. For example, clarifying the benefits each plan covers (such as psychotropic medications) and mechanisms for coordinating care and referrals becomes increasingly important.

Table 11.1. Characteristics of Bidding Areas.

Bidding Areas	Medicaid Eligibles FY92 and FY93	Bidders
A, B, D	38,618 42,781	CMHC Alliance (Consortia C)
E	8,936 9,461	CMHC
F	6,146 6,714	CMHC
H	13,438 14,909	CMHC
I	15,409 16,664	CMHC
J	10,075 10,971	CMHC
K	57,902 63,895	Not allowed to participate due to prior legal ruling
L	4,783 5,220	CMHC, MBH
M	28,041 31,003	CMHC, MBH
N	7,552 8,443	CMHC, MBH
P	6,968 7,555	CMHC
Q	4,409 4,550	CMHC
R	22,743 24,137	CMHC, MBH, Hospital
S	10,995 12,239	CMHC
T	4,648 5,083	CMHC, MBH

How Much of the State Should Managed Care Organizations Be Allowed to Compete For?

This question is fundamentally about how rapidly state governments should implement new programs. The Division of Mental Health wanted to retain flexibility with respect to the number of geographical areas included in the pilot program. In particular, the state wanted to phase in the program according to the interest and ability of contract agencies and the state (Colorado Department of Institutions, 1992, p. 7; Colorado Department of Social Services, 1993, pp. 12–13). However, several sections of the feasibility study and HCFA waiver provide some insight into the original scope of the program. The feasibility study stated, "It is anticipated that perhaps four geographic areas of the state will be covered during the pilot phase" (Colorado Department of Institutions, 1992, p. 19). The HCFA waiver stated that the state would operate the program in a portion of the state (Colorado Department of Social Services, 1993, pp. 5, 13).

How Will Managed Care Organizations Compete?

Considering these other pieces of information, organizations decide how they will compete for the state's business. In addition, the state has to decide how to select organizations for contract awards.

Table 11.1 shows the variation in the size of the fifteen bidding areas. CMHCs in the smaller bidding areas realized that it might not be actuarially sound to accept full risk, given the total number of eligibles in the area and its historical penetration rates (that is, the percent of Medicaid eligibles receiving mental health services). In addition, they realized that they might not possess the financial resources to become mental health HMOs. As a result, seven CMHCs formed voluntary consortia to bid on the RFP. Four CMHCs formed a consortium largely in the southern portion of the state (Consortia A), and three others formed a consortium in the western portion of the state (Consortia B). Three other CMHCs that were in the mental health service planning areas combined by the state in the RFP formed a third consortium (Consortia C).

Table 11.2 shows the regions that comprise these consortia as well as the number of Medicaid eligibles they contained in FY 1993. Based on the geographic coverage of the consortia as well as the number of Medicaid eligibles, the advantages of forming consortia are clear. It reduced risk for individual centers (particularly small, rural centers), allowed CMHCs to combine and share resources (such as money, programs, and information systems), and capitalized on natural geographical boundaries. However, it also posed a challenge for state agencies, because it consolidated providers and bidding regions, resulting in fewer and larger bidding areas.

In addition to these voluntary consortia, a competing proposal for four of the areas participating in the two voluntary consortia was submitted by a private, for-profit managed behavioral health firm operating out of Virginia. Founded in 1986, MBH had limited experience with the Medicaid population. It had been involved in a Medicaid demonstration project in Florida, in which it joined with CMHCs to provide services in the Tampa Bay area (Florida's District 6 Medicaid population), but the program did not become operational until after Colorado's program began. Its managed behavioral health care experience was mostly with the military, state employees of Maryland and Massachusetts, and county employees in Fulton County, Georgia.

MBH bid on three of the regions in the Consortia A (N, R, T) area and one of the regions in the Consortia B (L) area. As Figure 11.1 indicates, the MBH bid split the other two consortia that were forming for the purpose of bid submission. In the Consortia B area, MBH bid on the middle region (L), isolating the other two (H, Q). In the Consortia A area, MBH bid on three of the four regions, excluding one (P). Along with its proposal for these four regions, MBH bid on two areas independently, M and R (see Table 11.1 and Figure 11.1).

The only other competing proposal was submitted by a community hospital with a large inpatient psychiatric unit. It bid for area R. In total, thirteen proposals were submitted: ten for independent regions (including competing proposals from MBH and the community hospital) and three for consortia covering multiple areas. All CMHCs submitted proposals, either independently

Table 11.2. Consortia Formation and the Pooling of Risk.

Name and Composition of Consortia	Medicaid Eligibles FY 93
Consortia A	
N	8,443
P	7,555
R	24,137
T	5,083
Consortia Total	45,218
Consortia B	
H	14,909
L	5,220
Q	4,550
Consortia Total	24,679
Consortia C [A, B, D]	42,781
MBH Bid [N, R, and T from Consortia A and L from Consortia B]	
N	8,443
R	24,137
T	5,083
L	5,220
Bidding Area Total	42,883

or through a consortium. The RFP specified the proper proposal format and the information to be contained in it.

Proposals were scored by an evaluation committee. Once the proposals were scored, the results were submitted to the Department of Human Services purchasing director. The purchasing director reviewed the scores and then submitted them to the Division of Mental Health. A management team from the Division of Mental Health and the Office of Health and Rehabilitation selected the awardees using the rules described in the RFP (Colorado Department of Institutions, 1994a, pp. 90–91).

Who Wins?

On January 3, 1995, the notices of intent to award contracts were announced. Table 11.3 summarizes the results of the initial bidding process. Every proposal submitted by MBH was initially chosen; its consortium proposal (which included one geographical area that it also bid on separately [area R]) and its proposal for the other single bidding area (M)were accepted. Nine bidding areas, and eleven former mental health regions, were capitated (four urban and five rural).

MBH won its contracts on the basis of its technical score and cost score. The committee scored its technical proposals high relative to most of the CMHC proposals. In addition, its cost proposals were consistently scored higher than any cost proposal submitted by a CMHC or CMHC consortia (that is, the price that it bid was consistently lower).

Two aspects of the award are noteworthy. First, approximately 60 percent of all Medicaid eligibles are included in the capitation program (see Table 11.3). Second, the state had awarded two contracts—and the majority of the geographical bidding areas included in the pilot program (five of nine)—to an out-of-state, for-profit provider. Twenty-eight percent of all Medicaid beneficiaries, and 48 percent of those included in the pilot program, would be covered by MBH contracts. This posed a major threat to the CMHCs. Not only might individual CMHCs have difficulty surviving as subcontractors, but MBH could potentially prevent the voluntary consortia from functioning and hence from competing in the future.

In response to the announcement, the CMHCs that lost the bid, together with the community hospital, filed an appeal with the Department of Administration, the agency responsible for purchasing, and contracting for, mental health services in the state of Colorado. The RFP directed bidders who wished to protest the process to appeal to this agency. There were multiple bases for the CMHCs' appeal. The Department of Administration did not view many of the CMHCs as reasonable or applicable, but it did rule that the evaluation process had been unfair due to a procedural issue.

Table 11.3. Capitated and Noncapitated Bidding Areas: Initial Awards Compared with Final Agreement.

INITIAL AWARD		NEGOTIATED AGREEMENT
CAPITATED		
A, B, D [Consortia C]		Same
E [CMHC]		Same
I [CMHC]		Same
M [MBH]		MBH-CMHC Joint Venture [Health Network]
S [CMHC]		Same
		MBH -Consortia A Joint Venture [Health Network]
N, R, T, and L [MBH Combined Bid]		MBH-Consortia B Joint Venture [Health Network]
TOTAL BIDDING AREAS CAPITATED	9	12
TOTAL MBH BIDDING AREAS	5	8
TOTAL CAPITATED ELIGIBLES	155,031	182,045
TOTAL MBH ELIGIBLES	73,886	100,900
NONCAPITATED		
F		Same
H		MBH-Consortia B Joint Venture [Health Network]
J		Same
K		Same
P		MBH-Consortia A Joint Venture [Health Network]
Q		MBH-Consortia B Joint Venture [Health Network]
TOTAL BIDDING AREAS NONCAPITATED	6	3
TOTAL MEDICAID ELIGIBLES NONCAPITATED	108,594	81,580
PERCENTAGE MEDICAID ELIGIBLES CAPITATED	58.8	69.1
PERCENTAGE MBH CAPITATED	47.7	55.4
MBH PERCENTAGE OF TOTAL STATE	28.0	38.3

Along with the appeal filed with the state, the CMHCs filed a lawsuit in civil court. (As discussed previously, legal battles are not unusual in the wake of contract award announcements; see Mayberg, 1995; Patullo, 1995; Ray, 1995.) Both the appeal and the lawsuit threatened to halt the implementation of the program, potentially requiring a reevaluation of the bids and delaying implementation. The state, however, was planning to move forward with implementation in the noncontested sites.

The CMHCs, Community Hospital, MBH, and the Division of Mental Health negotiated a settlement over the course of the next several months. Legally, MBH was awarded the contract, so the bidding process would not have to be repeated. As part of the settlement, however, MBH formed joint ventures with Consortias A and B and with the CMHC in area M, creating three limited-liability companies (referred to as Health Network). Finally, the community hospital became the provider of first choice for general, inpatient psychiatric care for area R.

This settlement had several important consequences. First, the number of areas included in the pilot program expanded. Under this new arrangement, the number of areas increased from nine to twelve, and the number of beneficiaries increased from 155,031 to 182,045 (see Table 11.3). Seventy percent of all Medicaid eligibles were now included in the pilot program. Second, the role of public providers was significantly changed. The settlement resulted in the CMHCs' becoming partners with MBH, as opposed to being subcontractors to it. Finally, the settlement led to unique organizational arrangements. What exists presently is a diversity of mental health finance and delivery structures with different degrees of financial and delivery integration: freestanding CMHCs, consortia, and joint ventures.

Conclusion

State governments are under enormous pressure to reduce the costs of their Medicaid programs. In addition, there are problems with existing Medicaid programs that state policymakers and providers believe managed care initiatives may improve. As a result, the states have pressed the federal government for more flexibility in administering the Medicaid program. One area in which states have pressed for increased flexibility is the use of managed care. Can state governments successfully borrow and implement managed care techniques developed in the private sector, becoming aggressive purchasers of managed care?

On the surface, the answer is a resounding yes. However, several assumptions underlie this belief, and on closer examination these assumptions prove to be more complex than anticipated. As I have discussed, state governments have a unique role in ensuring and providing care to the poor. Consequently, their ability to borrow managed care strategies will be constrained. In particular, state Medicaid reform initiatives are subject to political processes and must be balanced against other goals (access and equity).

Despite these constraints, state governments have a unique ability to shape managed care programs for public beneficiaries. Through their institutional and economic power, state governments are already shaping the emerging managed care market. As discussed, the two general strategies state governments can employ involve very different roles for state government and for traditional public providers. Market, political, and legal forces play a significant role in determining which strategy and approach state governments ultimately pursue. However, legal forces are increasingly playing a role. Two important policy questions emerge from this discussion.

First, should governments pass on financial risk to private entities? Clearly this is a financial strategy for reducing costs and providing incentives for organizations to alter inefficient patterns of care. But what implications does this strategy have for the government's social welfare role?

Second, to what extent should the public sector be buffered from market forces? On the one hand, many believe that traditional public providers are not operating efficiently (Clark, Dorwart and Epstein, 1994). On the other hand, those providers evolved because the government had difficulty compelling private firms to participate in the Medicaid program. Private plans are currently interested in the Medicaid market, but what are the long-term prospects of these firms' remaining in the market?

Finally, implementing managed care programs is challenging, involving many technical and organizational challenges. This is particularly true for new and innovative programs, like the one in

Colorado, that involve services for Medicaid beneficiaries with mental illnesses of varying severity. As discussed, the formulation of the managed care program for mental health services was in part precipitated by the anticipated entry of HMOs. A question for future research is how managed care initiatives for AFDC and low-income women will affect the development of programs for other populations. In addition, special populations, by definition, include a smaller subset of Medicaid eligibles with unique needs. If states select capitation as a strategy, the smaller number of eligibles in a special population may result in the emergence of several competing large plans or providers. In this case, monitoring contracts and plan performance becomes even more important. In general, the distinctive features of mental illness increase the need for state agencies to develop more effective means of monitoring access, measuring quality, and ensuring consumer advocacy. These challenges are not intractable. However, they do suggest that the path to success will require the best technical, organizational, and policy expertise available.

Notes

1. The Division of Mental Health was reorganized and renamed during the implementation of the managed care legislation. However, throughout this chapter I refer to the Division of Mental Health because during the period discussed here the division was primarily responsible for implementing the capitation pilot program.

2. Readers generally interested in sociological perspectives on the role of government in the economy or the role of the welfare state in the economy are referred to Block (1994) and Esping-Andersen (1994), respectively.

3. The actual term used was coordinated assessment and service agency (CASA), but this was later changed to mental health assessment and service agency (MHASA).

References

Balz, D., and Brownstein, R. *Storming the Gates: Protest Politics and Republican Revival.* Boston: Little, Brown, 1996.

Block, F. "The Role of the State in the Economy." In N. J. Smelser and R. Swedberg (eds.), *The Handbook of Economic Sociology.* Princeton, N.J.: Princeton University Press, 1994.

Bloom, J. R., and others. "An Analysis of Capitation for Mental Health Services." *Policy Studies Journal,* 1994a, *22*(4), 681–691.

Bloom, J. R., and others. *Colorado's Capitation Plan: An Analysis of Capitation for Mental Health Services.* Working Paper no. 1–94. Berkeley, Calif.: Institute for Mental Health Services Research, 1994b.

Bloom, J. R., and others. "Colorado's Medicaid Capitation Demonstration Project and Its Implementation." In K. Wittemore (ed.), Current State Policies for Mental Health Services. Des Moines: Greenwoood, 1996.

Bluford, J. W. "A Public-Sector HMO in a Competitive Market: Ensuring Equity for the Poor." *Journal of Health Care for the Poor and Underserved,* 1994, *5*(3), 192–198.

Campbell, J. L., Hollingsworth, J. R., and Lindberg, L. N. (eds.). *Governance of the American Economy.* New York: Cambridge University Press, 1991.

Chamberlain, R., and Rapp, C. A. "A Decade of Case Management: A Methodological Review of Outcomes Research." *Community Mental Health Journal,* 1991, *27,* 171–188

Cheeks, D. "Mental Health Group Facing Antitrust Probe." *The Tennessean,* June 11, 1996, p. A1.

Christianson, J. B., and Gray, D. Z. "What CMHCs Can Learn from Two States' Efforts to Capitate Medicaid Benefits." *Hospital and Community Psychiatry,* 1994, *45*(8), 777–781.

Christianson, J. B., and others. "Use of Community-Based Mental Health Programs by HMOs: Evidence from a Medicaid Demonstration." *American Journal of Public Health,* 1992, *82*(6), 790–798.

Clark, R. E., Dorwart, R. A., and Epstein, S. S. "Managing Competition in Public and Private Mental Health Agencies: Implications for Services and Policy." *Milbank Quarterly,* 1994, *72*(4), 653–678.

Colorado Department of Institutions, Division of Mental Health. *Capitating Medicaid Mental Health Services in Colorado: A Feasibility Study.* Denver: Colorado Department of Institutions, 1992.

Colorado Department of Institutions, Division of Mental Health. *Request for Proposals, Amendment No. 2.* Denver: Colorado Department of Institutions, 1994a.

Colorado Department of Institutions, Division of Mental Health. *Request for Proposals: Colorado Medicaid Mental Health Capitation and Managed Care Program.* (RFP# SF402015) Denver: Colorado Department of Institutions, 1994b.

Colorado Department of Social Services. *Colorado Medicaid Mental Health Capitation and Managed Care Program: Request for Federal Waivers.* Denver: State of Colorado, 1993.

Cook, F. L., and Barrett, E. *Support for the Welfare State: The Views of Congress and the Public.* New York: Columbia University Press, 1992.

Coughlin, T. A., Ku, L., and Holahan, J. *Medicaid Since 1980: Costs, Coverage, and the Shifting Alliance Between the Federal Government and the States.* Washington, D.C.: Urban Institute Press, 1994.

Dangerfield, D., and Betit, R. L. "Managed Mental Health Care in the Public Sector." *New Directions for Mental Health Services,* no. 59. San Francisco: Jossey-Bass, 1993.

Esping-Andersen, G. "Welfare States and the Economy." In N.J. Smelser and R. Swedberg (eds.), *The Handbook of Economic Sociology.* Princeton, N.J.: Princeton University Press, 1994.

Folland, S., Goodman, A. C., and Stano, M. *The Economics of Health and Health Care.* New York: Macmillan, 1993.

Frank, R. G., and Gaynor, M. "State Government Choice of Organizational Structure for Local Mental Health System: An Exploratory Analysis." *Advances in Health Economics and Health Services Research,* 1993, *14,* 181–196.

Frank, R. G., McGuire, T. G., and Newhouse, J. P. "Risk Contracts in Managed Mental Health Care." *Health Affairs,* 1996, *14*(3), 50–64.

Freund, D. A. *Medicaid Reform: Four Studies of Case Management.* Washington, D.C.: American Enterprise Institute Press, 1984.

Freund, D. A., and Hurley, R. E. "Medicaid Managed Care: Contributions to Issues of Health Reform." *Annual Review of Public Health,* 1995, *16,* 473–495.

Graham, J. "The Medicaid Dilemma: Switch to HMOs Leaves Poor in Flux." *Denver Post,* Feb. 4, 1996, p. 1.

Grob, G. N. "Government and Mental Health Policy: A Structural Analysis." *Milbank Quarterly,* 1994, *72*(3), 471–500.

Hadley, J. R., Schinnar, A., and Rothbard, A. "Managed Mental Health in the Public Sector." In S. Feldman (ed.), *Managed Mental Health Services.* Springfield, Ill.: Charles C. Thomas, 1992.

Health Care Financing Administration, Department of Health and Human Services. "Medicaid Program: Demonstration Proposals Pursuant to Section 1115 (a) of the Social Security Act; Policies and Procedures." *Federal Register,* 1994, *59*(186), 49249–49251.

Hurley, R. E., Freund, D. A., and Paul, J. E. *Managed Care in Medicaid: Lessons for Policy and Program Design.* Ann Arbor, Mich.: Health Administration Press, 1993.

Kaiser Commission on the Future of Medicaid. *Medicaid and Managed Care: Lessons from the Literature.* Washington, D.C.: Kaiser Commission on the Future of Medicaid, 1995.

Kennedy, C., and Manderscheid, R. W. "SSDI and SSI Disability Beneficiaries with Mental Disorders." In R. W. Manderscheid and M. A.
Sonnenschein (eds.), *Mental Health, United States, 1992*. Department
of Health and Human Services pub. no. SMA 94–3000. Washington,
D.C.: U.S. Government Printing Office, 1994.

Lindblom, C. E. *Politics and Markets*. New York: Basic Books, 1977.

Lurie, N., and others. "Does Capitation Affect the Health of the Chronically Mentally Ill?" *Journal of the American Medical Association*, 1992,
267, 3300–3304.

Lutterman, T. C. "The State Mental Health Agency Profile System." In
R. W. Manderscheid and M. A. Sonnenschein (eds.), *Mental Health,
United States, 1992*. Department of Health and Human Services pub.
no. SMA 94–3000. Washington, D.C.: U.S. Government Printing
Office, 1994.

Manderscheid, R. W., and Sonnenschein, M. A. (eds.) *Mental Health,
United States, 1992*. Department of Health and Human Services pub.
no. SMA 94–3000. Washington, D.C.: U.S. Government Printing
Office, 1994.

Mayberg, S. "Causes and Effects of Litigation in Medicaid Managed
Behavioral Healthcare Ventures." *Behavioral Healthcare Tomorrow*,
1995, *4*(2), 40–43.

Mechanic, D., and Aiken, L. (eds.). *Paying for Services: Promises and Pitfalls
of Capitation*. New Directions for Mental Health Services, no. 43. San
Francisco: Jossey-Bass, 1988.

Mechanic, D., Schlesinger, M., and McAlpine, D. D. "Management of
Mental Health and Substance Abuse Services: State of the Art and
Early Results." *Milbank Quarterly*, 1995, *71*(1), 19–55.

Mechanic, D., and Surles, R. C. "Challenges in State Mental Health Policy and Administration." *Health Affairs*, 1992, *11*(3), 34–50.

Montesano, M. T. "Managing Medicaid: Community Plan Finding Success in Lancaster." *Pennsylvania Medicine*, 1995, *98*(9), 18–20.

Oss, M. "More Americans Enrolled in Managed Behavioral Care: Annual
Market Share Survey Reports an Increase in Managed Behavioral
Health Enrollees in 1994." *Open Minds*, 1995, *8*(12), 12.

Patullo, W. "Is Believing You Have a Case a Good Enough Reason to Sue?"
Behavioral Healthcare Tomorrow, 1995, *4*(2), 40–47.

Physician Payment Review Commission. *Annual Report to Congress*. Washington, D.C.: Physician Payment Review Commission, 1995.

Ray, C. "Casualties of Litigation: Trust, Credibility, Political Equilibrium,
Cost-Effectiveness." *Behavioral Health Care Tomorrow*, 1995, *4*(2),
40–47.

Rovner, J. "The Safety Net: What's Happening to Health Care of Last Resort?" *Advances,* 1996 (Special Suppl. no. 1).

Shonick, W. *Government and Health Services: Government's Role in the Development of U.S. Health Services, 1930–1980.* New York: Oxford University Press, 1995.

Skocpol, T. *Protecting Soldiers and Mothers: The Political Origins of Social Policy in the United States.* Cambridge, Mass.: Harvard University Press, 1992.

Speckman, Z. *The Medicaid Experiment: Utah's Prepaid Mental Health Plan.* Salt Lake City: Utah Department of Health, 1992.

Steinwachs, D. M., Kasper, J. D., and Skinner, E. A. "Patterns of Use and Costs Among Severely Mentally Ill People." *Health Affairs,* 1992, *11,* 178–185.

Surles, R. C., Blanch, A. K., and Shern, D. L. "Case-Management as a Strategy for Systems Change." *Health Affairs,* 1992, *11*(1), 151–163.

Chapter Twelve

Messing with Medicare

Markets and Politics in the 104th Congress

John D. Wilkerson

The federal government is a major purchaser of health care services. In 1994 the Medicare and Medicaid programs alone accounted for nearly one-third of all health care spending in the United States and more than 17 percent of all spending by the federal government. Whereas real spending in other major areas, such as defense, has remained level or declined in recent years, spending on Medicare continues to increase at a rate of 10 percent per year. As tens of millions of Baby Boomers begin to enter the program around 2010, the cost of the program promises to rise even more dramatically.

Medicare reform was not a priority among Republican candidates in the 1994 election season, but it was clear to political insiders that other promises made in the campaign could not be kept without making substantial reductions in future Medicare spending. Democrats believed that Republicans had backed themselves into a corner, and they looked forward to returning the licking they had received in the court of public opinion during their own health care reform effort. An opportunity for Republicans to avoid such a licking occurred in April 1995, when Medicare trustees reported that the hospital trust fund (Part A of Medicare) would run out of money by 2002. Congressional Republicans "seized" on this report as a way to reframe the debate from one in which they would be accused of cutting a popular program to pay for tax cuts and reduce the deficit to one where they would be seen as attempting to save a popular program from imminent bankruptcy (Rosenbaum, 1995c).

Short-term cost control is the primary goal of the proposed congressional reforms to the Medicare program. The $270 billion in projected savings was based on what House Republicans needed to balance the federal budget in seven years while reducing taxes, rather than what was needed to restore the hospital trust fund to solvency ($90 billion) (Rosenbaum, 1995b). The reforms would introduce a much wider range of private health plan options for enrollees. Any insurer that is willing to accept a fixed payment per enrollee from the government and that meets state-mandated standards would be eligible to offer its services to Medicare enrollees. And health plans could offer cash rebates to enrollees who choose limited coverage, in addition to charging supplemental premiums for increased flexibility or more comprehensive benefits.

Proponents argue that these changes will "save and strengthen" the Medicare program by introducing the efficiency gained through market competition (Horn, 1995, p. 1). However, the reforms also include provisions that would dramatically alter the structure and purpose of the program over the long term, moving it away from an entitlement program providing mainstream health care services and toward an income-subsidy or voucher program with much greater variation in access, coverage, and quality of care. The Republican reforms would put the federal government in a better position to limit Medicare spending, but they are being promoted with deceptive claims about their real effects.

Background

Medicare provides health care coverage for approximately 34 million Americans sixty-five years of age or older and approximately 5 million disabled younger Americans (Health Care Financing Administration, 1995, p. 47). The program is divided into two parts that correspond roughly to insurance coverage for inpatient hospital care (Part A) and for outpatient physician services (Part B). Inpatient care accounts for about two thirds of the approximately $160 billion in current program spending (Health Care Financing Administration, 1995, p. 243). In the absence of major reform, total Medicare spending is expected to rise to about $340 billion by 2002 (Rosenblatt, 1995).

The two parts of the program are financed differently. All workers are required to participate in Part A by contributing 1.45 percent of their wages to it; this contribution is matched by their employers. These contributions are directed to a trust fund that finances the program. Individuals can choose not to participate in Part B. If they do choose to participate (more than 90 percent do), they must pay a monthly premium while they are receiving benefits (Health Care Financing Administration, 1995, p. 46). By law this premium is currently set at 25 percent of the program's costs. Because program costs have increased less quickly than projected in recent years, enrollee premiums currently cover 31.5 percent of costs (in 1994 the monthly premium was about $47). The remainder of Part B's costs are financed through general revenues. (For an excellent summary of program benefits and costs, see Davis and Burner, 1995.)

The divided structure of the Medicare program is easier to understand from a historical and political perspective than in terms of efficient health care delivery. In 1965 private health insurance primarily covered hospital services. Early Medicare proponents wanted to provide the elderly with "mainstream" health care coverage similar to what many employers were providing for their employees (Ball, 1995, p. 68). This was the purpose of Part A. The program's designers did not intend to provide coverage for physicians' services outside of hospitals, in part to avoid a confrontation with the American Medical Association (p. 68).

Part B was added to the program by House Appropriations Chairman Wilbur Mills, who hoped to use it to diminish seniors' expectations about what the government would provide (Marmor, 1973). Part B was originally intended to be a voluntary private insurance program that seniors could participate in if they wanted to be covered for outpatient physician services as well as inpatient care. Reformers soon discovered, however, that the costs of this insurance would be prohibitively high for older seniors unless younger seniors also participated (voluntarily). Government subsidies were introduced to lower the Part B premium to the point where younger seniors would also choose to participate (Ball, 1995).

Economists see health insurance as socially desirable because it provides peace of mind by reducing the risks of catastrophically high charges for an unexpected illness or accident. The Medicare program was originally envisioned as a limited insurance program. Only hospital services were targeted, because they tended to be the most financially catastrophic for the elderly (Fein, 1986, p. 63). Medicare enrollees had to make a substantial out-of-pocket payment before government reimbursement kicked in, and even then the government paid only part of all subsequent costs.

Today, most of the health insurance purchased in the United States is not the insurance of economic theory. It is "prepaid" health care—most enrollees expect that once they or their employer has paid the premium, they are entitled to be reimbursed for most or all of their health care expenditures. Medicare has also evolved over the past thirty years to become much more like prepaid health care and much less like the insurance described by economists. This has occurred incrementally, as additional benefits were added and as deductibles and premiums were not adjusted to keep pace with inflation and rising program costs. If today's enrollees were required to pay the same proportion of the costs of Part B as they were in the early years of the program, their annual deductible would be $1,000 rather than $100. Their annual premiums would be about $1,000 per year rather than about $600 (Davis and Burner, 1995, p. 232). In addition, most enrollees (89 percent) now have private or public supplemental insurance coverage that expands their Part A and Part B benefits and reduces their out-of-pocket expenses even further (p. 237).

The Politics of Medicare Reform in the 104th Congress

It is always misleading to refer to a group of individuals as having identical goals. Nevertheless, the proposed Medicare reforms can be best understood by assuming that members of the Republican congressional majority share three central goals: to promote an ideology of less government and increased individual responsibility, to promote the virtues of private market approaches to government programs, and to win reelection.

Reducing Government and Promoting Individual Responsibility

In many respects the current battle over Medicare is part of a larger ideological contest that has been under way for decades (Shonick, 1995; Fein, 1986). Conservatives are more likely to believe that individuals are responsible for their own circumstances. Liberals are more likely to believe that factors beyond individuals' immediate control have a great deal to do with their circumstances. As a result, many Republicans oppose entitlement programs not only because they redistribute wealth but also because they are thought to discourage individual responsibility and initiative.

The Republican reforms would create a precedent for varying individuals' Medicare payments according to their economic need. The overall cap on program spending would put beneficiaries and providers, rather than the government, at financial risk if program costs increased more quickly than expected. And because health care plans would not be required to provide the Medicare benefits package in exchange for government payments, all beneficiaries might eventually have to pay much more to maintain the benefits the government currently guarantees.

Promoting Efficiency Through the Market

Congressional leaders point out that after national health care reform failed, some large employers reduced their health care costs, but Medicare costs continued to rise. Many Republicans appear to believe that the Medicare program would benefit from an injection of market competition similar to what is seen in the private insurance market today. Some conservatives also believe that overuse of expensive services with small or no health benefits is an important source of health care inflation (Butler, 1996; Cutler, 1996).

The reforms would allow virtually any insurer to market its services to Medicare enrollees and would place few restrictions on the range of alternatives it could offer or the prices it could charge.

The government's payment would be fixed by law, but plans could compete on the basis of price (by offering cash rebates to enrollees) and on the basis of service (by offering more comprehensive benefits or provider choice).

Medicare beneficiaries would be encouraged to enroll in private managed care plans, which give insurers and providers a financial incentive to limit inappropriate utilizations, and to open medical savings accounts (MSAs), which are thought to give individuals a financial incentive to consider the costs of their care (Meyer, 1995; Pauly and Goodman, 1996). MSAs are also attractive to conservatives because consumers, rather than insurers or providers, decide whether a particular service is worth the cost.

Winning Reelection

In politics, ideas are of little consequence if one is not in a position to promote them. Congressional Republicans learned this lesson during their forty years of minority status in the House of Representatives. Although Medicare's biggest challenge will come when millions of Baby Boomers begin retiring around 2010, the focus of congressional efforts has been on reducing Medicare spending over the next seven years. This short-term focus stems from a campaign pledge that many Republican candidates took during the 1994 elections. The "Contract with America" promised lower taxes and a balanced budget without touching Social Security. Many congressional Republicans see their party's ability to meet these promises as central to their success in the 1996 elections.

With Social Security "off the table," members of the newly elected Republican majority knew that it would be extremely difficult to balance the budget and lower taxes without addressing the spiraling costs of the Medicare program. According to conservative writer David Brooks, they "went after" Medicare because "if you care about the deficit foremost, you go after the biggest programs first" (Weisskopf and Maraniss, 1996, p. 23). At the same time, Republicans were aware of the program's widespread popularity. In June 1995 House Speaker Gingrich predicted that if Republicans "solve Medicare, we will govern for a generation. If we don't, we're going to have a big fight next year" (McGinley, 1995a, p.

A18). Gingrich was referring, of course, to solving the *political* problem of tampering with one of the two untouchable social programs (the other being Social Security) (Clymer, 1995). His pollster, Frank Luntz, predicted that Medicare would be "a textbook case of political communications" (Hunt, 1995). Democrats predicted that Republicans had grabbed a tiger by the tail, and that it was now going to bite them.

Republican Strategy

Republican strategists considered a range of approaches to reducing the costs of the program without arousing the concerns of seniors, providers, and the public. Polls indicated widespread public support for the benefits of Medicare but also that many people believed that the program was too costly and in financial trouble (Blendon and others, 1995). Most seniors also believed that the program's troubles stemmed primarily from excessive charges by providers and from outright fraud rather than from an expanding Medicare population, overutilization, and increasingly expensive technologies. Although there was widespread opposition to cutting Medicare to reduce taxes or the deficit, there was also a widespread belief that these (desirable) goals could be achieved with cutting Medicare and that Medicare could be saved without raising the payroll tax or increasing premiums (Blendon and others, 1995, p. 1646; Rosenbaum, 1995a).

House Speaker Newt Gingrich (R-Ga.) and Senate Majority Leader Robert Dole (R-Kans.) first hinted that cuts in Medicare were on the table in early 1995 (Chen, 1995a; Rogers, 1995) and announced their intention to save Medicare from imminent bankruptcy in mid April. Neither chamber revealed any details of its proposed reforms until mid September, however. This long delay was due to the technical difficulty of achieving almost $300 billion in cost reductions while keeping an early pledge by Gingrich to do it "without significantly affecting anyone now enrolled in the program" (Wines, 1995). It was also due to a desire to keep the details out of the public spotlight for as long as possible (McGinley, 1995b). By law the 1996 budget had to be passed by October 1, the beginning of the next fiscal year. Republican leaders hoped that President Clinton would be forced to choose between compromising with the Republicans on a balanced budget bill (which included the Medicare reforms) and shutting the government down, before the sweeping Medicare changes became a public issue (Chen, 1995b).

Many, but not all, of the most visible features of the reforms adopted by Congress were consistent with public perceptions and attitudes (Hook, 1995). Enrollees could choose to remain in the fee-for-service program and would not be forced to join private managed care plans. The House bill was titled the Medicare Preservation Act of 1995, to underscore the Republicans' claim that the goal of the bill was to save Medicare rather than to fund tax cuts and deficit reduction. The compromise reached by the House and Senate specifically required that revenues from any increases in beneficiaries' Part B premiums go directly to the Part A trust fund.

Most of the savings came from reduced payments to fee-for-service providers rather than from higher out-of-pocket costs for enrollees or increased taxes on employers and employees. And when the Congressional Budget Office (CBO) estimated that the House proposal fell $80 billion short of its $270 billion goal, the House adopted a "fail-safe" provision that required the secretary of health and human services to impose additional, unspecified cuts in the future to meet the goal (Rosenbaum, 1995b). Congressional Republicans would later specify that any additional cuts would be borne by fee-for-service providers only.

The final bill did not increase deductibles or copayments. It did increase beneficiaries' Part B premiums, however. For 95 percent of enrollees, premiums would be about $20 per month more than projected under existing law by 2002. The richest beneficiaries would have to pay as much as 100 percent of costs. These premium increases have since become the focus of Democratic opposition.

The reforms also reflected efforts to win political and financial support—or at least reduce opposition—from organized interest groups, particularly those that had proven pivotal in the failure of health care reform during the 103rd Congress (1993–94). House leaders pursued a dual strategy of inviting a wide range of interests to present their views, while threatening to exclude the concerns of groups that sought to undermine their efforts (Chen and Rosenblatt, 1995). The most visible example of a concession occurred after the American College of Surgeons complained that the House reforms would reduce surgical payments by 10 to 12 percent the next year (Pear, 1995a). The day after Speaker Gingrich announced that he would revise the language so that physicians' payments would not decline, the American Medical Association announced that it was supporting the House bill (Pear, 1995b).[1] Additional provisions were not as easily characterized as quid pro quos, but they nonetheless represented important concessions to key players.

Some important interest groups were clear winners, such as large and small private insurers represented by the Health Insurance Association of America and the American Association of Health Plans (formerly the Group Health Association of America). The American Medical Association, on the other hand, lost many of the provisions that had led to its early support, including malpractice reform, antitrust waivers, and weaker financial solvency standards for networks organized by doctors. Although the American Association of Retired Persons complained that the cuts were "too much too soon," the reforms included provisions allowing it and other associations to market Medicare services to enrollees directly.

The Republican strategy was less successful publicly. The original threat of an impending Medicare "train wreck" appeared to backfire as Republican leaders' own words undermined their claim that the reductions were needed to save and strengthen the program. On October 24, 1995, in a speech before the American Conservative Union, Senate Majority Leader Dole said that he had been there "fighting the fight, voting against Medicare—one of twelve [legislators]—because we knew it wouldn't work in 1965." The next day, in a speech before a Blue Cross–Blue Shield conference, House Speaker Gingrich said that Republicans "didn't get rid of it in round one because we don't think that's politically smart and we don't think that's the right way to go through a transition. But we believe it's going to wither on the vine" (Vobejda and Harris, 1995).

By December, according to "pollsters on both sides, a substantial segment of defectors to the GOP in 1994 [were] drifting back to the Democratic fold in large part because of the Medicare debate" (p. 23). Ironically, the public appeared to oppose the

Republican reforms for the same reasons it had opposed President Clinton's Health Security Act and voted against Democratic incumbents in 1994. Although there was widespread agreement that something needed to be done, the public opposed both reforms because of a perception that they would lead to less choice, higher costs, and lower-quality health care.

Democratic Strategy

In October 1995 Congressional Democrats "wheeled out a 14-foot-high papier-mâché Trojan horse" to underscore their claim that the Republican reforms were not really intended to "preserve and protect" Medicare. At the same time, a senior Gingrich aide "paraded about with an eight-foot-tall ostrich—a living symbol, supposedly, of the Democratic head-in-the-sand refusal to save Medicare from bankruptcy" (Chen, 1995c, p. A1). More appropriate metaphors for the Republican and Democratic strategies would be hard to find.

In the first half of 1995 President Clinton proposed Medicare reforms that would have reduced future spending by almost $190 billion. By June he was proposing only $124 billion in reductions. By July Republicans were declaring the President "AWOL" during the budget process, and President Clinton was telling voters "I got the message in 1994, and I'm not going to let the government mess with your Medicare" (Richter and Rosenblatt, 1995).

This remarkable transition reflected a growing belief among Democratic politicians that Medicare could be the Republicans' Achilles' heel. In 1994 Republican strategist William Kristol had advised congressional Republicans to stop trying to work with Democrats on national health reform and to do everything possible to defeat it. In an ironic reversal, Democrats appeared to be pursuing the same strategy in 1995. In 1994 Majority Leader Dole had publicly doubted whether the health crisis that Democrats were trying to solve even existed. Democrats were now criticizing the Republicans for fabricating a Medicare crisis. In 1994 Representative Bill Archer (R-Tex.) was calling President Clinton's proposed $238 billion in Medicare reductions "cuts" that would "devastate . . . quality of care and availability of care" for the elderly

(Priest, 1995, p. C3). As chairman of the House Ways and Means Committee in 1995, Representative Archer authored the Medicare Preservation Act, which he claimed would "slow the growth" of Medicare spending by $270 billion over seven years.

While Republicans needed to persuade voters that Medicare cuts were not simply intended to make seniors pay for tax cuts for the rich, Democrats needed to counter the growing public perception that the entire Medicare program was about to go bankrupt and that Democrats were acting irresponsibly by not acknowledging it (hence the Trojan horse and the ostrich).

Details of the Medicare Preservation Act of 1995

The Medicare Preservation Act was included in a much larger appropriations bill, the Balanced Budget Act of 1995 (H.R. 2491).[2] The Republican reforms would reduce the rate of increase in projected Medicare spending from 10 percent to about 7 percent per year over the next seven years (Congressional Budget Office, 1995, p. 2). By 2002 spending would be 23 percent less than what it is currently projected to be (Gold, 1995). The CBO has said that this rate of increase would still allow for real growth in program spending (from increased use of services or more expensive services) after controlling for general inflation and enrollment increases (p. 22). That rate of growth would be much lower than it has been in the past, however.

Premiums, Deductibles, and Covered Benefits

The reforms would not increase beneficiaries' deductibles, and they maintain the Part B premiums at their current level of 31.5 percent of costs for all but the wealthiest 3 percent of enrollees (H.R. 2491, Section 8511).[3] Single persons earning more than $110,000, and couples earning more than $150,000, would be required to pay 100 percent of their Part B insurance coverage (H.R. 2491, Section 8512). The list of benefits covered by Medicare (and that all health care plans would be required to provide) would not be altered.

Fee-for-Service Medicare

House Speaker Gingrich claimed that he was referring to the Health Care Financing Administration when he said that he expected "it to wither on the vine" (Clymer, 1995). This seems unlikely. Liberal observers have used Gingrich's words to argue that Republicans are secretly planning to kill off the entire program (Dreyfuss and Stone, 1996, p. 24). A more plausible explanation is that Gingrich was referring to fee-for-service Medicare, which *is* likely to wither and die if the reforms become law.

Nine out of ten Medicare enrollees currently opt for the traditional program rather than for a federally approved Medicare health maintenance organization (HMO). The reforms do not explicitly force enrollees out, but they are clearly designed to make fee-for-service Medicare less attractive compared to prepaid options. According to the CBO, nearly two thirds of the expected $270 billion in savings over seven years in the GOP plan would come from reducing future payments to physicians, hospitals, and other facilities participating in fee-for service Medicare (Congressional Budget Office, 1995, table 1).

As discussed, if any additional cuts in spending are required to achieve the $270 billion in savings, those cuts will also be targeted at fee-for-service providers and not at the private plans operating under the new Medicare Plus program (H.R. 2491, Section 8631). As health care economist Uwe Reinhardt put it, "Medicare enrollees won't leave fee-for-service Medicare, but doctors will" (McGinley and Georges, 1995, p. A1). Increasingly, enrollees will find that they must enroll in a private Medicare Plus plan if they hope to continue seeing their own Medicare doctor.

Medicare Plus

While fee-for-service Medicare is being made less attractive, the Republican reforms create a new Medicare program in which the government offers a fixed, or capitated, payment to a private health plan in exchange for providing all the covered services an enrollee may require. The Medicare Plus program would differ from the existing Medicare HMO program in several important respects. A much wider range of providers would be permitted to market services to Medicare beneficiaries, and would have to meet standards established by state insurance commissioners rather than the federal government. Any insurance company with at least five thousand enrollees would be eligible to market its services if it is willing to accept prepayment from the government (H.R. 2491, Section 1851 [a]2). Private plans would no longer have to be composed primarily of non-Medicare enrollees. As discussed, plans could charge supplemental premiums even if they did not provide supplemental benefits, and they could offer cash rebates (Fraley, 1995a, p. 3536).

Employers would be permitted to include retirees in their company plans, as long as the plans accept government prepayment. Other associations, such as the American Association of Retired Persons, would be permitted to market plans to enrollees if they were not organized solely for the purpose of selling insurance (H.R. 2491, Section 1853). And networks of physicians and hospitals with at least 1,500 enrollees (so-called provider-sponsored organizations) would be permitted to offer their services directly to Medicare enrollees, instead of having to contract with an insurer.

The current payment methodology for Medicare HMOs would be altered from 95 percent of the fee-for-service adjusted average per capita cost (AAPCC), adjusted for the age and sex of the enrollee, to a "blended capitation" rate that would gradually reduce regional differences (H.R. 2491, Section 1854). The AAPCC formula has been criticized for placing too much weight on regional differences in medical costs that have little to do with differences in individual patients' health status (see Wennberg, Freeman, and Culp, 1987). The reforms would limit payment increases to private prepaid plans at about 5 percent per year on average and establish minimum monthly payments ($300 in 1997 and $350 in 1998) to attract prepaid plans to areas where there has been little penetration to date (General Accounting Office, 1996). (In 1995 AAPCC monthly payment rates ranged from a low of $177 to a high of $679 [General Accounting Office, 1996, p. 31]). The CBO estimates that these changes will reduce average payments on behalf of beneficiaries by $2,000 (about 25 percent) by 2002.

Medical Savings Accounts

The Medicare Plus program also includes a special high-deductible medical savings account option. Beneficiaries who choose this option would use government payments to purchase a private insurance policy with a deductible as high as $6,000 and deposit the remainder into a personal savings account. The funds would be used to pay for medical services incurred below the deductible. Once the deductible had been reached, the insurance plan would be required to pay 100 percent of the costs of all future covered services. Funds that remained in the savings account at the end of the enrollment period could be rolled over for future medical expenses (tax free) or used for any other purpose.

Partisan Differences

The main differences between the Republicans and Democrats on Medicare are largely philosophical and political rather than financial. In many respects the Republican proposals are similar to what President Clinton has proposed in the past. The president has proposed reducing the rate of increase in Medicare spending to 8 percent per annum, compared to about 7 percent for the Republicans. Clinton would also obtain most of his savings from reducing payments to providers and from encouraging beneficiaries to shift from fee-for-service Medicare into private managed care plans.

However, in dollar terms the president's plan would reduce spending by less than half of what the Republicans have proposed over seven years ($124 billion as of February 1996). It would set individuals' Part B premiums at 25 percent of costs rather than 31.5 percent, as the Republican proposal would. It would not include medical savings accounts, and it would more closely regulate private providers. Most significantly, the president's plan would not limit overall spending in the program, as the Republicans propose, and would require private plans to provide a specific set of benefits in exchange for the government's payment.

While Clinton's concept of health care is to "guarantee coverage for everyone and use the government to ensure quality and availability," Republicans ultimately "want seniors to select the coverage they can afford and let market competition control costs"

(Fraley, 1995b, p. 3664). If costs increase more quickly than expected, the Republicans' plan would require enrollees and providers to cover the difference. In contrast, the president's plan would require taxpayers to cover the difference.

Implications of the Proposed Market for Medicare Services

Republican leaders claim that free-market principles are the centerpiece of their Medicare reforms. Politically, free-market principles are rhetorically attractive because they suggest a self-regulating system that will "work automatically to contain costs and reduce misallocations, maximize producer and consumer freedom, encourage change, be responsive to new discoveries (both technological and organizational), and allow for diversity" (Fein, 1986, p. 174). Seen in this light, government regulation and supply seem archaic, cumbersome, and unnecessary.

How well is the market for Medicare services proposed by the Republicans likely to perform in providing quality health care services to all seniors for less cost? To what extent do the reforms address sources of health care market failure? Will they promote increased competition among buyers and sellers? Will they address inefficiencies resulting from imperfect information and negative and positive externalities?

Savings from Increased Efficiency?

The first thing to note about the reforms is that the source of most of the savings is reduced payment rates to fee-for-service providers rather than increased competition among private managed care plans. According to the CBO's estimates of the House bill, $180 billion of the $270 billion in savings (66 percent) would come from fee-for-service reductions ($147 billion in specific cuts and $33 billion in additional cuts to keep spending under the seven-year cap). Another $54 billion (20 percent) would come from requiring enrollees to pay higher premiums.

Only $34 billion of the savings (12 percent) would come from the introduction of the Medicare Plus program. Most of that ($29 billion) would come from reducing the government's payments to prepaid plans for existing enrollees. The additional eleven million beneficiaries who would be expected to enroll in Medicare Plus plans over the next seven years would save only $5 billion, while the Medical Savings Account option is predicted to *increase* the costs of the program by $4 billion over seven years as two million beneficiaries choose them (Congressional Budget Office, 1995).

The actual distribution of savings will certainly be different. The CBO's estimates are based on an assumption that Medicare managed care enrollment will increase to 14 percent of beneficiaries by 2002 without any reform and to 23 percent if the Republican reforms are adopted. In fact, Medicare managed care enrollment increased by almost 50 percent in 1995 alone (from about 6 percent to almost 10 percent of enrollees). At the current pace, enrollment will exceed 14 percent by the end of 1996. But even if *all* current Medicare enrollees were to switch to Medicare Plus plans, the CBO's estimates suggest that the additional savings would still be modest.

A Competitive Market for Medicare Services?

As discussed, the Republican reforms would dramatically increase the potential for competition among providers in the Medicare market and make Medicare enrollees more financially attractive to prepaid plans in historically neglected areas (General Accounting Office, 1996). However, increased competition does not by itself lead to increased efficiency if other sources of market failures remain unaddressed. The reforms also include numerous provisions intended to address well-known health care market failures, from providing seniors with guides for comparing health plan benefits and performance to providing financial incentives for enrollees to report fraudulent providers and subsidizing hospitals that train physicians and care for large numbers of uninsured patients. Instead of considering all of the potential sources of market failure, I will focus on what is likely to be the most costly if it is not adequately addressed—the tendency of people to choose health plans based on their current health status.

Adverse Selection and Risk Selection

Adverse selection refers to the tendency of individuals to shop for insurance based on their expected health status. If insurers know less about an individual's health status and assume that people only purchase insurance if it is a good deal, those who offer more comprehensive policies risk attracting individuals who expect to use more services. It makes sense to raise premiums based on this expectation, but this only makes the policy even less attractive to healthier individuals. In what economists call a "death spiral," premiums continue to rise until comprehensive coverage becomes unaffordable or unavailable (Ackerloff, 1984, chap. 2).

There are real risks for insurers who attract too many high-cost Medicare enrollees. In 1994 ten percent of Medicare enrollees incurred about 70 percent of all Medicare costs. These enrollees cost the program more than $28,000 each on average, compared to less than $1,500 on average for the other 90 percent of enrollees (Moon and Davis, 1995, p. 39). When plans receive about $3,600 a year on average, the bottom line difference between attracting a healthy enrollee and an unhealthy one can be dramatic.

Risk selection refers to insurers' efforts to design their policies or their marketing efforts to attract healthier individuals and avoid sicker ones. The tactics used range from portraying enrollees in advertisements as active, young, and happy (rather than ill but well cared for) to offering benefits (such as fitness club memberships) that are likely to appeal only to healthier people, offering plans that provide only limited coverage for costly chronic conditions, and developing a reputation as "sticky and nitpicky" when it comes to paying high-cost claims (Scism, 1994).

Private plans have already succeeded in attracting healthier Medicare enrollees (and deterring less healthy ones). Brown and his colleagues (1993) determined that enrollment of approximately 6 percent of Medicare beneficiaries in private Medicare HMOs caused the overall costs of the program to *increase* by 5.7 percent. Although Medicare HMOs are paid only 95 percent of the average fee-for-service rate in a given area, they are actually overpaid, because their enrollees tend to be much healthier (and thus less costly) than fee-for-service patients; thus the capitated payments they receive more than offset their expenses.

Adverse selection and risk selection can be mitigated by requiring insurers to offer the same minimum benefits package; by requiring longer-term contracts, so enrollees do not choose policies based on their expected health care needs and insurers do not drive sicker individuals out of their plans; by requiring insurers to offer the same choices to all individuals; and by adjusting payments to plans so that insurers with healthier enrollees receive less and those with sicker enrollees receive more (Cutler, 1996, p. 35; Moon and Davis, 1995, p. 42).

The Republican reforms would require managed care plans to provide the same minimum benefit package that fee-for-service enrollees are eligible to receive. They would establish annual enrollment periods to eliminate the current thirty-day waiting period for switching between fee-for-service and private plans. Insurers would be required to offer the same plan to all potential enrollees. And payments to plans would be adjusted for regional differences in costs and the age and sex of enrollees. Because prior research suggests that age and sex are poor predictors of variations in health care expenditures (Newhouse, 1993), the reforms also require the government to evaluate the "need to . . . take into account the health status of beneficiaries" as well (Section 1805 [b]2).

Critics believe that these safeguards will not be sufficient to deter plans from focusing on attracting healthier enrollees instead of on offering better services at lower cost, as efficiency implies (for example, see Enthoven and Singer, 1996). Most of the criticism has been directed at MSAs, but it might be applied to other prepaid options as well. MSAs are advocated as a way to lower health care costs by giving consumers a financial incentive to seek less costly forms of care (Pauly and Goodman, 1996). However, the limited evidence on their performance in private markets suggests that MSAs attract much healthier populations than do other insurance options (White, 1995; Mechanic, 1995).

The CBO assumes that MSAs will attract healthier beneficiaries with the prospect of substantial cash rebates and deter sicker individuals with the prospect of substantial out-of-pocket costs. The CBO also assumes that payments to MSA enrollees will not be adequately adjusted for their lower risks and that as a result, Medicare resources will be diverted from plans with higher-than-average costs that care for sicker enrollees and into the pockets of healthier enrollees with lower-than-average costs.

There are political reasons to support the CBO's assumptions. If Republicans hope to shift large numbers of content Medicare fee-for-service enrollees into private plans, they need to make private plans more attractive and fee-for-service Medicare less attractive. If healthier beneficiaries are attracted to private plans, private plans will be overpaid, and fewer dollars will be available to pay for the care of enrollees in fee-for-service Medicare (recall the fail-safe provision that requires any additional spending cuts to come from the fee-for-service sector). At least in the short term, individuals who choose private plans will receive better services, or private plans will make more money. Both effects would accelerate the decline of fee-for-service Medicare (while demonstrating the "superiority" of the private market).

Conclusion

Economic theory takes the existing distribution of resources as a given and evaluates alternatives according to whether they make individuals better off or worse off *compared to their starting position*. Economic theory does not tend to be concerned with how equitably resources or economic gains are distributed in the first place or after the fact. A society, in contrast, might favor making some individuals worse off in order to make others better off, even if this might lead to a decline in overall economic efficiency.

The proposed Medicare reforms need to be evaluated for their redistributive consequences (that is, how they may alter access and coverage for individuals with health and income differences) as well as for their impact on economic efficiency (that is, whether they will reduce the costs of providing the same set of services). Health insurance policy is appropriately political, because values besides efficiency are involved. As discussed, insurance is valued from the perspective of economic efficiency, because it allows individuals to reduce the uncertainty associated with unpredictable, high-cost events. If the distribution of health insurance is left to the market, individuals will pay different rates depending on the insurer's expectations about their use of services.

A central motivation for the establishment of the Medicare program was the fact that many elderly Americans (who tended to be sicker and poorer than the rest of the population) could not afford private health insurance. The proposed reforms would mean that Medicare beneficiaries who can afford to pay more would have better coverage, access, and quality of care. Enrollees who opt for MSAs would be able to see any provider they choose and can afford, at a time when fewer providers would agree to accept fee-for-service enrollees in exchange for the government's payment. (Existing limits on what Medicare providers can charge for their services would not apply to Medicare MSAs.) New managed care options that permit enrollees to go to any physician they choose if they are willing to pay more (such as point-of-service plans) would also be available to those who can afford them, while fee-for-service enrollees would face the prospect of fewer provider options, longer waits, and (possibly) lower-quality care.

The poorest elderly would also be adversely affected if the Medicaid program is reformed. Currently, 30 percent of Medicaid spending goes to provide services (primarily nursing home care) for the 11 percent of Medicaid recipients who are elderly. The legislation passed by the House and Senate would provide states with fixed grants for Medicaid to spend as the states prefer. As is the case with Medicare, future spending on the program would be cut so that states would have less, at a time when the number of uninsured Americans is increasing. It seems likely that many states will require seniors who are currently receiving Medicaid subsidies to join lower-cost managed care plans.

Unfortunately, the political debate has focused on less consequential (but more salient) aspects of the reform. Republicans have sought to focus attention on averting a short-term fiscal problem that could be addressed with much smaller cuts in spending (or increases in revenues), without discussing how other features of the reform might alter the existing commitment to mainstream health benefits for all seniors. Democrats have sought to focus attention on the fact that the reforms would modestly increase most beneficiaries' premiums over the next seven years, without offering responsible alternatives for ensuring the long-term financial viability of the program.

The unanswered questions about Medicare reform are whether the unknown efficiency gains of increased market competition would offset reductions in government payments to both fee-for-service providers and private plans, and who would reap the benefits of any efficiency gains. Can the recent success of many businesses in lowering their health care costs translate into long-term savings in Medicare? If there are widespread overutilization and waste in the program, will the proposed reforms eliminate them?

Will the government have the political will to enforce provisions in the legislation that mitigate market failures, if doing so would be unpopular and costly to important constituencies and might lead to higher costs for government?

The 1996 elections will play a central role in shaping the future of the Medicare program. As this chapter is being completed (April 1996), Congress and the president have reached a short-term agreement on a budget for fiscal year 1996, but it does not appear likely that any agreement on long-term Medicare reform will be reached before the fall. If presumptive Republican presidential nominee Dole (who has touted his original opposition to the program) is elected to the presidency and Republicans retain control of Congress, a market-based reform bill will surely be passed, and the program will move incrementally toward a subsidy program based on financial need—despite widespread public support for the current entitlement. If President Clinton is reelected and the Democrats regain control of Congress, the outcome will probably be interpreted (to varying degrees) as a rejection of Republicans' efforts to "gut" important federal programs, and verification of the dangers of "messing with Medicare" and other popular entitlements. It seems unlikely that the government will tackle the long-term reforms needed to reduce the existing program's unsustainable redistribution of wealth from future generations to today's seniors.

Ironically, the best prospects for long-term reform may be if the outcome of the election is less decisive. If President Clinton is reelected but Republicans retain control of Congress, both sides will have an incentive to move the debate beyond the current political impasse. In the past, bipartisan commissions have been used effectively to hammer out agreements on controversial issues like Social Security reform and military base closings when policymakers agreed that something needed to be done but were reluctant to do it publicly. There does appear to be broad agreement between Clinton and the Republicans that the soaring costs of the Medicare program need to be addressed. A stalemate might lead Republicans to the table with the realization that they will not be able to accomplish their goals without the president's support. And the president might support a bipartisan commission as a less visible and more credible way to impose costs on constituencies in his own party.

What kind of agreement might be reached? In a recent issue of *Health Affairs,* liberal and conservative academics independently recommended converting Medicare to a "defined contribution program" (Butler and Moffit, 1995; Aaron and Reischauer, 1995). The government would select a limited set of private plans (based on price and quality) that would be permitted to market services to Medicare beneficiaries. Enrollees would select from among the government-approved alternatives. If the plan's premium was more than what the government paid, the beneficiary would be required to cover the difference. The government's payment would be based on market prices instead of being capped by legislative fiat, as is the case in the current Republican proposal.

This approach would be similar to current efforts by private and public purchasing groups to "manage competition" among private plans, as discussed in previous chapters. Politically, it would allow Republicans to claim victory in introducing free-market cost controls, and allow Democrats to claim that they had prevented Republicans from throwing seniors to the for-profit wolves.

Notes

1. Specialist physicians' reimbursement rates had been calculated using a larger multiplier than that used for primary care physicians. The reform would have actually cut the current rate for specialists rather than simply slowing the rate of increase, as was the case for primary care physicians. Democrats suggested the compromise was worth billions of dollars to doctors, while Republicans countered that it was worth no more than $400 million (Pear, 1995b).

2. Several versions of the bill were passed. This chapter focuses on the details of the House-Senate compromise sent to the president.

3. The 31.5 percent rate is based on the actual proportion of costs that enrollees are currently paying. Although existing law sets the rate at 25 percent of costs, the costs of the program have not increased as quickly as forecasted. In the past, Part B premiums have been as high as 50 percent of the costs of the program.

References

Aaron, H. J., and Reischauer, R. D. "The Medicare Reform Debate: What Is the Next Step?" *Health Affairs,* 1995, *14*(4), 8–30.

Akerlof, G. A. *An Economic Theorist's Book of Tales.* New York: Cambridge University Press, 1984.

Ball, R. M. "What Medicare's Architects Had in Mind." *Health Affairs,* 1995, *14*(4), 62–72.

Blendon, R., and others. "The Public's View of the Future of Medicare." *Journal of the American Medical Association,* 1995, *274*(20), 1645–1648.

Brown, R. S., and others. "Do Health Maintenance Organizations Work for Medicare?" *Health Care Financing Review,* 1993, *15*(Fall), 7–23.

Butler, S. M. "The Conservative Agenda." In H. J. Aaron (ed.), *The Problem That Won't Go Away: Reforming U.S. Health Care Financing.* Washington, D.C.: Brookings Institution, 1996.

Butler, S. M., and Moffit, R. E. "The FEHBP as a Model for a New Medicare Program." *Health Affairs,* 1995, *14*(4), 47–61.

Chen, E. "Dole, Gingrich Take Cautious Aim at Medicare." *Los Angeles Times,* Jan. 31, 1995a, p. A1.

Chen, E. "GOP's Lid on Medicare Proposals May Backfire." *Los Angeles Times,* July 25, 1995b, p. A15.

Chen, E. "GOP Plan Advances on Bumpy Road." *Los Angeles Times,* Oct. 1, 1995c, p. A1.

Chen, E., and Rosenblatt, R. A. "AARP Declaring War on GOP Medicare Plan." *Los Angeles Times,* Oct. 10, 1995, p. A4.

Clymer, A. "Of Touching Third Rails and Tackling Medicare." *New York Times,* Oct. 27, 1995, p. A11.

Congressional Budget Office. *Cost Estimates for H.R. 2485, the Medicare Preservation Act of 1995.* Report submitted to Representative Bill Archer, Oct. 18, 1995.

Cutler, D. M. "Public Policy for Health Care." Paper prepared for "Fiscal Policy: Lessons for Economic Research" conference, University of California, Berkeley, February 1996.

Davis, M. H., and Burner, S. T. "Three Decades of Medicare: What the Numbers Tell Us." *Health Affairs,* 1995, *14*(4), 231–243.

Dreyfuss, R., and Stone, P. H. "Medikill: Inside Newt's Plan to Gut Medicare and Enrich One of His Biggest Contributors." *Mother Jones,* Jan.–Feb. 1996, pp. 22–27.

Enthoven, A. C., and Singer, S. J. "Market-Based Reform: What to Regulate and by Whom?" In H. J. Aaron (ed.), *The Problem That Won't Go Away: Reforming U.S. Health Care Financing.* Washington, D.C.: Brookings Institution, 1996.

Fein, R. *Medical Care, Medical Costs: The Search for a Health Insurance Policy.* Cambridge, Mass.: Harvard University Press, 1986.

Fraley, C. "GOP Scores on Medicare but Foes Aren't Done." *Congressional Quarterly Weekly Report,* Nov. 18, 1995a, pp. 3535–3538.

Fraley, C. "Clinton, GOP Are Far Apart as Medicare Talks Begin." *Congressional Quarterly Weekly Report,* Dec. 2, 1995b, p. 3664.

Friedman, M. "A Way Out of Soviet-Style Health Care." *Wall Street Journal,* April 17, 1996, p. A20.

Fuchs, V. R. "Economics, Values, and Health Care Reform." *The American Economic Review,* 1994, *86*(1), 1–24.

General Accounting Office. *Medicare HMOs: Rapid Enrollment Growth Concentrated in Selected States.* GAO report no. B-232994. Washington, D.C.: General Accounting Office, Jan. 18, 1996.

Gold, S. D. "Cuts That Grow and Grow." *New York Times,* Nov. 14, 1995, pp. A15, A25.

Health Care Financing Administration. *1995 Data Compendium.* HCFA pub. no. 03364. Baltimore, Md.: U.S. Department of Health and Human Services, 1995.

Hook, J. "GOP Medicare Proposals Win Broad Support." *Los Angeles Times,* Sept. 21, 1995, p. A1.

Horn, S. *Report from U.S. Representative Steve Horn: California's 38th Congressional District.* [Bulk-mail pamphlet.] Washington, D.C.: U.S. House of Representatives, 1995.

Hunt, A. R. "The Duplicity Wars on Medicare." *Wall Street Journal,* Sept. 21, 1995, p. A23.

Marmor, T. R. *The Politics of Medicare.* Chicago: Aldine, 1973.

McGinley, L. "Gingrich's Many Parleys: Long Days on Medicare Link His Political Health to an Explosive Issue." *Wall Street Journal,* June 29, 1995a, p. A18.

McGinley, L. "Medicare Plan by House GOP Is Short of Goal." *Wall Street Journal,* Sept. 11, 1995b, p. A18.

McGinley, L., and Georges, C. "Medicare Bill Would End Egalitarian Approach." *Wall Street Journal,* Oct. 20, 1995, p. A1.

Mechanic, R. E. "How Would MSAs Work in the Real World?" *Business and Health,* November 1995, pp. 29–37.

Meyer, H. "The Conservative Agenda: Pushing Business out of Health Care." *Business and Health,* June 1995, pp. 23–25.

Mitchell, A. "White House Lists Budget Priorities." *New York Times,* Nov. 25, 1995, p. 1.

Moon, M., and Davis, K. "Preserving and Strengthening Medicare." *Health Affairs,* 1995, *14*(4), 31–46.

Newhouse, J. *Free for All? Lessons from the RAND Health Insurance Experiment.* Cambridge, Mass.: Harvard University Press, 1993.

Pauly, M. V., and Goodman, J. C. "Using Tax Credits for Health Insurance and Medical Savings Accounts." In H. J. Aaron (ed.), *The Problem That Won't Go Away: Reforming U.S. Health Care Financing.* Washington, D.C.: Brookings Institution, 1996.

Pear, R. "Retirees and Doctors Attack Republican Medicare Plan." *New York Times,* Oct. 6, 1995a, pp. A11, A22.

Pear, R. "Doctors' Group Says G.O.P. Agreed to Deal on Medicare." *New York Times,* Oct. 12, 1995b, p. A1.

Priest, D. "Dressing for Success: The Parties Trade Medicare Gowns." *The Washington Post,* Oct. 1, 1995, p. C1, C3.

Richter, P., and Rosenblatt, R. "Clinton Slams GOP on Medicare Plans." *Los Angeles Times,* July 26, 1995, p. A4.

Rogers, D. "Dole Suggests New Cutbacks in Health Programs to Balance Budget." *Wall Street Journal,* Feb. 16, 1995, pp. A16, A18.

Rosenbaum, D. E. "'Leave Benefits Alone' Is Cry at Retiree Enclave in Florida." *New York Times,* June 2, 1995a, p. A1.

Rosenbaum, D. E. "Savings and Smoke." *New York Times,* Sept. 15, 1995b, p. A1.

Rosenbaum, D. E. "The Medicare Brawl: Finger-Pointing, Hyperbole, and the Facts Behind Them." *New York Times,* Oct. 1, 1995c, p. Y13.

Rosenblatt, R. A. "The Cost of Fixing Medicare." *Los Angeles Times,* June 7, 1995, p. A5.

Scism, L. "Picking Cherries: Health Insurer Profits by Being Very Choosy in Selling Its Policies." *Wall Street Journal,* Sept. 20, 1994, p. A1.

Shonick, W. *Government and Health Services: Government's Role in the Development of U.S. Health Services, 1930–1980.* New York: Oxford University Press, 1995.

Vobejda, B., and Harris, J. "Democrats Pounce on GOP Medicare Comments." *Washington Post,* Oct. 27, 1995, p. A4.

Weisskopf, M., and Maraniss, D. "Endgame: The Revolution Stalls." *Washington Post* (National Weekly Edition), Jan. 29–Feb. 4, 1996, pp. 6–24.

Wennberg, J. E., Freeman, J. L., and Culp, W. J. "Are Hospital Services Rationed in New Haven or Over-Utilized in Boston?" *Lancet,* 1987, *8543*(1), 1185–1189.

White, J. *Medical Savings Accounts: Fact Versus Fiction.* Brookings Occasional Paper. Washington, D.C.: Brookings Institution, 1995.

Wilensky, G. "The Score on Medicare Reform—Minus the Hype and Hyperbole." *New England Journal of Medicine,* 1995, *333*(26), 1774–1777.

Wines, M. "Gingrich Promises Big but Painless Cuts in Medicare." *New York Times,* May 8, 1995, p. A1.

Chapter Thirteen

Lessons for the United States
Britain's Experience with Managed Competition

Donald W. Light

This chapter offers a different perspective on the unmanaged competition between managed care corporations that is now transforming the American health care system, a perspective informed by Great Britain's attempt to transform an entire health care system so that cost shifting to weaker purchasers is not possible. This perspective lends itself to a three-step conclusion. First, if one is going to rely on economic price competition in health care, one must overcome the inherent forms of market failure in health care. Otherwise, competitors will "win" by selecting lower risks, providing fewer services, substituting cheaper or worse services for better ones, or simply being lucky in how cases turn out, given the high levels of variability and uncertainty in what patients need and how they respond. The facts that only 10 percent of the population generates 72 percent of the health care costs, that the seller (the doctor) is the buyer's agent, and that this seller controls all the esoteric, complex knowledge needed to decide what is worth paying for create mighty temptations to exploit patients and purchasers alike, even if they are organized into cooperatives.

An earlier generation of economists understood why markets do not work well in health care, especially when treating the seriously ill (Arrow, 1963; Boulding, 1958, p. 255; Buchanan, 1960, pp. 400–401; Ginzberg, 1954; Klarman, 1965; Samuelson, 1955, p. 122;

Stigler, 1952, pp. 219–220; summarized in Light, 1993). The reasons that markets fail in health care might lead one to hypothesize that employers, Medicare, and Medicaid are saving money because they are buying less service or access for their enrollees or employees, although the large profits of managed care corporations suggest that they are paying too much for what they are getting. If a roomy Toyota Camry with an automatic transmission, air conditioning, and electrical everything costs $20,000, and a little Corolla with a stick shift, no air, and crank-down windows costs $15,000, America's health benefit purchasers have gotten the Corolla, at the "bargain" price of $18,000. The corporate packagers who put together deals like this are smiling all the way to the bank.

These problems led Enthoven to his finest work (1988), a model of *managed* competition with specific rules, provisions, and oversight so that sellers must compete on price, efficiency, and value. Enthoven's model includes universal coverage and a uniform benefits package, so competitors cannot select or deny enrollees based on risk; the organization of services into managed care systems, so that much of the variability and uncertainty inherent in health insurance is smoothed out through volume contracts; widely available information on price and performance; and other safeguards against market failure.

The second step in a conclusion based on the British experience is that if you do introduce price competition with most of the necessary safeguards in place, you will find that it costs a lot to run. It also entangles the government, health alliance, or other market manager in heated politics concerning which services are being cut, which facility is being closed, and whose ox is being gored. High barriers to entry and exit remain. Annual contracts pit providers against one another and against purchasers, and they require a great deal of time and effort just to carry on with treating sick patients. "Caveat emptor" replaces "confidat emptor," thus undermining the trust on which medical care relies (Mechanic, 1996). And not much competition can take place if everyone is to get good, equitable services. All this leads to the final step of the conclusion, that what an employer, community, or society needs is strong, cooperative purchasing ability and providers who are actively seeking to meet the health needs of their population in the most cost-effective way.

This is a far cry from what seems to be a tragic hurtling in the United States toward large, investor-driven health care corporations that reduce services to suffering and sick enrollees and play doctors and hospitals off one another. These health care packagers are locking in their market shares to minimize competition, and they routinely extract 15 to 25 percent from their revenues for marketing, contracting, institutional (not clinical) management, and profits—all at the expense of clinical services. They pass a fraction of the savings they realize back to employers, but they increasingly control the supply and provision of vital services. Future profits will have to come either from providing less care for high-risk sick people or from expanding demand (even though they claim to accomplish the opposite). The main effect of competition in modern history, employers and payers should remember, has not been to do the same things more efficiently but to spur economic growth through new products, new "needs," and new markets. Turning health care into a for-profit industry has enabled companies to make a great deal of money since it began twenty-five years ago, without slowing down overall costs much at all. Despite some savings in some places during this shakeout period, it looks like health care will be a growth industry in the United States for a long time to come, even as employers and the government organize to get more for their money.

Managed Competition for an Entire Health Care System

While private and public U.S. health policy aspires to true managed competition, in fact it can only achieve bits and pieces of it, because the United States does not possess some of the basic safeguards required by the model. By contrast, Britain and many other countries have those basic safeguards in place. These include universal health coverage, independent of age, health condition, or risk; equitable financing; equitable access and distribution; and a systemwide infrastructure that can be mobilized to sponsor or manage the markets, provide market information, track quality, and track value (Light 1995b, 1995c). Besides these, Prime Minister Thatcher had other advantages. She had one of the most equitably distributed systems in the West, thanks to years of centralized planning. She started with a strict national budget (something Enthoven does not favor but probably should, given the ways providers and competitors can expand the market). This budget was allocated to regional health authorities and then to district health authorities. Mrs. Thatcher started with an administrative overhead that was among the lowest in Europe and seven years of a new program to strengthen management. She also started with a kind of geographical health maintenance organization (HMO) design that—with district health authorities providing specialty, hospital, and community services for a defined population—was undergirded by a strong, efficient primary care system that gave every resident a personal physician to control all referrals except emergencies. The national contract with these general practitioners (GPs) was (and is) an ingenious balance of straight pay, fee for service, and capitation, so incentives were balanced and risks kept low (Fry, Light, Rodnick, and Orton, 1995). Thus, while managed competition would aim to correct the distortions of market competition in the United States, managed competition in the United Kingdom was used to introduce market forces into a state-administered system that was among the cheapest, most comprehensive, and most equitable in the West.

With this roughly described starting point, let us turn in more detail to five positive and six negative lessons from the British experience with managed competition. The concluding section of this chapter draws three lessons from recent tendencies of the National Health Service (NHS) to shrink back from the hazards and costs of managed competition and to move toward community-based purchasing (Light and May, 1993). Essentially, I will argue that while the British have improved on the American model of managed competition in several ways, the limited competition allowed in Britain has increased both demand and costs. It is creating inequalities, dislocations, and fragmentation. What the British are realizing is that most of the benefits come from *purchasing* cooperatively and wisely for the health needs of communities.

Five Positive Lessons from Designing Managed Competition British-Style

The NHS started off meeting nearly all of Enthoven's requirements (1988) for avoiding the many forms of market failure in health care. By turning every health authority from an administrative office into a purchaser and every hospital, specialist, and community or home health service into a seller, Mrs. Thatcher leapfrogged pallid manifestations of the Enthoven model in Minneapolis and Los Angeles, where unmanaged competition among managed care corporations prevailed (and still does). Rarely has an organization with a million employees and a $60 billion budget been redesigned so rapidly into something so profoundly different from what it had been. Given the natural tendencies of markets to differentiate by cost, complexity, and price, this framework was vital, because it contained those tendencies within a relatively equitable and universal system, as Enthoven (1988) advocated.

To compensate for the higher costs of treating people who are poor, old, at high risk, or living in rural areas, providers are paid more for them. To minimize skimping and underservice, the NHS version of managed competition includes significantly increased professional and consumer checks: medical audits of treatment effectiveness, a patient's charter of rights, an expanded complaints system, and comparative assessment of performance. The emphasis on local, community-based, and small-scale practices of what might be called primary managed care maximizes possibilities for communication, accountability, and coordination with other community-based services and public health efforts.

1.   *Have supply-side competition within a fixed budget.* Theoretically, competition should not work within a budget limit (Alain Enthoven has repeatedly emphasized that his concept of managed competition should not be subject to budget limits). The economic expression of preferences, as buying and selling take place, results in a natural total that Enthoven says would be distorted by a limited budget. But British leaders did not dare (and their treasury would not allow them) to drop the key feature that has held NHS expenditures in check. Why not create markets of competitive contracts among doctors and hospitals within budget limits? The resulting design is called "the internal market." Since firms outside the NHS hold contracts too, a more accurate term is supply-side competition, with budgets set at the national and district level.

2.   *Allocate funds based on needs; choose services based on effectiveness.* This is ultimately the most profound feature of British-style

managed competition, one that is now transforming the reformed health care system itself. While HMOs and Enthoven's model of managed competition are implicitly based on the health needs of enrollees, intense annual competition between buyers distorts this goal. Market-induced demand and advertising campaigns take precedence over the considerable needs of patients with chronic disorders, who are costly and to be avoided in a competitive market, where buyers seek to attract only the healthiest customers.

The British approach of supply-side managed competition allocates to district health authorities a population-based budget roughly adjusted by risk. This leveling of the playing field means that past inequities between affluent and poorer areas are now being rectified. Since implementing this formula all at once would mean that some regions would experience serious budgetary reductions from their historical budgets based on utilization and politics, the change is being phased in gradually. When one gets down to the small scale of primary care practices, the variations in practice budgets from years of differences determined by social class, politics, and area are still greater and more inequitable. In response, the NHS is about to transform these primary care budgets by using needs-based capitation as well, so that the variations reflect needs rather than clinical practice styles and historic biases in funding (Healthcare Financial Management Association, 1993, pp. 6–10; Appleby and others, 1994).

In British supply-side managed competition, each district has a single purchasing authority with the long-term responsibility of maximizing the health, well-being, and functioning of that area's population. This differs profoundly from annual competition for the healthiest subscribers. It eliminates all the gaming observed among American health insurers (Reinhardt, 1982; Light, 1992; Stone, 1993; Woolhandler and Himmelstein, 1994). It establishes a strong commitment to the health of a stable population. In the context of American policy debates, it would be called single-payer managed competition, a combination not usually considered.

Within the first two years of the reforms, the British started using the term *commissioning* to connote that district purchasing authorities should do more than purchase existing services "off the shelf." Commissioning focuses on how best to spend allotted funds to meet a population's needs with new, more cost-effective configurations of clinical and other services. It also focuses on reducing future needs by addressing their causes—by teaching better skills to young mothers, for example, or providing adult caregivers to the disabled and the infirm. Sometimes it involves discouraging harmful behaviors in individuals, like smoking and drinking; sometimes it is ecological or community-based, addressing such concerns as poor housing, dangerous neighborhoods, and pollution.

For a health care system built up around hospitals, major academic centers, and the elaboration of subspecialized medicine, the implications of a needs-based health care budget based on a stable population are more radical than Enthoven's model of managed competition. The center of *medical* care becomes the periphery of *health* care, the services of last resort after one does as much as possible to prevent or diminish problems in the first place. And when one does turn to medical care, one uses all the resources of primary care and home care first, before turning to specialty or hospital care (Light, 1991).

When medical services are necessary, the goal is to use effective ones. Like the United States, the United Kingdom is going through a long, research-based process to define what "results," "outcomes," and "effectiveness" mean to different people under different circumstances, to figure out how to measure them, and to see how well different approaches work. The British call it "evidence-based medicine." The point here is that needs-adjusted limited budgeting for a stable population aligns priorities and incentives in fundamentally new ways aside from managed competition itself.

3. *Have competition among professional agents at the "wholesale" level.* Although the American model of managed competition focuses on "retail" consumers (patients) choosing among health plans by price, quality, and the fruits of efficiency, a good argument can be made that the complex, esoteric, and contingent nature of health care calls for professional agents to compare alternate services and buy the best services in volume ("wholesale") for groups of consumers.

The British version of managed competition uses this "wholesale" approach to purchasing health care. The buyers' agents are basically the district health authorities, though larger GP practices have been given funds to buy some specialty and community services for their much smaller, local patient panels (see below). This approach is supported by evidence indicating that British patients are a long way from being the informed, smart buyers that health authorities and physicians are—or that the American model of managed competition assumes they are (Rice, Brown, and Wyn, 1993; Light, 1995b). One is struck by the results of surveys showing how few British even know what the transformation of budgets, incentives, organization, and power is about or have any idea about its impact on their care (Mahon, Wilkin, and Whitehouse, 1994; Jones, Lester, and West, 1994). Nor do patients have much interest in looking or traveling beyond their local area for better care (Mahon, Wilkin, and Whitehouse, 1994, pp. 118–121). Even among patients who had waited for more than a year for an elective procedure, three-quarters were unwilling to travel more than ten miles. After the reforms, only one patient in twenty asked his or her physician about other hospitals to which he or she might go. Two thirds did not know which specialist their GP had referred them to until they received an appointment letter with his or her name on it. Most patients are focused on their customary doctor and nearby hospital and put their faith in them. Even if this were not so, there are serious questions about how much time patients would be willing to devote to the kind of quantitative, systematic review of competing services that full-time professionals do. For these reasons, the British adoption of a wholesale model of managed competition seems an improvement.

4. *Set up small, local, physician-run primary care "HMOs."* Besides making health authorities into purchasers responsible for the health needs of a population, the NHS reforms set up a program by which qualified GP groups with nine thousand or more patients (subsequently reduced to five thousand) could receive and manage the budget for a specific list of low- and mid-risk patients, specialty and hospital services, prescriptions, home health care, community services, dietetic and chiropody services, and services for people with many outpatient mental health problems and learning disabilities (Glennerster, Matsaganis, Owens, and Hancock, 1994, p. 76; Ham, 1994, p. 20).

Essentially, GP fundholding creates mini HMOs run by GPs. It is one of the few truly new innovations in health services design since World War II (Fry, Light, Rodnick, and Orton, 1995). It addresses a number of frustrations and wishes of GPs that might be pertinent to primary care in other systems. British physicians said that they wanted to hold funds in order to coordinate services and improve quality, select the specialists and hospitals they work with, develop a better on-site constellation of services, and have the budgets to develop their own comprehensive primary care service (Glennerster, Matsaganis, Owens, and Hancock, 1994, pp. 83–86).

GP fundholding practices have distinct advantages over American-style full-service HMOs, and some disadvantages. They are small, local, and personal. They are run by the GPs themselves—encouraging clinically, as opposed to administratively, managed care—who are directly accountable to their patients (Fry, Light, Rodnick, and Orton, 1995). They allow GPs to make their patient services more comprehensive.

One implication of GP fundholding is that competitive contracts do not have to cover all services or all risks, as American policymakers mistakenly believe (Fry, Light, Rodnick, and Orton, 1995, chap. 8). It is the all-services, all-risk approach to managed competition in the United States that is forcing doctors and patients into large managed care corporations, for nothing smaller can deliver the full range of services and absorb all the financial risks. This approach thus effectively reduces choice of plans to a few large plans per area. By contrast, GP fundholding or primary managed care gives GP groups the funds for a wide range of relatively low-risk services, and risk is limited to $7,500 per patient per year. After that, costs are absorbed from a reserve fund held by the area commissioning authority.

The concept of a primary care mini HMO is ideally suited to meeting the major challenges of the 1990s. It provides a base for prevention and for extending health promotion upstream. It coordinates the growing number of short-stay and ambulatory care procedures. It reflects the shift from institutions to households. Primary care HMOs develop shared care and the management of chronic health problems, coordinating health care with other local services.

Four principles underlie GP fundholding from an American point of view (Fry, Light, Rodnick, and Orton, 1995). One is to design a comprehensive primary care contract and give it to clinicians. This gives patients and the system a foundation of clinically managed care rather than "MBA managed" care, and much more choice in small cities, large towns, and even semirural areas. Fundholding also brings GPs into the center of the NHS. They are responsible for and interact with other segments of the health care system more than they had to do under independent national contracts.

The second principle is to pass on enough risk to motivate people, but not so much risk that they can make or lose large sums. This contrasts with the American tendency to pass on as much risk as possible to providers, forcing them to cut services, raise barriers to access, avoid sicker patients if possible, and join large corporate entities with deep pockets who can bear the risk. In the NHS, there is the added reality that a poorly run practice cannot actually lose real money, even if it goes over budget (which few do). GP fundholders do not physically hold the money; it is held in their account at the district level. If a practice "loses money"—its account shows a negative balance—the area authority must replenish it. Before that happens, however, financial and management teams go out and review all aspects of the practice in order to turn it around.

The third principle is that profits must be plowed back into the practice. If GP fundholders try to pocket the profits personally, it is a criminal offense. Fundholders tried to start personal for-profit corporations to which they referred their own patients; but unlike in the United States, this practice was quickly outlawed. Use of surpluses must be reviewed and approved. This too minimizes the conflict of interest inherent in providers' receiving capped prepayments.

The fourth implicit principle is continuity of care. In Britain health care is locally integrated by one's personal physician.

GP fundholding profoundly changes the organization and power structure of medicine, giving GPs the power of the purse over some specialty and hospital services. GPs are getting specialists to work more closely with them and to be more responsive to the needs of both their patients and themselves (Glennerster, Matsaganis, and Owens, 1992; Farmer, 1993, pp. 62–63). They are also more invested now in developing good ways to care for the disabled and for people with chronic problems, so they can reduce hospital admissions and specialty consultations.

Despite these design advantages of GP fundholding, they create serious hazards (Light, 1995c). It eliminates the purchaser-provider split that is the foundation of managed competition and the NHS reforms. It compromises the commitment of GPs to their patients. Conflicts of interest are inherent. The organization of specialty services can easily become fragmented as different fundholders make purchasing decisions that do not add up. So far fundholding decisions are uncontrolled, and no quality checks have been put in place, though the situation is likely to change soon. Systematic evaluation is minimal; the success of fundholding is "running on anecdotes," as one senior official put it. Decentralized services and administration are inherently more costly, even if they have other clinical and political advantages. A number of the GPs feel swamped with managerial work, and overall stress is high (Light, 1995a). GPs vary greatly in their managerial competence, and none is trained for the job. Inevitably, some practices are not well run (though only one has gone into receivership). More serious, GP fundholding creates a two-class system in which some patients are "sponsored" by real funds, while patients in non-fundholding practices are not financially sponsored so clearly. GPs need practice managers (which they are getting), and specialists need more stability in their budgets and professional lives than this transitional period provides. But the concept of clinically managed primary care HMOs nevertheless has benefits for patients and physicians, and it lowers costs.

The British government is currently extending the idea so that all GP practices can be fundholders or part of fundholding groups, and a number of different arrangements are happening in the field that might interest American policymakers. These include small practices attaching themselves to a larger practice so they can fundhold, small practices combining in order to qualify as a fundholder, practices hiring a common bargaining agent to negotiate fundholding terms with the health authority, and practices widening their range to include more high-risk secondary services.

5. *Use local, nonprofit, community-based services.* The limited-risk primary care contracts and the emphasis on using NHS resources when possible have kept managed competition largely local and nonprofit. While the NHS reforms were clearly intended to create a level playing field for private, for-profit providers and hospitals,

for-profit medicine has not won much of the main business in acute care.[1] Appleby found that in 1991–92 only 0.5 percent of purchasers' contracting partners were from the private sector (Appleby and others, 1994, pp. 51–52). In 1992–93 private contractors accounted for only 0.04 percent of providers' contracts.

NHS facilities—now "self-governing trusts"—have natural advantages in competitive markets, and they have learned quickly how to use them. Being old, their capital debt is small, and they are usually more fully staffed and equipped than are private institutions. It has been NHS staff and teams who do most of the private work anyway, down the street in a private hospital. For these reasons, plus old ties, values, and customs, the local, community facilities and groups have gotten the lion's share of the business. Vertically integrated managed care systems could form, as in the United States, but they would have to be sufficiently more efficient to pay for the system's overhead and management costs to win contracts from local providers in a nearly zero-sum game. It is unlikely that even the best American managed care systems could match the cost-effectiveness of current NHS arrangements.

Let us pause to reflect on these five adaptable policy lessons. The tendency, despite the fundamental flaws of competition and even managed competition, to allow the market to expand in the United States leads to the first policy lesson: hold the line on one's budget. The second lesson implies that employers and other purchasers should not allocate by demands but by needs—a lesson that is being slowly realized, with many reversals, in the United States. Choosing services based on effectiveness is a lesson that is being learned rapidly in the United States as purchasers, managed care companies, and the federal government develop outcome measures and clinical protocols. Concerning the third lesson, there is a fair amount of competition taking place at the wholesale level (for example, between employers and managed care providers). The British approach suggests that this is the direction in which we should be heading. Concerning the fourth lesson, primary managed care (Fry, Light, Rodnick, and Orton, 1995) has been suggested for the United States but not taken up. It would provide more choice, reflect the variety of communities and tastes that make up the nation, and keep most managed care in the hands of local physicians rather than distant executives. It is an idea that employers, insurers, and other contractors of services could use to avoid large-scale corporations' forming oligopolies. Finally, the fifth lesson suggests that the United States is going in entirely the wrong direction, toward large for-profit corporations and away from a structure that can address the epidemiological needs and risks of the population in the twenty-first century.

Six Negative Lessons of Implementation with Managed Competition

The British have had more experience with managed competition than any of the nations that are considering its systematic implementation. Managed competition has been costly and disruptive. Many of the improvements attributed to it are continuations of earlier trends, and most innovations (such as GP fundholding) have significant drawbacks. Six lessons are drawn here from studies, observations, and interviews over the past several years.

1.   *To preserve equity and to avoid political embarrassment, the British system allowed little competition.* The British experience with managed competition is sobering for any country that (unlike the United States) really does behave as if it has limited funds. Since managed competition began, the British have had to find more and more funds to pay for more managers, more consultants, more data, more marketing, more consumer pressures, more consumer complaints, more underbudgeted areas, and more demands for high quality.

Very quickly the government realized that competition unleashed very powerful forces, forces that historically have been used to promote economic growth, not restraint. The government also realized from the poor business plans of the first self-governing trust hospitals and from the inability of health authorities to purchase that the reform to which it was committed could quickly become a disaster. In response, the government took a number of actions to minimize the very competition it was boldly promising.

By December 1990 the secretary of state for health had admitted that the government had been carried away in its application of business thinking to health care. A sea change took place behind the scenes, one that had become evident by 1991 in various changes in language. "Buyers" became "purchasers" and then "commissioners." "Sellers" became "providers," acknowledging their distinct and central role in medicine. "Budgets" became "funds" or "amounts." Most important, "marketing" became "needs assessment." Ever since, the government has found itself in the awkward position of setting up the structure for a highly competitive market, yet denying to an anxious public and suspicious press that any such thing has taken place.

Behind these actions, the policy of managed competition was a command performance by a powerfully centralized government. One might call it *dictated* competition (perhaps a contradiction in economic theory but not in politics). In effect, Mrs. Thatcher announced that on a certain day, hospitals and specialists in one of the world's largest welfare organizations would compete for their budgets rather than receive them.[2] Ironically, however, politically dictated competition meant that actual competition was minimized. The collectivity of ministers, the management executive, and the Department of Health, referred to by some NHS employees as the Kremlin, subsequently issued orders, directives, executive letters, and advisories by the hundreds specifying the terms by which competition would take place.[3] First, the government required a practice year of "shadow purchasing," in which the provider units and their administrative offices were required to provide the same services from the same sources with nearly the same budgets but make up pretend or "shadow" contracts for practice. Next, the government required that the first year of real contracts must go largely to the same providers, hospitals, and so on, for nearly the same services, so that there would be a "steady state" and a "smooth take-off" as the health service was transformed from an administered service to an internal market. There followed hundreds of pages of terms, guidelines, and prohibitions from the management executive and the Department of Health. All this meant that a huge restructuring took place with hardly a patient or ball being dropped. But it also meant that the competing parties settled into stable, barely competitive relationships before the real contracting began after the practice year.

The chairs of all health authority boards and most of the chief executives of trusts were (and are) appointed by the secretary of state for health and thus the prime minister. Both became personally involved in major regional appointments and in responses to criticism or crises. This eliminated the famous civil service professionalism and tenure of Great Britain, and it replaced it not with survival of the fittest but survival of the politically loyal. Thus, even low-level staff personnel in the second and third years explained in confidential interviews that they felt they must either submit "doctored" data on the success of the reforms, so that their superiors would have their expectations confirmed by "facts," or be criticized for turning in "bad" reports.

Finally, the government quickly reined in the ability of trust hospitals to borrow money, and it imposed performance requirements that made it difficult for them to take risks that might lead to failure. Trust hospitals had to earn a 6 percent return on assets in use, stay within their external financing limit, set prices equal to average costs, have no cross-subsidization between services, make no capital investment that could not be demonstrated to be fully recovered from contract income, not dispose of their surpluses, and obtain most of their income from contracts with NHS authorities and fundholders (Bartlett and Le Grand, 1994). Trusts cannot go bankrupt. Bartlett and Le Grand concluded that "the independence and autonomy available to trusts is highly circumscribed, and the incentives to improve performance, which might be expected to be associated with an ability to retain financial surpluses earned through improved management performance, are eliminated" (p. 56). They also concluded that the financial success of better-performing trusts was largely an artifact of their being financially stronger and having lower costs before they became trusts. Strong initial performance was largely the result of one-time declines in real estate values that gave hospitals operating returns significantly above the 6 percent requirement.

On the purchasers' side, systematic evidence shows that they altered past funding patterns only at the margins and often at variance with their declared priorities (Klein and Redmayne, 1993, p. 17). They were able to free up less than 1 percent of their budgets for purchasing decisions, and ironically they moved more money toward acute services and away from community services. On the whole they handled "priority overload" by spreading the money around to many small initiatives (Klein, 1993, p. 73). This national study found "no agreement as to what should be included in a purchasing plan" (p. 6). Some plans had detailed analyses of demographics and needs, while others plunged into the details of contracts with providers. Time pressures and lack of good data made this almost inevitable.

In conclusion, the government's decisions to dictate competition, make managers accountable to political leaders, and eliminate most competition (because it can be so damaging) raise serious doubts about the wisdom of managed competition. The government's conservative requirements for a practice year and "steady state" contracts were responsible and sensible, but they greatly limited competition. A large number of unanticipated problems and complexities were addressed during that time. Without failed competitors' exiting, there cannot be much real competition (and in most national health care systems that are trying to contain costs there is not much entry of new competitors, either). Moreover, a national system with a history of tight budgets and taut supply or limited choice means that little can change. If there is barely enough money to do a job and everyone is being used to the hilt, especially when there are new entrants or few are exiting from the scene, there is very little room to maneuver.

The lesson, or question, for other countries drawn to the theory of managed competition is whether they dare let health care markets run freely. Are they ready to watch as competitors drop unprofitable services, expand profitable ones to oversupply, and drive less well managed hospitals into bankruptcy? For if they are not, then they will end up with all the extra costs of competition and few of its potential savings.

2.   *The system lacked good market information and effective purchasers.* At the outset, the government neglected the obvious fact that effective competition depends on good market information and strong purchasers. Surveys in 1991 and 1992 of NHS managers found high agreement that the "information required was limited, non-existent, inaccurate, or late" (Appleby and others, 1994, pp. 34–35). Eighty percent of the purchasers surveyed said they had difficulty obtaining comparable cost data in 1991. Sixty-five percent said they also lacked data on patient flows. Over 70 percent of provider-sellers surveyed also said that obtaining cost data was a problem (pp. 42–43).

As a result, health authorities had no choice but to purchase largely by means of block contracts with hospitals and units, hardly what advocates had in mind as competition. By 1992–93, 88 percent of all contracts were still block contracts, and only 10 percent had enough information to be based on costs per procedure (p. 40).

Closely related to the lesson that one needs to start with good market information and effective purchasers if competition is to improve the value of one's health care dollar is the need for good information on quality. The British immediately perceived this and made medical audits part of the reforms. But an independent assessment concluded that these audits, which are done by clinicians of their own work, are largely "an extension of the profession's current self-management arrangements" (Kerrison, Packwood, and Buxton, 1994, p. 157). Audit funds go specifically to senior doctors, not purchasers or even managers. They define what aspects of medicine are to be audited (mainly technical aspects) and by what measures. Yet the research team found that no vision or guidelines exist to inform these decisions. Also, the amount and quality of data at most sites are wholly inadequate. The results of audits are not tied to purchasing decisions, and clinicians do not emphasize resource use as an important focus of the audit.

3. *The system turned providers into entrepreneurs and potential monopolists.* The reforms rewarded providers who converted from thinking of themselves as public servants to thinking of themselves as entrepreneurs and exploiting their monopolistic advantages. Overall, there are few sellers competing with one another in the NHS. Ironically, one needs choice, and therefore slack, in a market for competition to make producers more efficient. In the case of the NHS, careful planning and tight budgeting over the previous decades had kept duplication to a minimum, so introducing competition strengthened the hand of provider-sellers rather than of buyers. In short, competition in taut, highly imperfect markets can backfire and turn carefully budgeted providers into active monopolists. The dangers of monopolistic action by provider-sellers are abetted by several factors: their natural advantages in health care markets; the weakness of buyers, as discussed before; the disinclination of patients to travel very far, so markets are de facto kept small; and the natural forms of professional behavior

that are regarded by economists as anticompetitive, such as restrictive collegial behavior (Light, 1994a, p. 363).

Often the "product" being bought and sold is difficult to define, because medical services are emergent and contingent (Light, 1993). The "product" being bought emerges as the diagnosis and treatment unfold, and it is contingent on information and responses to previous efforts. It is not even clear who is buying and who is selling, because the seller-providers often decide what is to be done (bought) and serve as the buyer's (patient's) agent. Independent information on what is being bought (however that gets defined) is difficult and costly to gather. Moreover, the seller-providers control much of the information needed to decide what to buy, and they can easily manipulate this information if given the incentive to do so. All of these problems became evident within the first year of the British reforms, and several still plague them.

So far, entrepreneurial exploitation by British doctors has been minimal, in part because the government has severely restricted such behavior and in part because the cultural shift to a commercial ethos takes many years, as it has in the United States since the end of World War II (Starr, 1982; Light, forthcoming). But the dangers of commercialism may well increase. GPs have now been given a strong economic stake in a wide array of services, and while they may not pocket the profits, there are ways of plowing them back into their practice so that the doctors benefit. Consultants (chiefs of services) have had to become small businessmen and increasingly market their services to a wider range of purchasers. Trust hospitals have only begun to exercise their powers to alter staff mix, compensation, and contracts.

4.   *The system created new inefficiencies, costs, and dislocations.* Even though it is supposed to save money overall, competition in health care creates new inefficiencies, costs, and dislocations. In the United Kingdom they have cost the government considerable funds. First, very large costs went into constructing the basic market itself—defining what the products are, determining costs, setting prices, gathering market information, contracting, monitoring—because the British had few itemized costs or prices beforehand, only budgets. Second, there has been a wide and diverse effort to obtain data on every aspect of productivity, quality,

and cost-effectiveness. The cost of collecting all these data was estimated early on to subtract about 10 percent of the budget from clinical services, unless compensatory efficiencies resulted (Light, 1990a). Third, large sums were invested in computer systems and data systems that did not work, did not provide the necessary information for purchasing, or were not compatible with one another. As of 1995 the majority of trust hospitals still lacked the information necessary to assess their cost-effectiveness and thus to make competition a viable enterprise. Regulations have had to increase in proportion to the variety of market imperfections discussed above and the dangers that accompany them.

The following are some of the new inefficiencies that come with competition in health care:

- *Managerialism*
  Managerial power versus clinical responsibility
  Bossing instead of facilitating
  Front office overstaffing
- *Datamania*
  Forms, data, and accounting beyond what can be digested
    and used
- *"Accountability" as an end*
- *Disruptions and inefficiencies from having underused losers and overused winners*
- *Ethos of commercialism replaces ethos of service*
  Gaming
  Favorable selection
  Cost shifting
  Service dilution

Savings must more than make up for these new costs if change is to be worthwhile. One of them (the fourth in our list here) concerns the effects when the winners win and the losers lose. Winning institutions find themselves swamped with more business than they can handle. Their quality and efficiency may decline because they won! Meanwhile, losers become still more inefficient as their unused capacity rises. Because it is extremely difficult to shut down a health care facility, the increased inefficiencies of the losers are dragged along in the system for some time and make up part of everyone's costs. In short, winning and losing do not produce efficiencies if markets clear slowly and if the costs of losing institutions have to be carried. Such costs are the "price of progress" in dynamic, open markets like those for personal computers or cars, but within a tight, closed budget that just pays for treating all the sick, such progress is difficult to attain, and a nation may be left just with the costs.

Also contributing to the costs of competition was the granting of new freedoms and power to qualified hospitals as "self-governing trusts." This gave those deeply entrenched institutions, which consume a large percent of the national budget, more powers and more incentives to persist and grow, even when the nation wanted to dehospitalize its system and reallocate the large sums locked up in hospital-based services. The theory of competition, some British leaders emphasize, required that hospitals be made into independent sellers that would sink or swim in the marketplace. But up to six weeks before the reforms were announced, only a diluted version of trusts was being explored (Butler, 1994; see also Appleby and others, 1994, p. 48). In reality, the government preselected the winners (Bartlett and LeGrand, 1994), and at nearly every point when they have appeared to be in trouble, it has stepped in. In any case, strong trust hospitals lock in large sums that need to be redirected toward community care, prevention, or primary care.

Another new cost is management itself. In the first three years of competitive markets, it appears that managerial costs in the NHS have approximately doubled, from 5 to 11 percent. The number of managers in the system has approximately tripled, in large part to handle the complex and relentless requirements of contracting. The increased number is due partly to supervising nurses' being reclassified as "managers," a principal way for them to make more money—managerial salaries have been rising two to three times faster than doctors' salaries or nurses' salaries. Although by American standards the proportion and cost of managers in the NHS may seem low, it is their rate of increase that is notable.

An unanticipated consequence is that managers have organized themselves into powerful political associations. They become entrenched, like a union. Satisfying the managers becomes an end in itself. All this is done in the name of improved efficiency and productivity, though the data are lacking to support this claim, and

U.S. data indicate that the managerial revolution here has primarily benefited managers (Woolhandler and Himmelstein, 1994). One can expect competition to increase significantly the size and cost of management teams, and the question is whether they make back their cost or more by improving the cost-effectiveness of services.

Finally, another new cost stems from destabilizing institutions and providers by putting them at risk of losing some of their revenues. In a given competitive market, fear of losing part of one's business seems much more prevalent than the expectation of winning. In either case, many institutions believe that hiring the best management team possible will ensure success. As a result, the number of managers, their compensation, and their power increase. The sheer pace of the reforms and the frequency with which the rules—and even the structure—of managed competition have changed have produced a widespread perception of new costs in mistakes, low morale, and confusion. The lack of an articulated vision of what one is rushing toward has added to the distress.

Turning to dislocations, some are good in the sense that they show the market is working. Perhaps the largest and most successful have been the decisions by purchasers in communities outside London to buy specialty services nearby rather than to send patients to the very expensive, major academic hospitals in London. This has certainly highlighted the inefficiencies, waste, and oversupply of academic medical centers, but the size and scope of dislocations are so great that the government is essentially administering the situation in an old-style state-planning mode of closing or consolidating facilities by administrative fiat. One issue is that increased use of local secondary care has left major tertiary care centers in financial crisis—an example of how regional planning falls victim to the market.

An example of the dislocations and costs of competition within a closed budget is the financial side of GP fundholding. The generous allocations to GP fundholders are depleting the budgets of district health authorities, so that some cannot pay for nonemergency care. This, in turn, has created a two-tier market between the "sponsored" patients of fundholders and the unsponsored patients of GPs who do not hold funds. It has also created "budget refugees," known as extracontractual referrals, because some patients see consultants not under contract with their home authority or GP.

GP fundholding has created a related dislocation, the conflict between health authorities' purchasing all services for an area's population and GP fundholders' purchasing selected services for their patient panel. The level and character of the purchasing differ significantly. Moreover, money siphoned off from the health authorities for the fundholders punches holes in the authorities' budgets, so they cannot carry out their overall, integrating mandate.

5. *The system substitutes ideological conviction for evaluation.* It is widely believed in Britain that using competition to solve the problems of health care is a tactic based more on ideology than on the reality of the health care system (May, 1993; Webster, 1993). By international standards, British health care had one of the lowest administrative overheads and smallest budgets per capita in the Western world. If efficiency is measured by services delivered per million dollars, then the NHS was among the most efficient. Although Mrs. Thatcher declared that crises due to underfunding were due to inefficiencies (which managed competition would rectify), there is considerable evidence that underfunding itself was (and is) a major source of inefficiency. Beds and services routinely had to be closed down because a given hospital or unit ran out of money before the year's end. In fact, underfunding may be one of the major sources of inefficiency in the NHS, because units have to carry the deadweight costs of underused capacity (Light, 1990c, 1991).

Compared to the previous two decades, funding for units of service slowed down during the 1980s (Robinson and Judge, 1987). Yet costly technological advances, rising expectations, and the burdens of an aging population all accelerated the volume of services. The Thatcher administration was repeatedly attacked in the late 1980s for underfunding and letting desperately ill patients wait for treatment and even die while waiting (Butler, 1994). Wards were closed on an unprecedented scale. An editorial in the *British Medical Journal* declared the NHS to be in terminal decline (Smith, 1988). Thus a strong case can be made that many of the problems, and certainly the ones that pushed Mrs. Thatcher into the political corner that prompted the market reforms, were largely due to underfunding. Efficiency gains from the managerial reforms and the contracting out of services during the earlier part of the 1980s meant that "there was little more scope within the existing system for greater yields without the addition of further resources" (Webster, 1993, p. 19).

The government chose ideology over reality by not examining closely the character of the inefficiencies it wished to reduce in order to decide whether competitive markets would reduce them and, if so, how the markets should be structured. In fact, the government did not review or analyze the nature of inefficiencies at any time, either before or after declaring that competition would make the NHS more efficient. Had they done so, they would have found that many of the inefficiencies were embedded in professional standards, clinical habits, the organization of work, the division of labor, hierarchies of power, and organizational rules (Light, 1991). Thus, introducing competitive contracting would not alone dislodge and eliminate them. The following lists some embedded inefficiencies found in the NHS at the start of managed competition:

- *Purchasing*
  Underfunding or overfunding of services
  Fragmented and duplicative purchasing
  Funding unneeded and ineffective services
  Lack of health services research to evaluate unneeded, ineffective, or inefficient services
- *Provider dominance*
  Overuse of hospitals and technology
  Overspecialization and overcertification of doctors and
    nurses
  Underuse of primary care and prevention
- *Entrenched civil service staff*
  No incentives to be productive and perform well
  Short work week and work year
  Low staff morale
  Pilfering
  High staff turnover

- *Managerial imperialism*
  Managerial authority divorced from clinical responsibility
  Overmanaged, top-heavy bureaucracy that perpetuates itself

To this list can be added wasted bed days, underused theater (operating room) time, overused theater time, subspecialists' being embedded in hospitals, high staff turnover, uncoordinated staff leaves, bureaucratic elaboration, and the overuse of hospitals (Light, 1990b). If only competitive bidding is established, embedded inefficiencies are likely to be carried forward within the calculations of costs and the structure of contracts as part of the taken-for-granted nature of the work.

Finally, the government did not commission empirical studies of the services or the markets they were creating, because independent evaluation of performance was not considered necessary. Further, they changed the ways in which data were collected or classified so that comparisons between prereform and postreform NHS services, finances, and efficiencies would be difficult. The ideology of competition would not tolerate good market information on performance (Smith, 1994). This antiempirical stance seems to have softened in 1995; yet as recently as December 1994 the *British Medical Journal* published details of suppressed data, obstructed access to other data, use of the Official Secrets Act to block information about services, gag clauses in trust contracts that prohibit doctors from saying anything critical about the quality of medicine they observed, and political control over health care professionals (Smith, 1994).

In these ways, the British policies advocating competition to bring tough-minded realism to health care were not rooted in reality. More deeply, they were not anchored in a vision of where the NHS wanted to go and a strategic plan for getting there. After summarizing the central elements of the reforms, Butler (1994, pp. 19–20) asks, "Yet what was it all for? What were the goals or purposes or objectives of the white paper? . . . What was the theory underlying the Government's belief in the capacity of the internal market to enhance the efficient use of resources?"

6. *The system politicized rationing and suppressed criticism.* The ideology of competition promises to depoliticize cost containment

(Enthoven, 1985). Instead, health care services have become more politicized at the same time that market forces have come into play. The choice, then, is politicized health care without economic competition or with it (Klein, 1993). With it, the political stakes get considerably higher, because risks are higher and services get destabilized.

The implication of choosing an ideological solution to real problems that unleashes dangerous forces is that a government will unintentionally generate political crises and embarrassment for itself. The British government's response to these dangers has been to announce "Success by Declaration." This involves three notable policies. One requires that no one in a national position speak critically of government actions. This in effect produces a blackout of realistic exchange about real problems that need solving. This "we can do no wrong" posture greatly limits what can be done to repair a decision that is not working.

The second way in which the government attempted to hide failures and mistakes and minimize criticism was to commission virtually no independent evaluations, to minimize data collected on the performance of providers and units, and to reclassify data that exists so that evaluations of how the reforms have affected services are very difficult to make (Radical Statistics Health Group, 1992). The devolution of management has increasingly fragmented national data, a point that raises basic questions about the relationships between markets and measured quality or efficiency. All the senior health economists and health service researchers confirm this situation (see essays in Light and May, 1993; Robinson and Le Grand, 1994). Most of the studies cited in this report are small in scale and limited, but there is little else.

The third indirect but important way that feedback on problems and criticism is minimized is to minimize consumer involvement in markets. Of course, consumerism appears to be one of the basic platforms of the market reforms; the key document is entitled *Working for Patients* (Secretaries of State for Health, 1989). Yet the government has commissioned little research on the role and dynamics of patient preferences, and a good case can be made that working "for" patients means that consumer choice is irrelevant, because the NHS will provide the best possible care for everyone (Mahon, Wilkin, and Whitehouse, 1994). The goals of higher quality and efficiency are assumed to respond to patients' preferences. Moreover, medical services do things *to* people rather than *for* them, and they have little or no power of exit. Patients are little involved in choosing a hospital or consultant, yet they seem highly satisfied with the choices made.

Looking over these six negative lessons, one might summarize that if one cannot have good competition in health care that produces lower prices, better services, and greater value without sacrificing equity, don't do it. The negative lessons have taken us deeply into the British experience itself in order to explain them. We have learned that, contrary to the image of an invisible hand sorting out the problems of health care, competition is as highly politicized as administrated services. Its strong tendency to increase inequalities and create political embarrassment means that a nation interested in avoiding both will allow little competition to take place, even as it trumpets its virtues. Competition also legitimates demands, which are greater than needs, and promotes consumerism. The result is pressure to spend more, not less. Moreover, purchasing may be hard to separate from selling in health care, and the amount of managing of markets needed forces governments back into a strong administrative posture.

One point made clear by the negative lessons is that smart, informed purchasing is what makes competition work. Yet the service providers and packagers have the natural advantages in health care, and competition alters their values and behavior toward commercialism and maximizing their self-interest. These and other points made above suggest that the United States is heading for greater costs, dislocations, and inequities as its relatively unmanaged markets expand and the entire system gets locked into dependence on corporations aiming to maximize the quarterly returns to their investors.

Beyond Managed Competition: Three Positive Lessons

As the analysis above has indicated, the British are struggling with their own conflicts and contradictions and with the locked-in inefficiencies of a hospital-dominated budget. Yet they are clearly moving beyond managed competition to something better:

1.   *Focus on purchasing more than on competition.* By the second year of managed competition, many district and regional executives and purchasers began to express in interviews their exasperation with competing against one another, especially in markets that the central management was constantly altering. Wasn't the point of needs-based purchasing to work *together* to figure out how best to spend a limited budget and help people with their health problems? Didn't this mean that the act of purchasing—or even better, commissioning—was what really mattered (Light, 1994b)?

The conversion of administrative authorities into purchasers with budgets for the health care of a fixed population has transformed thinking and services from a focus on clinical intervention to a focus on prevention, health maintenance, new configurations, and accountability. Competition is secondary and gets in the way. Purchasing or commissioning promotes accountability, greater value, and a structured process of reflecting on what one is doing; administering services does not. For instead of service groups' getting this year's budget based on last year's budget, they must come together over a common needs-based budget and think through more cost-effective ways to reconfigure their services and reallocate their funds.

This seems to be the principal lesson that has emerged from the British experience with systemwide managed competition: *almost all the benefits of the health care reforms have stemmed from the act of purchasing, and almost all the hazards, inequities, and cost increases have come from competing.* This conclusion may seem strange, even contradictory—how can one purchase without competition resulting? Certainly some competition is inherent in purchasing, but it can be minimal, and the policy focus makes a great difference. The paradox of purchasing without much competition is solved by setting rules for equity, universality, and cost containment that have the net effect of minimizing supply-side economic competition in a market prone to distortions and market failure. Bilateral monopolies, like the Kaiser HMO's annual contract with its separately incorporated physicians, provide each party with an occasion to review their goals, relationship, and performance.

Cooperative purchasing between parties or enterprises that have a common goal (like maximizing the health of a people) is like the Japanese approach to economic growth, in which protected entities (like health authorities) have long-term relationships with the best producers they can find and work with them to improve their service or product (Best, 1990; Johnson, 1995). This neglected, nineteenth-century method of achieving economic growth differs markedly from Anglo-American ideas about competition (Fallows, 1993). Competition focuses on the process of buying and selling between individuals. It *assumes* that this process will increase wealth for everyone. Cooperative and regulated purchasing focuses on maximizing production (in this case, of health) for the entire community. Ironically, the United Kingdom used this approach to become the strongest industrialized nation in the world and then started losing its strength when it shifted to laissez-faire, Adam Smith–style competition (Lazonick, 1991; Fallows, 1993). Competition is short-term and unplanned, with a roller coaster of profits and losses. Cooperative and regulated purchasing is long-term and planned. Competition assumes there will be more and more money and wealth—everyone can keep winning. In a zero-sum situation like a health care budget, however, competition maximizes losers and disruption in a frustrating contest of everyone against everyone else. For these reasons, some of the leading health policy analysts in the United States are warning against the current rush to competition and advocating cooperation instead (Coile, 1995): "The ultimate goal for health care's stakeholders is to create healthy customers and communities. . . . Only if all parties agree to cooperate in reducing demand and optimizing resources can America provide affordable health care to its 250 million residents" (p. 7).

2.   *Focus on needs-based commissioning, including prevention and community care.* The focus on long-term purchasing within limited budgets leads inexorably to "promoting the health of the population, involving it in a wide range of relationships extending beyond the NHS itself" (Functions Analysis Group 7, 1994, p. 1). Purchasing for the health needs of a population fundamentally alters one's framework from budgeting for medical services to asking, "How can we best spend this money to meet the health needs of our area?" That question, in turn, quickly forces one into complex but important debates about what "need" means, how to measure it, and how to decide priorities. All this has led the British to reconceptualize purchasing as "commissioning"—that is, the creative rethinking (like "commissioning a building") of what kinds of services will best maximize the health of a population

or community. Needs-based commissioning, in turn, calls for *joint* commissioning—that is, the joining together of hospital and community services with primary care, and both with social services, so that integrated plans can be carried out. Joint commissioning centers on the creative process of figuring out how best to spend limited funds to maximize the health of a population. It is now the revolutionary force in the NHS.

As early as the second year, purchasers were advocating joint commissioning (Ham and Heginbotham, 1991). Purchasers found that they could best assess their populations' health needs together. They found that it made more sense to work jointly in providing care to patients with chronic conditions. Top administrators started forming joint commissioning authorities (even though they were illegal, because each partner was required to purchase only in its own domain). The senior managers developed elaborate informal procedures and accounting mechanisms to obey the letter of the law while breaching it in reality. Parliament hastily began to write a law to make the inevitable legal. As these and other developments have strengthened purchasing, GPs and trusts have combined organizationally and politically to match the size and power of the joint authorities. The fragmenting effects of GP fundholding on needs-based purchasing and on addressing the overall needs of a population also require coordination.

Yet, although joint commissioning is obvious, it is not easy. For professionalism and battle-hardened tactics of turf protection require a complex, long, and sometimes painful effort to reconcile quite different visions of needs, concepts of clients or patients, and notions about which interventions are most effective. Hospitals and traditional expenditures, as noted before, are deeply entrenched. Further, GP fundholders operate at a local, clinical level, which somehow has to be put in the context of overall health needs. "The dilemma here is that health authorities and fundholders offer a starkly contrasting approach to purchasing. . . . In simple terms, the choice is between needs-based purchasing for large populations and demand-based purchasing for small populations" (Ham and Spurgeon, 1992, p. 32). Yet all agree that it is the larger goals of preventing illness and death to which all purchasing should be directed.

Joint commissioning also refers to joining these two with the budget for community care services that is now part of the local or municipal budget for social services. This is very complicated and politically charged, for NHS services are not means-tested, but local services are. Is nursing home care a social service, a part of public housing with a nurse or doctor coming in now and then, or a part of health care? Similar questions can be and are being raised about many other kinds of maintenance services for people with chronic conditions. Joint commissioning can also refer to joining the budgets and efforts of public health with those of clinical services. The British, like many peoples, have a master plan for prevention. But given the integrated hierarchical structure and culture of the NHS, its master plan for prevention gets built into priorities for funding and decisions about the reorganization involved in joint commissioning. Community health and social services are part of this integration. Many interesting and original models for integrating these agencies and programs are being developed. The obvious need to work with authorities involved in reducing crime and violence, providing safe and adequate housing, generating more jobs, and training the workforce widens that circle still further. In short, the British have discovered that the underlying agenda of managed competition for cost-effective medical services is to prevent illness and death, promote health, and mobilize community-based health programs.

3. *Emphasize long-term responsibility and continuity.* The lesson for American managed competition is that multiple purchasers competing to maximize profits in fluid markets are unlikely to address the most pressing health needs or to well serve those who are most needy. In fact, if they do they will lose money and thus the investor confidence they need to survive. Given that so much of the cost is for the care of so few very sick people (about 72 percent of health care dollars are consumed by only 10 percent of a population), incentives are intense to avoid them or disenroll them.

The British are now focusing on joint purchasing authorities that have a long-term responsibility for improving the well-being of a resident population and the services offered it. Trust and accountability are maximized, in contrast to the high rates of switching and the spot markets that characterize the most "advanced" American markets. In the case of health care, almost everyone agrees that improvement should center on the health status and functioning of the population.

Conclusion

In many ways, these last three adaptable policy lessons reinforce the goals and vision with which the NHS started, which were only partly implemented after 1948. Through the transformation from budgeting services to purchasing for health gain and maintenance, the NHS has sharpened its focus on the reasons for its existence—the *health* of the people, not medical services themselves. The first eleven adaptable policy lessons, together with these last three, can help to prepare the NHS, or any other nation, to address the tidal wave of chronic conditions that will begin to swell in the next decade and extend well into the twenty-first century. For the United States, they suggest that a basically different policy orientation is urgently needed if it is to meet those needs without consuming still more of its GNP. The American system already consumes 14 percent of GNP for health care, up from 9 percent when it started using competition to contain costs in the late 1970s—and still with massive uninsured populations and underinsured employees. By the end of the 1990s, as its unmanaged markets expand and its undying faith in competition prevails, will its health care expenditures consume 18 percent of GNP?

Notes

1.   Private for-profit and nonprofit providers have become a major presence in the care of the elderly, the mentally handicapped, and the mentally ill, thanks to a funding door Mrs. Thatcher opened to the treasury. As a result, expenditures have risen over one hundred–fold in these areas, not quite what Mrs. Thatcher had in mind when she championed the efficiency of the private sector.
2.   American readers need to appreciate that "announcing" a reform in a system where the prime minister always has a majority in Parliament (and this prime minister held particular sway) is tantamount to ordering it. I was amazed to watch, between announcement and the passage of the law many months later, that nearly everyone began implementing the reforms as if they were already law.
3.   See the extraordinary set of brief articles assembled by the editor of the *British Medical Journal* entitled "The rise of Stalinism in the

NHS" (Smith, 1994). The management executive is formally part of the Department of Health, but the position is so powerful that it has become at least parallel to, if not greater than, that of the department.

References

Appleby, J., and others. "Monitoring Managed Competition." In R. Robinson and J. Le Grand (eds.), *Evaluating the NHS Reforms*. London, England: King's Fund Institute, 1994.

Arrow, K. "Uncertainty and the Welfare Economics of Medical Care." *American Economic Review*, 1963, *53*, 941–973.

Bartlett, W., and Le Grand, J. "The Performance of Trusts." In R. Robinson and J. Le Grand (eds.), *Evaluating the NHS Reforms*. London, England: King's Fund Institute, 1994.

Best, M. H. *The New Competition: Institutions of Industrial Restructuring*. Oxford, England: Polity Press, 1990.

Boulding, K. E. *Principles of Economic Policy*. Englewood Cliffs, N.J.: Prentice Hall, 1958.

Buchanan, J. W. *The Public Finances*. Homewood, Ill.: Irwin, 1960.

Butler, J. "Origins and Early Development." In R. Robinson and J. Le Grand (eds.), *Evaluating the NHS Reforms*. London, England: King's Fund Institute, 1994.

Coile, R. C., Jr. "Managed Cooperation, Not Competition: A Proposal for Implementing National Health Reform." *Frontiers of Health Services Management*, 1995, *10*(3), 3–28.

Enthoven, A. C. *Reflections on the Management of the National Health Service: An American Looks at Incentives to Efficiency in Health Services Management in the UK*. London, England: Nuffield Provincial Hospitals Trust, 1985.

Enthoven, A. C. *Theory and Practice of Managed Competition in Health Care Finance*. Amsterdam, The Netherlands: North-Holland, 1988.

Fallows, J. "How the World Works." *The Atlantic Monthly*, 1993, *272*(6), 61–87.

Farmer, A. "The Changing Role of General Practice in the British National Health Service." In D. Light and A. May (eds.), *Britain's Health System: From Welfare State to Managed Markets*. New York: Faulkner & Gray, 1993.

Fry, J., Light, D. W., Rodnick, J., and Orton, J. *Reviving Primary Care: A US-UK Comparison*. New York: Radcliffe Medical Press, 1995.

Functions Analysis Group 7. *Local Strategy and Purchasing*. London, England: NHS Management Executive, 1994.

Ginzberg, E. "What Every Economist Should Know About Health and Medicine." *American Economic Review,* 1954, *44,* 104–119.

Glennerster, H., Matsaganis, M., and Owens, P. *A Foothold on Fundholding.* London, England: King's Fund Institute, 1992.

Glennerster, H., Matsaganis, M., Owens, P., and Hancock, S. "GP Fundholding: Wild Care or Winning Hand?" In R. Robinson and J. Le Grand (eds.), *Evaluating the NHS Reforms.* London, England: King's Fund Institute, 1994.

Ham, C. *Management and Competition in the New NHS.* Oxford, England: Radcliffe Medical Press, 1994.

Ham, C., and Heginbotham, C. J. *Purchasing Together.* London, England: King's Fund College, 1991.

Ham, C., and Spurgeon, P. *Effective Purchasing.* HSMC Discussion Paper 28. Birmingham: Health Services Management Centre, 1992.

Healthcare Financial Management Association. *Introductory Guide to NHS Finance in the UK.* (2nd ed.) London, England: Healthcare Financial Management Association, 1993.

Johnson, C. *Japan: Who Governs?* New York: W. W. Norton, 1995.

Jones, D., Lester, C., and West, R. "Monitoring Changes in Health Services for Older People." In R. Robinson and J. Le Grand (eds.), *Evaluating the NHS Reforms.* London, England: King's Fund Institute, 1994.

Kerrison, S., Packwood, T., and Buxton, M. "Monitoring Medical Audit." In R. Robinson and J. Le Grand (eds.), *Evaluating the NHS Reforms.* London, England: King's Fund Institute, 1994.

Klarman, H. E. *The Economics of Health.* New York: Columbia University Press, 1965.

Klein, R. "Rationality and Rationing: Diffused or Concentrated Decision Making?" In M. Tunbridge (ed.), *Rationing of Health Care in Medicine.* London, England: Royal College of Physicians, 1993.

Klein, R., and Redmayne, S. *Patterns of Priorities: A Study of the Purchasing and Rationing Policies of Health Authorities.* Birmingham, England: National Association of Health Authorities and Trusts, 1993.

Lazonick, W. *Business Organization and the Myth of the Market Economy.* New York: Cambridge University Press, 1991.

Light, D. W. "Biting Hard on the Research Bit." *The Health Service Journal,* 1990a, *100*(5224), 1604–1605.

Light, D. W. "Labelling Waste as Inefficiency." *The Health Service Journal,* 1990b, *100*(5223), 1552–1553.

Light, D. W. "Learning from Their Mistakes?" *The Health Service Journal,* 1990c, *100*(5221), 1470–1472.

Light, D. W. "Effectiveness and Efficiency Under Competition: The Cochrane Test." *British Medical Journal,* 1991, *303,* 1253–1254.

Light, D. W. "The Practice and Ethics of Risk-Rated Health Insurance." *Journal of the American Medical Association,* 1992, *267,* 2503–2508.

Light, D. W. "Escaping the Traps of Postwar Western Medicine." *European Journal of Public Health,* 1993, *3,* 223–231.

Light, D. W. "Health Care Systems and Their Financing." In J. Walton, G. Owen, and P. Rhodes (eds.), *The New Oxford Medical Companion.* Oxford, England: Oxford University Press, 1994a.

Light, D. W. *Strategic Challenges in Joint Commissioning.* London, England: Northwest Thames Regional Health Authority, 1994b.

Light, D. W. *The Future of Fundholding.* London, England: Institute for Health Services Management, 1995a.

Light, D. W. "*Homo Economicus:* Escaping the Traps of Managed Competition." *European Journal of Public Health,* 1995b, *5,* 145–151.

Light, D. W. "Managed Competition: Policy Lessons from the British Experience." Report to the Physicians Payment Review Commission, 1995c.

Light, D. W. "The Restructuring of the American Health Care System." In T. J. Litman and L. S. Robins (eds.), *Health Politics and Policy.* (3rd ed.) Albany, N.Y.: Delmar, forthcoming.

Light, D., and May, A. (eds.). *Britain's Health System: From Welfare State to Managed Markets.* New York: Faulkner & Gray, 1993.

Mahon, A., Wilkin, D., and Whitehouse, C. "Choice of Hospital for Elective Surgery Referral: GPs' and Patients' Views." In R. Robinson and J. Le Grand (eds.), *Evaluating the NHS Reforms.* London, England: King's Fund Institute, 1994.

May, A. "Thatcherism, the New Public Management, and the NHS." In D. Light and A. May (eds.), *Britain's Health System: From Welfare State to Managed Markets.* New York: Faulkner & Gray, 1993.

Mechanic, D. "Changing Medical Organization and the Erosion of Trust." *Milbank Quarterly,* 1996, *74*(2), 171–190.

Radical Statistics Health Group. "NHS Reforms: The First Six Months— Proof of Progress or a Statistical Smokescreen?" *British Medical Journal,* 1992, *304,* 705–709.

Reinhardt, U. E. "Table Manners at the Health Care Feast." In D. Yaggy and W. G. Anlyan (eds.), *Financing Health Care: Competition vs. Regulation.* New York: Ballinger, 1982.

Rice, T., Brown, E. R., and Wyn, R. "Holes in the Jackson Hole Approach to Health Care Reform." *Journal of the American Medical Association,* 1993, *270,* 1357–1362.

Robinson, R., and Judge, K. *Public Expenditures and the NHS: Trends and Prospects.* London, England: King's Fund Institute, 1987.

Robinson, R., and Le Grand, J. (eds.). *Evaluating the NHS Reforms.* London, England: King's Fund Institute, 1994.

Samuelson, P. A. *Economics.* (3rd ed.) New York: McGraw-Hill, 1955.

Secretaries of State for Health. *Working for Patients.* London, England: Her Majesty's Stationary Office, 1989.

Smith, R. "The Rise of Stalinism in the NHS." *British Medical Journal,* 1994, *309,* 1640–1645.

Smith, T. "New Year Message." *British Medical Journal,* 1988, *296,* 1–2.

Starr, P. *The Social Transformation of American Medicine.* New York: Basic Books, 1982.

Stigler, G. J. *The Theory of Price.* (Rev. ed.) New York: Macmillan, 1952.

Stone, D. A. "The Struggle for the Soul of Health Insurance." *Journal of Health Politics, Policy and Law,* 1993, *18,* 287–318.

Webster, C. "The National Health Service: The First Forty Years." In D. Light and A. May (eds.), *Britain's Health System: From Welfare State to Managed Markets.* New York: Faulkner & Gray, 1993.

Woolhandler, S., and Himmelstein, D. U. "Giant H.M.O. 'A' or Giant H.M.O. 'B'?" *The Nation,* Sept. 19, 1994, pp. 265–266.

The Potential and Limits of Competitive Managed Care

John D. Wilkerson, Kelly J. Devers, Ruth S. Given

The preceding chapters provide "snapshots" of recent changes in the health care marketplace that are having or will have important consequences for the efficiency and equitable distribution of health care in the United States. What does the future hold? Will the trend toward price competition among private managed care organizations continue? If so, what consequences will it have for health care financing and delivery and for the nation's health? While it is not possible to predict the answers to these questions with certainty, it is possible to identify and discuss the key variables that will shape the future of health care in the United States.

In this Conclusion we propose and discuss a model that, while not predictive, is nevertheless useful for identifying the broader social and environmental forces that will influence how the system develops and the consequences for what should be the ultimate objective of any health care system—better health.

Goals of a Health Care System

According to the World Health Organization, "Health is a state of complete physical, mental, and social well-being, and not merely the absence of disease or injury" (Evans and Stoddart, 1994, p. 28). Clearly, health is determined by many things that have little to do with access to affordable health care, from genetic predispositions to environmental pollutants, family environment, and cultural influences and expectations. Even if one's definition of health is limited to "the absence of disease or injury," in terms of bang for the buck, innovations in medical care have had much less of an impact on improving the health of Americans over the past century than have innovations in public health such as sanitation, immunizations, and changes in lifestyles and behaviors (Fuchs, 1974; McGinnis and Foege, 1993).

It would be wrong to conclude from the previous paragraph that medical care has not been beneficial to individuals and to society as a whole. Access to medical care and technological improvements has reduced mortality and improved quality of life for many individuals. The point is that from the perspective of a society, additional investments in medical care may not be the best way to use limited resources to promote health and improve quality of life. A market that efficiently allocates resources to produce health care *services* (the focus of this book) may not be efficient at producing *health*. But what does it mean to efficiently produce health?

From a social perspective, health care markets should contribute to three ultimate goals. The first is to provide an optimal level of health for society. The second is to distribute that health equitably. The third is to produce it efficiently.

Optimal Level of Health

A society may be said to have achieved its optimal level of health when it expects that more total social benefits would accrue from spending additional resources on things other than additional improvements in health. We could devote all of our resources to improving our health status, but we probably would not want to. Currently, one seventh of the nation's income (gross domestic product) is spent on health care services. How does a society decide that the health status of its citizens is "good enough?" And how does it decide that it is not willing to spend any more on improving health?

Equitable Distribution of Health

Health is equitably distributed when a society is no longer willing to make additional investments, economic or political, to redistribute resources to improve the health of certain members. Americans' health status varies greatly, as does their access to health care services. But health status will always vary, if for no other reason than that illnesses and accidents can be capricious. How does a society decide that an existing distribution of health or access to health care is unfair or fair (Schroeder, 1996)? And how does it decide that it is or is not willing to further redistribute resources to make health outcomes or access to health care more fair?

Thus, the optimal level and equitable distribution of health in a society cannot be determined without involving trade-offs among competing values that must be resolved through political channels. Many societies have explicitly limited overall spending on health care services while still guaranteeing access to affordable care for all their citizens. Other societies, such as the United States, have consistently rejected caps on overall health care spending and (at least implicitly) decided that for all but the poorest and the elderly, health care will be rationed according to individuals' ability to pay.

Efficient Production of Health

Some approaches to achieving the same level and distribution of health or health care services are more costly than others. Ideally, a society would choose the least costly means, once it had decided on its optimal level and distribution of health. But this is a difficult task, for both technical and political reasons. Things other than health care services, such as education and income, appear to have much larger effects on health status than does access to health care (Fuchs, 1994, pp. 56–57). However, the benefits of an investment in heart surgery, for example, are immediate and measurable, while the benefits of a similar investment in college scholarships for inner-city teens would be distributed across individuals and over time. Even though the aggregate health benefits to society of the latter might be substantially larger, they would be more difficult to isolate technically and to defend politically.

Health and Health Care Services

If health care services are not the primary determinants of health, what are? A more complete perspective on the impact of the health care marketplace and other forces on health is proposed in Figure C.1. As mentioned, the objectives that are typically used in evaluations of health care systems—cost, coverage, quality, and access to services—are intermediate rather than ultimate goals.

Health

Health is influenced (both positively and negatively) by epidemiological and demographic characteristics, technological developments, economic and political circumstances, and sociocultural differences.

Some of these forces affect a society's health in ways that are largely independent of the performance of the health care market. Although the market may respond to demographic changes by, for example, developing new approaches (both services and products) to health care that address the special needs of an expanding elderly population, it is not likely that the market will be able to prevent overall health care costs from rising or the aging population's health from ultimately declining.

The effects of other forces, in contrast, *will* significantly depend on how both the market and public policymakers respond. Thousands of hemophiliacs became infected with HIV because blood suppliers were slow to introduce costly screening tests (Shilts, 1988). Many other Americans became infected after political considerations prevented the federal government and local communities from implementing prevention campaigns in the epidemic's early stages.

The effects of these forces on health will also depend on the responses of other markets, institutions, and actors that are not directly involved in providing, consuming, or regulating health care services. Shoe manufacturers, for example, may inadvertently produce positive (or negative) health consequences as they promote recreational sports to sell more shoes. Government regulators may require public utilities to install scrubbers on their smokestacks to reduce a by-product—air pollution—that has harmful health effects. Animal rights supporters may devote resources to increasing public awareness of the negative health consequences of eating meat in order to promote their (non–health related) goal of reducing animal suffering.

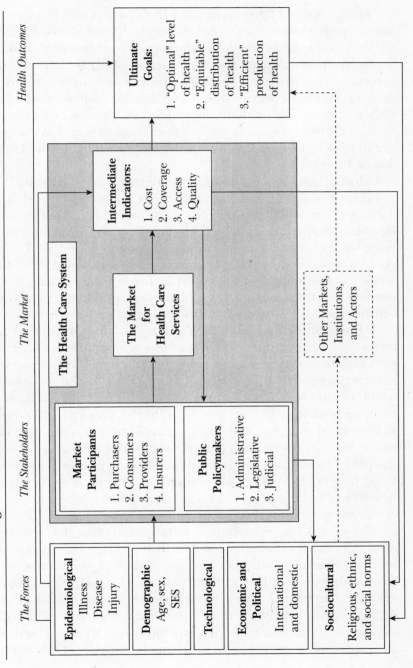

Figure C.1. Health-Related Forces and the Health Care System.

Epidemiological forces include all the diseases and injuries that are the proximate causes of differences in health status. The most striking examples of the consequences of epidemiological forces for health have involved the introduction of previously unknown infectious diseases, such as AIDS, and the development of drug-resistant strains of previously known diseases, such as tuberculosis. Other, less striking epidemiological forces, such as heart disease, various chronic respiratory conditions, and cancer, have a much greater impact on overall morbidity and mortality in the United States, however.

Most of the focus of the health care system is on treating these proximate causes of illness, although it is not always clear that this focus is the most efficacious for society as a whole. The large dollar amounts spent on finding a medical cure for AIDS might have been better spent on social education programs designed to prevent its transmission (Hay, Osmond, and Jacobson, 1988; Stipp, 1996). The same argument could be made for spending less on treating heart disease and lung cancer and spending more on preventing the behaviors, such as smoking, that cause them.

Although the social benefits of emphasizing prevention may be easy to demonstrate, public interests are not always congruent with private interests. Traditionally, the American health care market has not provided the level and scope of preventive services that would be optimal for society as a whole. The explanation is simple from an economic perspective. Most health plans do offer extensive prenatal care, because gains are realized almost immediately, in the form of fewer birth complications and thus lower costs to the plans. In contrast, the benefits of smoking prevention, though large, may not be realized for decades, so a health plan that invests heavily in smoking cessation programs will not realize most of the economic gain from those programs.

Demographic forces include general population characteristics associated with differences in health status, including age, sex, income, education, and occupation. Although the link between demographics and health is not always clear, changing demographics can have a major impact on overall population health. Aging is clearly one of the most important natural causes of declining health status. For example, morbidity due to the presence of chronic conditions increases substantially with age. Only 9.2 percent of the U.S. population between fifteen and forty-four years of age suffered from a chronic condition in 1991, compared with 44.2 percent of those seventy-five years of age or older. Health status also varies by socioeconomic status (income, education, and occupation) (Pinkney, 1994). When asked to assess their own health status, only 3.9 percent of individuals with incomes above $50,000 reported it to be fair or poor, compared with 19.9 percent of individuals earning less than $14,000 (National Center for Health Statistics, 1995).

In the United States, demographic changes over the coming decades will have dramatic consequences for health and health care spending. By 2025, one quarter of the population will be sixty-five years of age or older (up from about 15 percent today). There is also evidence of increasing inequality in incomes (Silverstein, 1996; Murray, 1996). The effects of these changes will depend in part on how America's health care system responds to the challenges they raise. Because of the aging of the population, we can expect many more people with chronic conditions, which are often very expensive to treat. The ability to maintain current standards of care will depend either on even higher rates of spending on health or on dramatic improvements in the efficiency of the health care system.

Technological forces can also have large positive or negative consequences for health. Emissions from industry and vehicles have large adverse effects on health (Morris, Naumova, and Munasinghe, 1995). A recent study of 239 metropolitan areas, for example, indicates that cardiopulmonary deaths caused by airborne particulates exceed the number of deaths caused by automobile accidents or by AIDS and breast cancer combined (Cone, 1996). Other technologies, such as modern agriculture, have almost certainly produced a net improvement in health. As is true for the other forces already discussed, the impact of these technological forces on health typically has little to do with the health care system.

How the health care system responds to technological developments can also have large effects on health. HMOs claim that they are uniquely positioned to promote prevention, but their willingness to lobby for reducing environmental pollutants will depend on the extent to which they will profit from a benefit that accrues not only to their enrollees but also to the general community. Economic theory suggests that because the benefits will be distributed broadly, such preventive services will be undersupplied.

Other technological forces do suggest real opportunities for improving health through the health care system. Rapid advances in computer technology, in combination with the recent deregulation of the telecommunications industry, are expected to stimulate the development and use of health care information systems that can both increase efficiency and improve quality of care (Skolnick, 1996). Such systems could serve a number of purposes, including providing patient-level clinical data for tracking medical outcome–based quality of care within specific institutions; allowing better access to providers, via "telemedicine," for residents of rural areas; and improving the availability of up-to-date clinical research and general health information to providers and consumers through the Internet (Ziegler, 1995; Pitta, 1996).

In the medical technology arena, the development of new screening techniques will make it possible to detect some diseases earlier, when they are less expensive to cure (Naj, 1996; "Ultrasound Breast Cancer Test Approved," 1996). In such cases, earlier diagnosis can allow the use of less invasive surgical techniques, simultaneously reducing costs and improving outcomes.

However, it is also possible for technological innovations to lead to higher health care costs with little positive health benefits or raise other concerns (Cutler, 1996). Screening of asymptomatic patients is an area of technical innovation that may be expected to increase costs. Promotion of more and more sensitive diagnostic tests for the detection of breast and prostate cancer, for example, may result in much unnecessary treatment in the event of a high rate of false-positive results (Winslow, 1994; Kolata, 1996). Not only does excessive screening result in increased costs, but unnecessary treatment for these conditions (especially in the case of mastectomy and prostatectomy) can reduce quality of life for patients. Also, the development and adoption of better health care information systems raises concerns about safeguarding the confidentiality of highly sensitive patient information. Even if all of the technical problems inherent in such ambitious information systems are solved, concerns over system security and access to personal records may make implementation politically infeasible (Gorman, 1996).

Economic and political forces can also affect population health in ways that are largely independent of the functioning of the health care system. Studies have shown that unemployment due to business cycles is associated with higher rates of morbidity and possibly mortality from certain causes (Haan, Kaplan, and Syme, 1989; Catalano, 1991). Although some of this effect may be partly due to a corresponding reduction in health care coverage and access, much of it probably results from the increased stress associated with economic dislocation. Similarly, political events can have a large impact on health. In addition to the obvious impact of politically inspired events such as war, changes in political control of the government can inspire dramatic health-related reforms. In the 104th Congress, a newly elected Republican majority reduced federal spending on popular environmental programs. At the other end of the Washington Mall, Dr. David Kessler, a Bush appointee, announced that the Food and Drug Administration was considering regulating tobacco as a drug, even though there was little public support for increased government regulation of tobacco use among adults.

Economic and political forces also influence health through their effects on the health care system. As discussed in Chapter One, the federal government played a central role in encouraging the development of prepaid health plans during the 1970s, when there was little support among providers and little awareness among the public. National and international economic forces (especially increased global competition) have also played a central role in raising the cost-consciousness of U.S. employers and promoting the rise of price-competitive managed care. In the future, an improving economy would mean that employers would have more resources to devote to providing high-quality health care for their employees, and the government would have more resources to devote to its role as a safety net provider. The results of forthcoming elections will also shape the future roles and obligations of employers and of the federal and state governments in this health care system.

Sociocultural forces such as ethnicity, religion, and cultural norms can influence health by affecting how we behave and by altering our expectations about what it means to be healthy. With respect to behavior, activities that are not directly related to considerations of health often have health consequences. Teen-agers start smoking or drinking to impress their peers and because it gives them pleasure (Levin, 1996). Mormons abstain from alcohol and cigarettes for religious reasons (Fuchs, 1974). Recent immigrants from Mexico have been shown to have better health outcomes than those who have become acculturated to American society (Guendelman, Chavez, and Christianson, 1994). Individuals or groups who are more effective at influencing the political process are more likely to have their health concerns addressed by policymakers.

What a society considers to be relevant to health also affects the amount and distribution of resources devoted to health. Most Americans probably define health less broadly than the World Health Organization. At the same time, Americans probably include "quality of life" along with the "absence of disease or injury" when they think about health today, much more than they did in the past. Along the same lines, society's willingness to devote resources to address a health problem can depend importantly on prevailing beliefs about its causes. Many people were probably less concerned about AIDS when it was the "gay cancer" than when it began to increasingly affect heterosexuals and children.

Sociocultural forces can also have important consequences for the functioning of a health care system. The efficiency of a health care system can be improved by recognizing that people from different ethnic groups and cultures see health and interpret illness differently and respond differently to different treatments. While individuals may be diagnosed with an identical disease, the "illness" that they personally experience and their attitude toward it will be shaped by their past and present sociocultural surroundings (Conrad and Kern, 1994). More generally, a society's expectations about health (and health care) define the boundaries for what the health care system is expected to do. An ever-larger proportion of private and public health care spending will be devoted to caring for people with chronic conditions as the nation's population ages. The "high cost of dying" will raise important ethical questions about society's responsibility to the chronically ill. These questions will not be resolved by health care providers or public policy; they will be resolved by changing social expectations about the obligations of society to individuals, and individuals to society.

The Health Care Market

What is the likely effect of the health care market itself on health? The functioning of the health care market relies on the behavior and actions of the key stakeholders in the health care system. Figure 1 divides these stakeholders into two major categories, health care market participants and public policymakers. The market participants include private and public health benefit purchasers, health care consumers, providers, and insurers. The policymakers include elected and appointed officials in the legislative, judicial, and administrative branches of federal, state, and local governments with jurisdiction over health care issues. Since health care markets exhibit market failures of many types, there is a high degree of public intervention to attempt to improve efficiency and equity. As a result, public policymakers of all sorts play a particularly important role in the functioning of the health care market.

The behavior of the various stakeholders will depend on their goals, their resources, and their opportunities for shaping the system and its outcomes. Predicting how all of the different actions produced by these differences in goals, resources, and opportunities will converge to produce the "health care system" that exists at a particular point in time is obviously difficult, and probably impossible.

Nevertheless, it is possible to highlight a few general lessons about the ability of health care markets to address some of the challenges to health raised by these different forces. In some situations, health care markets can be expected to function relatively efficiently. In others, they are unlikely to play an important role in addressing important opportunities to improve health. Any action, if it occurs, will need to be initiated through other channels.

Markets work best when large numbers of buyers and sellers are competing for private goods and services that are easily valued by both buyers and sellers. Under these conditions, markets can be expected to allocate resources efficiently to produce health. However, in health care markets there is frequently little competition among providers, providers and consumers often cannot accurately value the services they are selling or buying, and the benefits of those services are sometimes broadly distributed.

Figure C.2 graphically describes the ability of markets to address a number of health-related issues. The core of the diagram represents the (small) realm of health care market activity that functions best in a totally free market setting. The rest of the figure identifies those areas where a free market would not produce the most efficient or equitable outcome and indicates, for each area, specific health-related issues and responses, if any, that can be used to address them.

Market failures may be addressed effectively through public (and sometimes private) interventions in the market. Many of these specific interventions have been discussed in this book. The goal of public or private attempts to manage competition between private health plans (through such things as required standard benefits packages and quality monitoring) is to reduce or eliminate prevalent market failures. However, the success of attempts to inject competition into a previously noncompetitive market depends not only on the validity and applicability of the underlying theory but also on the extent to which a strategy that is theoretically sound can actually be implemented. What emerges from the political process is often very different from what the original proponents of a reform had in mind, as the three previous chapters in this volume illustrate. And even if politics does not intervene in formulating or implementing policy, it is not clear that some health care market failures can be adequately addressed, for primarily technical reasons. An important example of this problem is the difficulty of measuring and monitoring quality of care in HMOs (Prager, 1996; see Chapter Five).

At some point it is probably more efficient to use other means than the private market to provide health care services and promote health. Information about the effectiveness of different treatments, for example, is very valuable both to providers and to society as a whole. It is also very expensive to produce. Once information is produced, it is very difficult to limit access to it. If firms cannot recoup their investment, there will be underproduction of such information despite its value to society. Another potential problem with using the market to provide information about the effectiveness of different treatments is bias. Drug companies often fund clinical research on their products, but many reserve the right to prevent publication of the results. In a recent case, a drug company asked that a *Journal of the American Medical Association*

**Figure C.2. The Ability of Health Care Markets
to Address Different Health-Related Issues.**

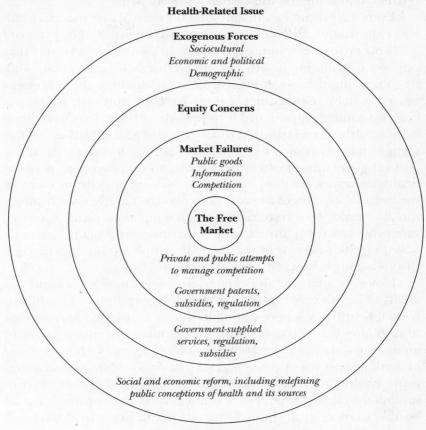

Health-Related Issue

Exogenous Forces
*Sociocultural
Economic and political
Demographic*

Equity Concerns

Market Failures
*Public goods
Information
Competition*

**The Free
Market**

*Private and public attempts
to manage competition*

*Government patents,
subsidies, regulation*

*Government-supplied
services, regulation,
subsidies*

*Social and economic reform, including redefining
public conceptions of health and its sources*

Health-Related Response

article reporting that one of the company's drugs was not significantly more effective than other, less costly substitutes be withdrawn prior to publication (King, 1996). Although the company claimed that the methodology was flawed, the fact that the drug generated approximately $400 million in annual revenues for this company probably contributed to the decision. Lack of confidence in firm-supported research provides a key rationale for using public funds for this purpose. While government-funded research is certainly not immune to political and economic pressure, both in terms of what gets funded and what gets reported (Stohlberg, 1996), the process is usually more open to public scrutiny and redress than would be the case in a private firm.

Even if a private health care market were always the most efficient alternative, intervention would still be justified to promote goals other than economic efficiency. In particular, a society that opposes distributing health care based strictly on individuals' ability to pay might favor intervention to redistribute these services more equitably. Governments alone have the authority to impose costs on some groups in order to provide benefits to others. Typically, wealth is redistributed through taxes and subsidies (in the form of payments or tax credits). In the health care context, the federal government offers tax credits to employers to provide health insurance for their employees and pays directly for many of the health care costs of the very poor and the elderly. Governments can also redistribute resources through regulations prohibiting private providers from, for example, discriminating against patients based on their race or ethnicity, or by supplying services directly through county hospitals and community clinics.

However, many health-related problems may be beyond the ability of health care markets, or even the government, to address. Even if health plans were willing to devote considerable resources to reducing tobacco consumption, the most effective approach, increasing the price of cigarettes, would appear to be beyond their immediate control. Although government could intervene to improve health and reduce health care costs related to tobacco consumption by taxing cigarettes, it is not clear that government would be able to successfully intervene to deal with other health-related concerns.

Violence has recently been identified as a serious and growing threat to public health in the United States (Shelton, 1995). The causes of violence, however, are complicated. When the roots of a problem are not well understood, a well-intentioned but misguided intervention can make a situation worse before it makes it better. In some cases, individuals will not respond as expected. In others, an intervention will lead to unanticipated and harmful side effects. Finally, of course, even when government intervention to address a health-related issue is feasible, there may be an absence of political will. In some cases policy initiatives stall because they would be harmful to particular stakeholders. More generally, they stall because of an absence of public support.

Potential and Limits of Competitive Managed Care

In the current environment, the focus of an increasing number of health plans has been on reducing costs to compete in an increasingly price-competitive environment. If their primary goal is to control costs or maximize profits, to what extent will managed care organizations' pursuit of these goals contribute to the ultimate goals of the health care system?

Before attempting to answer this question, it is important to recognize that the health care system continues to evolve rapidly in response to both private and public initiatives (Ginsberg, 1996). Mergers and alliances among providers, insurers, and purchasers are occurring at an almost breathtaking pace (Solomon, 1994). Historically unflappable HMO leaders such as Kaiser-Permanente have been set on their heels by leaner, aggressive for-profit competitors. To further complicate the picture, Congress and the president are on the verge of passing moderate health insurance reform, and they continue to debate major reforms to privatize the Medicare and Medicaid programs.

In the short term, the current emphasis on price competition is expected to spread across the nation. The 1995 Foster Higgins national survey of employer benefit costs provided powerful evidence that employers are currently controlling and even reducing their health benefit costs. In discussing these findings, Findlay and Meyeroff (1996) identify a number of contributing factors, including the continuing rapid shift to managed care and price competition among managed care plans. This environment has "produced sustained cost restraint only dreamed about in the 1980s" (p. 49). Although most evidence on the impact of price-competitive managed care has been based on the California experience, other areas of the country are now beginning to show similar results. Some large Philadelphia employers have seen declines in HMO premium rates, starting in 1995 (Johnsson, 1995a). A 1995 Milliman and Roberts survey of 376 HMOs indicated average national premium declines of 0.7 percent, with average declines in six of the nine U.S. Census regions in 1995. The largest average premium decline was 3 percent, in New England (Johnsson, 1995b).

The long-term prospects for competitive managed care are more difficult to diagnose. Obviously, a major national health care reform initiative could put an end to this movement. This seems unlikely, however. A more pressing question is what will happen when the dramatic cost savings that are currently being produced by taking advantage of a provider surplus are no longer available? To what extent will a price-competitive managed care system realize the efficiency gains popularly associated with the ideal of a population-based integrated health system? Our approach to considering these questions is to return to the ultimate goals of a health system discussed in the beginning of this chapter.

Optimal Level of Health

What impact is competitive managed care likely to have on the proportion of America's resources that are spent on health? This question has several components. The first relates to the ability of a health care system to limit overall spending on health. Many observers believe that the primary source of health care inflation over the past three decades has been the increased use of expensive medical technologies. Some of these technologies are cost-effective while others are not. However, being cost-effective is not the same thing as saving costs. As an example, some expensive approaches to treating myocardial infarctions are criticized as wasteful because, although patients are more likely to live for several more months compared with other treatments, they are not significantly more likely to live for another year (Cutler, 1996). To a health care plan, such a treatment does not save costs and is thus "inappropriate." To the patient or society, however, it may be seen as cost-effective, because although the treatment does not decrease (and actually may increase) costs, the benefit from the treatment also increases. Thus, from an individual or social perspective, the treatment is "appropriate."

A major challenge raised by competitive managed care is that, barring public intervention, a health plan's bottom line plays a central role in its judgments about the "appropriateness" of a treatment (Hiltzik, 1996). Competitive managed care is likely to slow the medical arms race by encouraging innovation in new technologies and drugs that save costs for health care plans and discouraging the development of new technologies and drugs that do not. However, this emphasis on cost savings may also have the effect of discouraging innovations that, while not saving costs for the plan, would be cost-effective for society and for patients if they were developed.

Health care costs are disproportionately incurred by the relatively small number of individuals who are seriously ill. In their pursuit of competitive prices for large purchasers, health care plans will make substantial efforts to avoid ending up with a higher-than-average proportion of chronically ill patients. For the chronically ill patients who are under their care, health plans will make substantial efforts to reduce the costs of that care.

The impact of their efforts on patient care will depend on how purchasers, patients, and providers react to these altered incentives. Purchasing groups and the government can play a central role in ensuring that plans maintain a certain level of care, rewarding plans that innovate in ways that improve quality of life (Magnusson and Hammond, 1996). With providers now acting as "double agents," patients' activism on their own behalf will also become an increasingly important predictor of the quality of their care, as will their ability to spend additional resources to access services and providers not covered by their plan. And the response of the physician double agents themselves, whether they are employees of an HMO or partners in a provider service organization, will critically affect the quality of care received by patients in an era of increased price competition (Johnsson, 1996).

Competitive managed care will create a health care environment where patients with "market power," whether gained through collective action, information and advocacy skills, or financial resources, will fare better. Patients who are chronically ill, less able to advocate for their own interests, and poor are most at risk of bearing the burden of competitive managed care's cost-saving efforts.

Equitable Distribution of Health

What impact is competitive managed care likely to have on the distribution of health care services and health in the United States? As has always been true, ability to pay will be the most important factor determining an individual's coverage and access and the quality of health care services received. In the abstract, competition and managed forms of care hold out the prospect of increasing access to affordable health care services by reducing the costs of the same quality of care. In practice, however, the evidence for cost savings through increased efficiency in the financing and delivery of care is limited.

Currently, most of the benefits of competitive managed care have gone to large employers who purchase health insurance for their employees. Managed care plans appear cheaper not only because they may operate more efficiently but also because they restrict service options. In effect, managed care has permitted employers to reduce costs by reducing benefits. Managed care plans are also cheaper because they have been able to negotiate lower prices with providers, who have traditionally shifted the costs of caring for uninsured patients onto insured patients (Preston, 1996). This change means that providers have fewer financial resources to care for the uninsured. Finally, competition among managed care plans has also reduced employers' costs by encouraging health plans to pay more attention to differences in expected utilization when setting premiums. Some of the reduced costs to employers have also come from imposing additional costs (in the form of higher premiums or reduced coverage) on purchasers with higher risks and less market power. Thus, many of the apparent benefits of competitive managed care for large employers have come from imposing new burdens on employees, safety-net providers (including the government), and other purchasers (Freudenheim, 1994).

At the same time, other economic and political forces are altering the landscape in ways that may adversely impact the individuals most affected by these changes. While private health insurance is becoming less affordable for many more individuals, governments are looking for ways to scale back their own health care–related spending. The distributive consequences of these cost-control efforts by employers and the government will ultimately depend on the extent to which managed forms of care are able to extract real efficiency gains from the health care system and the extent to which those gains are transferred to consumers rather than merely the shareholders of managed care companies.

Efficient Production of Health

What impact is competitive managed care likely to have on the efficient production of health? As discussed, the evidence for increased efficiency over the short term is mixed, particularly for the managed care plans that have been attractive in the current environment (IPA and PPO plans). Leaner forms of managed care (Alain Enthoven and Sara Singer [1996] refer to them as "carrier HMOs") may be better positioned to profit over the short term than plans that invest for long-term gains. Plans that invest in clinical and managerial research and many forms of prevention will be able to do so only to the extent that it gives them a competitive advantage (Pauly, 1996; Larson, 1996). In terms of short-term survival in an environment defined by price competition, these kinds of investments are akin to higher overhead costs. We should not expect plans to make substantial long-term investments unless they are rewarded financially for doing so in the short term, either through incentives offered by large private and public purchasers or by shareholders.

Over the longer term, the prospects for increased efficiency seem more promising. As opportunities to reduce costs by negotiating discounts with providers and shifting costs taper off—and there is evidence that this is already beginning to occur—health plans that develop more efficient approaches to care may be able to provide better outcomes for a lower cost (Johnsson, 1995a, 1995b). However, plans will continue to focus on approaches that promise certain short-term cost savings rather than approaches that offer less certain, longer-term savings or approaches that may be cost-effective but do not immediately reduce costs for the plan.

Managed care organizations can benefit from information on how to improve patient treatment outcomes, but it does not necessarily follow that they should be willing to participate in or support research and technology assessment. Because of information externalities, HMOs underinvest in such activities, from a societal perspective. The increasingly price-competitive environment has only exacerbated this problem. The head of the health technology group at Anderson Consulting commented on the current situation: "Ironically, the growth of managed care has highlighted the value and the need for technology assessment while diminishing the funds available to pay for it" (Borzo, 1995, p. 1).

Competitive Managed Care and the Health of the Community

Prepaid health plans certainly hold more promise for promoting health and preventing disease than the previous system, in which providers were reimbursed based on the quantity of services they provided. The extent to which this promise is realized will depend on the extent to which it is congruent with the financial interests of health plans and the extent to which plans are able to reorient providers, as well as consumers, toward promoting health instead of treating disease.

From a purely financial perspective, health plans will or will not decide to focus on health promotion based on a comparison of the expected costs and benefits. In other words, the question is whether preventive services will reduce costs for the plan, particularly over the short term. Most health plans offer prenatal preventive services because the expected benefits of avoiding birth complications are immediate and large, while the costs of these services are low. But what about other health-related behaviors? How far will the tentacles of competitive managed care extend into areas that have traditionally been beyond the boundaries of the private health care market?

The willingness of plans to emphasize prevention will depend importantly on the extent to which they are focused on surviving over the short term as opposed to investing for the long term. Even when they are focused on short-term survival, private and public purchasers with sufficient market power can induce them to offer preventive services. Purchasing groups can reward plans that offer preventive clinical services that do not save costs for the plan but are likely to result in improved health outcomes for enrollees. State and local governments can allocate Medicaid contracts based in part on a health plan's demonstrated commitment to improving health in a community.

To the extent that health care plans are oriented toward long-term investments, their willingness to invest in many forms of prevention would seem to depend on the extent to which their financial interests overlap with the health interests of the community. Ironically, the best arrangement for inducing plans to focus on many forms of prevention might be to have a single plan for each community (see Chapter Thirteen). The drawback, of course, is that any potential benefits in terms of an increased emphasis on prevention would be offset by the reduced efficiency of a monopoly provider (see Chapter Eight). On the other hand, in communities where there are multiple plans, each plan can expect to receive only part of the benefits of any investment it might make in community-based prevention.

The fact that managed care plans could mutually benefit from community-based prevention efforts suggests that over the longer term, health plans may play an increasingly important political role in coordinating collective action through the government to promote health and prevent disease. It would be a nice turn indeed if the power of the health care community were directed at initiatives that produced positive benefits for all concerned in terms of lower health care costs and improved health.

References

Borzo, G. "HMOs Value Research—If Others Pay for It." *American Medical News,* Nov. 20, 1995, pp. 1, 25–26.

Catalano, R. "The Health Effects of Economic Insecurity: An Analytic Review." *American Journal of Public Health,* 1991, *81*(7), 1148–1152.

Cone, M. "Grit in L.A. Air Blamed in 6,000 Deaths Yearly." *Los Angeles Times,* May 5, 1996, p. A1.

Conrad, P., and Kern, R. "The Social and Cultural Meanings of Illness." In P. Conrad and R. Kern (eds.), *The Sociology of Health and Illness: Critical Perspectives.* (4th ed.) New York: St. Martin's Press, 1994.

Cutler, D. "Cutting Costs and Improving Health." In H. J. Aaron (ed.), *The Problem That Won't Go Away: Reforming U.S. Health Care Financing.* Washington, D.C.: Brookings Institution, 1996.

Enthoven, A. C., and Singer, S. J. "What to Regulate and by Whom." In H. J. Aaron (ed.), *The Problem That Won't Go Away: Reforming U.S. Health Care Financing.* Washington, D.C.: Brookings Institution, 1996.

Evans, R. G., and Stoddart, G. L. "Producing Health, Consuming Health Care." In R. G. Evans, M. L. Barer, and T. R. Marmor (eds.), *Why Are Some People Healthy and Others Not? The Determinants of Health of Populations.* New York: Aldine de Gruyter, 1994.

Findlay, S., and Meyeroff, W. J."Health Costs: Why Employers Won Another Round." *Business and Health,* Mar. 1996, pp. 49–51.

Freudenheim, M. "To Economists, Managed Care is No Cure-All." *New York Times,* Sept. 6, 1994, p. A1.

Fuchs, V. R. *Who Shall Live?* New York: Basic Books, 1974.

Fuchs, V. R. *The Future of Health Policy.* Cambridge, Mass.: Harvard University Press, 1994.

Ginsberg, P. "A World in Transition." *Business and Health,* April 1996, pp. 60–62.

Gorman, C. "Who's Looking at Your Files?" *Time,* May 6, 1996, pp. 60–62.

Guendelman, S., Chavez, G., and Christianson, R. "Fetal Deaths in Mexican-American, Black and White Non-Hispanic Women Seeking Government Funded Pre-Natal Care." *Journal of Community Health,* 1994, *19*(5), 319–330.

Haan, M., Kaplan, G., and Syme, L. "Socioeconomic Status and Health: Old Observations and New Thoughts." In J. Bunker, O. Gomby, and B. Keher (eds.), *Pathways to Health: The Role of Social Factors.* Menlo Park, Calif.: Henry J. Kaiser Family Foundation, 1989.

Hay, J. W., Osmond, D. H., and Jacobson, M. A. "Projecting the Medical Costs of AIDS and ARC in the United States." *Journal of Acquired Immune Deficiency Syndromes,* 1988, *1*(5), 466–485.

Hiltzik, M. "Drawing the Line: An HMO Dilemma." *Los Angeles Times,* Jan. 17, 1996.

Johnsson, J. "West Meets East: Philadelphia HMOs Follow California into Price War." *American Medical News,* Feb. 13, 1995a, pp. 1, 7.

Johnsson, J. "HMO Price War Hits the East Coast." *American Medical News,* Nov. 11, 1995b, p. 11.

Johnsson, J. "Market Gains for Physicians." *American Medical News,* Apr. 1, 1996, p. 1.

King, R. "Bitter Pill: How a Drug Firm Paid for a University Study, Then Undermined It." *Wall Street Journal,* Apr. 25, 1996, p. A1.

Kolata, G. "Ability to Find a Tiny Tumor Poses Dilemma." *New York Times,* Mar. 27, 1996.

Larson, E. "The Soul of an HMO." *Time,* Jan. 22, 1996, pp. 45–52.

Levin, M. "Still Smoking." *Los Angeles Times,* Apr. 12, 1996.

Magnusson, P., and Hammond, K. H. "Health Care: The Quest for Quality." *Business Week,* April 8, 1996, pp. 104–106.

McGinnis, M. J., and Foege, W. H. "Actual Causes of Death in the United States." *Journal of the American Medical Association,* 1993, *270*(18), 2207–2212.

Morris, R. D., Naumova, E. N., and Munasinghe, R. L. "Ambient Air Pollution and Hospitalization for Congestive Heart Failure Among Elderly People in Seven Large US Cities." *American Journal of Public Health,* 1995, *85*(10), 1361–1365.

Murray, A. "Income Inequality Grows amid Recovery." *Wall Street Journal,* July 1, 1996, p. A1.

Naj, A. K. "Treadmill May Be Supplanted as Heart Test." *Wall Street Journal,* Mar. 11, 1996, pp. B3, B6.

National Center for Health Statistics. *Health, United States, 1994.* Hyattsville, Md.: U.S. Public Health Service, 1995.

Pauly, M. V. "Producing Research on Health Management and Managed Care: Market Failure or Success?" *Medical Care Research and Review,* 1996, *53*(Mar. Suppl.), s118–s131.

Pinkney, D. S. "Why Do Some People Get Sicker than Others?" *American Medical News,* Dec. 26, 1994, pp. 9–11.

Pitta, J. "Netscape Pioneer to Go Online with Health Site." *Los Angeles Times,* Mar. 5, 1996, pp. D1, D9.

Prager, L. O. "As Pressure Grows, Plan Performance Measures Move Toward Outcomes." *American Medical News,* July 1, 1996, pp. 1, 30.

Preston, J. "Hospitals Look on Charity Care as Unaffordable Option of Past." *New York Times,* April 14, 1996, p. A1.

Schroeder, S. "The Medically Uninsured—Will They Always Be with Us?" *New England Journal of Medicine,* 1996, *334*(17), 1130–1133.

Shelton, D. L. "L.A. County Tops Statistics for Gang-Related Crimes." *American Medical News,* Oct. 16, 1995, p. 5.

Shilts, R. *And the Band Played On.* New York: Penguin Books, 1988.

Silverstein, S. "Study Finds Gap Growing Between Rich, Poor in U.S." *Los Angeles Times,* Mar. 20, 1996, p. A1.

Skolnick, A. A. "Experts Explore Emerging Information Technologies' Effects on Medicine." *Journal of the American Medical Association,* 1996, *275*(9), 669–670.

Solomon, J. "With or Without You." *Newsweek,* Aug. 15, 1994, pp. 58–59.

Stipp, D. "The Gender Gap in Cancer Research." *Fortune,* May 13, 1996, pp. 74–76.

Stohlberg, S. "Activist's Battles Highlight Cigarette Firm's Firepower." *Los Angeles Times,* Apr. 14, 1996, p. A1.

"Ultrasound Breast Cancer Test Approved." *New York Times,* April 13, 1996, pp. 14, 29.

U.S. Public Health Service. *Health, United States.* Hyattsville, Md.: U.S. Public Health Service, 1992.

Winslow, R. "Prostate-Cancer Test May Be More Costly than Beneficial." *Wall Street Journal,* Sept. 14, 1994, p. B1.

Ziegler, J. "Telemedicine Starts to Pay Off." *Business and Health,* Oct. 1995, pp. 47–50.

The Editors

Kelly J. Devers is an expert appointee at the Agency for Health Care Policy and Research, Center for Organization and Delivery Studies. She received her B.A. from the University of Pennsylvania (1987) and her Ph.D. in sociology from Northwestern University (1994). From 1994 to 1996 she was a Robert Wood Johnson scholar in health policy research at the University of California, Berkeley. Dr. Devers's areas of interest include the organization and delivery of health care, its impact on access to and quality of care, and state Medicaid reform.

Ruth S. Given is director of the Department of Health Care Policy at the California Medical Association. She holds a B.A. from Stanford University (1975), an M.S. in health policy management from the Harvard School of Public Health (1985), and a Ph.D. in economics from the University of California, Berkeley (1994). Between 1985 and 1990 she worked for the southern California region of Kaiser-Permanente in a number of applied research positions. From 1994 to 1996 she was a Robert Wood Johnson scholar in health policy research at the University of California, Berkeley. Dr. Given's research interests involve the economics of managed care—specifically, the determinants of individual demand for health care services under managed care and regulation of the HMO industry.

John D. Wilkerson is assistant professor of political science at the University of Washington, Seattle. He received his B.A from Portland State University (1984) and his Ph.D. in political science from the University of Rochester (1991). From 1994 to 1996 he was a Robert Wood Johnson Scholar in health policy research at the University of California, Berkeley. Professor Wilkerson's areas of interest include legislative politics, political economy, and the politics of health care reform.

The Contributors

Linda A. Bergthold is vice president of the Lewin Group and head of the California office of Lewin. Her expertise is in state and national health care reform, medical benefit plan design, and managed care evaluation. Prior to joining Lewin, she worked for William M. Mercer, Inc., as a principal, assisting major employers with their health insurance purchasing strategies and programs. She also served as the cochair of the White House Health Care Reform Task Force's working group on benefit design in 1993. Dr. Bergthold was a Pew health policy fellow at the Institute for Health Policy Studies, University of California, San Francisco. Her book *Purchasing Power in Health: Business, the State, and Health Care Politics* was published in January 1990 by Rutgers University Press. Dr. Bergthold holds a Ph.D. and an M.A. degree in sociology from the University of California, Santa Cruz (1985), and a B.A. degree with honors from the University of California, Los Angeles (1962).

Andrew B. Bindman is associate professor of medicine, epidemiology, and biostatistics at the University of California, San Francisco. He earned his B.A. (1980) in psychology and social relations from Harvard College and his M.D. (1984) from the Mount Sinai School of Medicine. He is a Robert Wood Johnson Foundation generalist physician faculty scholar and the acting chief of the Division of General Internal Medicine at San Francisco General Hospital, where he teaches and practices internal medicine. In 1996 Dr. Bindman received the Young Investigator Award from the Association for Health Services Research.

Thomas C. Buchmueller is assistant professor in the Graduate School of Management, University of California, Irvine. He received his Ph.D. in economics from the University of Wisconsin, Madison

(1992), and his B.A. from Carleton College in Northfield, Minnesota (1985). His research focuses mainly on the labor market implications of employer-provided health insurance.

Leonard Finocchio is associate director for state health policy at the Center for the Health Professions at the University of California, San Francisco. He earned his B.A. degree (1985) in psychology at the University of California, Davis, and his M.P.H degree (1992) in health education and maternal and child health at the University of California, Los Angeles. Mr. Finocchio is also a doctoral student in health policy at the University of Michigan.

Jennifer Fishman received her master's degree (1996) from the School of Social Ecology at the University of California, Irvine, and is currently pursuing a doctoral degree in sociology at the University of California, San Francisco. Her research interests include women's health, medical sociology, and the structural organization of the health care system.

Donald W. Light is professor of comparative health care systems at the University of Medicine and Dentistry of New Jersey and is an adjunct senior fellow at the Leonard Davis Institute of Health Economics at the University of Pennsylvania. He has been working extensively on the British reforms in health care and on managed competition in the United States. Trained in sociology and history at Stanford (B.A., 1963), the University of Chicago (M.A., 1967), and Brandeis (Ph.D., 1970), Professor Light has been selected twice to be a visiting faculty fellow at Oxford University and has been made a fellow of the Royal Society of Medicine. He is coauthor, with John Fry and others, of *Reviving Primary Care,* published by Radcliffe Memorial Press (1995).

Harold S. Luft is Caldwell B. Esselstyn professor of health policy and health economics and director of the Institute for Health Policy Studies at the University of California, San Francisco. He earned his B.A. degree (1968) and Ph.D. (1973) in economics (specialization in health sector economics and public finance) at Harvard University.

Edward O'Neil is associate professor of family and community medicine at the University of California, San Francisco, where he also serves as codirector of the Center for the Health Professions. Since 1989 Dr. O'Neil has been the executive director of the Pew Health Professions Commission. Dr. O'Neil received his B.A. degree (1974) in humanities and M.A. degree (1975) in American studies at the University of Alabama. He received his M.P.A degree (1981) and his Ph.D. (1984) in American studies at Syracuse University. Prior to taking his position at UCSF, Dr. O'Neil was assistant dean for medical education at Duke University, where he was also associate professor in the Departments of Family Medicine and Public Policy.

Tracy M. Rodriguez is performance measurement manager for Kaiser Foundation Health Plan, Inc., headquartered in Oakland, California. She earned her B.S. degree (1981) in public health nutrition at the University of California, Los Angeles, and both her M.P.H. and M.B.A. (1992) at the University of California, Berkeley. Before joining Kaiser, she was director of quality at the Pacific Business Group on Health.

Helen Halpin Schauffler is associate professor of health policy, director of the joint program in public policy and public health, and principal investigator of the health insurance policy program at the University of California, Berkeley, School of Public Health. She earned her B.A. degree (1973) in biology and chemistry at Skidmore College, her M.S. degree (1976) in health policy and management from the Harvard School of Public Health, and her Ph.D. degree (1989) in health policy from Brandeis University, Florence Heller School of Social Welfare Policy.

Loel Scott Solomon is senior associate in the public policy and health care finance practice of the Lewin Group, a health care consulting firm located in Fairfax, Virginia. He earned his B.A. degree (1988) in political science at the University of California, Los Angeles, and his master of public policy degree (1992) at the University of California, Berkeley. Prior to joining the Lewin Group, Mr. Solomon served on the professional staff of the United States Senate Committee on Labor and Human Resources as health policy advisor to committee chairman Edward M. Kennedy. During his tenure with the committee, he also served on the president's task force on national health care reform as a member of the working group on cost control and employer-based financing.

Michael S. Sparer is assistant professor in the Division of Health Policy and Management in the Columbia University School of Public Health. He received a Ph.D. in politics from Brandeis University (1992) and a J.D. from the Rutgers School of Law (1980). Sparer spent seven years as a litigator for the New York City law department, specializing in intergovernmental social welfare litigation. He now studies and writes about the politics of health care, with an emphasis on the state and local role in the American health care system. He is the author of *Medicaid and the Limits of State Health Reform,* published by Temple University Press (1996), along with numerous articles and book chapters.

Howard Waitzkin is professor of medicine and social sciences and attending physician in internal medicine at the University of California, Irvine. He earned his B.A. degree in social relations (1966), Ph.D. degree in sociology (1972), and M.D. (1972) at Harvard University. His research focuses on patient-doctor communication, psychosocial issues in primary care, and comparative international health policy. Dr. Waitzkin's most recent book, *The Politics of Medical Encounters: How Patients and Doctors Deal with Social Problems,* was published by Yale University Press.

Name Index

Subject Index